Cardiopulmonary Transplantation and Mechanical Circulatory Support

T0202101

Oxford Specialist Handbooks published and forthcoming

Cardiopulmonary Transplantation and Mechanical Circulatory Support

EDITED BY
**Maziar Khorsandi, Steven Tsui,
John Dark, Alan J. Kirk,
Matthew Hartwig,
Mani A. Daneshmand, and
Carmelo Milano**

ILLUSTRATED BY
Jay LeVasseur

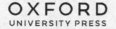

OXFORD
UNIVERSITY PRESS

OXFORD
UNIVERSITY PRESS

Great Clarendon Street, Oxford, OX2 6DP,
United Kingdom

Oxford University Press is a department of the University of Oxford.
It furthers the University's objective of excellence in research, scholarship,
and education by publishing worldwide. Oxford is a registered trade mark of
Oxford University Press in the UK and in certain other countries

© Oxford University Press 2022

The moral rights of the authors have been asserted

First Edition published in 2022

Impression: 1

All rights reserved. No part of this publication may be reproduced, stored in
a retrieval system, or transmitted, in any form or by any means, without the
prior permission in writing of Oxford University Press, or as expressly permitted
by law, by licence or under terms agreed with the appropriate reprographics
rights organization. Enquiries concerning reproduction outside the scope of the
above should be sent to the Rights Department, Oxford University Press, at the
address above

You must not circulate this work in any other form
and you must impose this same condition on any acquirer

Published in the United States of America by Oxford University Press
198 Madison Avenue, New York, NY 10016, United States of America

British Library Cataloguing in Publication Data
Data available

Library of Congress Control Number: 2022932691

ISBN 978–0–19–286761–2

DOI: 10.1093/med/9780192867612.001.0001

Printed in the UK by
Ashford Colour Press Ltd, Gosport, Hampshire

Oxford University Press makes no representation, express or implied, that the
drug dosages in this book are correct. Readers must therefore always check
the product information and clinical procedures with the most up-to-date
published product information and data sheets provided by the manufacturers
and the most recent codes of conduct and safety regulations. The authors and
the publishers do not accept responsibility or legal liability for any errors in the
text or for the misuse or misapplication of material in this work. Except where
otherwise stated, drug dosages and recommendations are for the non-pregnant
adult who is not breast-feeding

Links to third party websites are provided by Oxford in good faith and
for information only. Oxford disclaims any responsibility for the materials
contained in any third party website referenced in this work.

To my parents Shahin and Ali Khorsandi, MD and to the memory of Edward "Ted" Brackenbury, FRCS

Foreword

When people speak of vitality, it is often with reference to cardiorespiratory function. Indeed, throughout human history people have intuitively associated heart and lung function with one's life, virtue, and soul. Thus, when heart and lung transplantation emerged in the 1960s, it captured the world's attention far more than kidney or liver transplantation. After all, we associate ourselves with every heartbeat, every breath; not so much with urine and bile. It was as though successful replacement of the heart and lungs forced us to consider our humanity, and thus seemed more miraculous than technical.

The past 60 years have led the elements of pulse and breath to be characterized so well that they are now regularly exchangeable. The world is approaching its 100,000th cardiopulmonary transplantation, and mechanical support devices are rapidly becoming commonplace. With such prevalence, one would think that cardiopulmonary replacement might have lost its lustre. Yet every time I think about a heart or lung transplant, or a left ventricular assist device deployment, it still seems like a miracle to me—not because the mechanics and biology are mysterious, but rather because they are now so well defined. To be sure, it is immensely technical, and it is the enormity of what we now know about this practice that makes it so impressive. Assembling that knowledge into a usable format is increasingly important and challenging.

In saying that transplantation is technical, it is not to imply that it is amenable to rote education. There is really no transplant procedure that is exactly like another. Each case has its unique physiology, immunology, and histocompatibility, the latter of which literally defines individuality. There are so many reasons that this should not work, yet it does, almost routinely. I believe this is a tribute to the dedicated people who try to make sense of each case and derive and curate generalizable insights. *Cardiopulmonary Transplantation and Mechanical Circulatory Support* is a collection of those insights, to be used in the adept navigation of each improbable success. This is a concise resource to help practitioners quickly refresh the relevant information needed to recognize problems and deal with them. This is not a comprehensive treatise, as each chapter could warrant a book in and unto itself. Rather, this is a means of practical guidance, placing clinical challenges into the broad contexts of cardiopulmonary physiology and transplant immunology. It will be particularly useful to trainees, and to nurses, advanced practice providers, intensivists, and hospitalists caring for transplant patients and needing quick reference. This is a resource to provide order to the rapidly accumulating practical information needed to routinely transform lives, one miracle at a time.

Allan D. Kirk, MD, PhD, FACS
David C. Sabiston, Jr. Distinguished Professor of Surgery,
Immunology and Pediatrics
Chairman of the Department of Surgery
Duke University Medical Center
Durham, NC, USA

Foreword

Cardiopulmonary Transplantation and Mechanical Circulatory Support will serve as a valuable resource for residents, fellows, and advanced care practitioners. Thirty-eight chapters cover a variety of important topics, representing several years of effort by an international slate of authors and editors. While much of what we do in surgery for advanced heart and lung failure is evidence based, a substantial amount of it is also based on personal opinion, consensus, and institutional preference. What is presented here falls into the latter category. However, trainees require a foundational understanding of key concepts and techniques to begin their education in the field. This handbook is a practical guide and an excellent starting point for individuals learning to practice in this field. By no means is this intended as a definitive treatment on this topic but rather to lay the ground work for lifelong learning. Managing Editor Maz Khorsandi will be updating this handbook to ensure content remains current.

Those who possess a highly-developed awareness of this field and knowledge of related literature may take issue with some of the points made in the text. However, authors have attempted to simplify the concepts in order to make them more approachable to the reader. The best use of this handbook would be for study preparation by trainees with directed follow-up discussion with their attending providers, as well as focused literature searches to enhance and refine their depth of understanding. As these fields continue in their inevitable evolution, the stewardship of continued learning will require humility and receptiveness to new concepts and ideas that challenge existing notions, concepts, or dogma. This handbook is a starting point that is very readable, approachable, and useful. As such, it should inspire readers to engage in this complex and rapidly-evolving field and serve as a catalyst for advanced learning.

Michael S. Mulligan, MD
Professor and Chief, Division of Cardiothoracic Surgery
Endowed Professor in Lung Transplant Research
Director, Lung Transplant Program
University of Washington

Preface

As I approached the final stretch of my specialty training in cardiothoracic surgery, I felt that there was a paucity of a quick reference manual for my subspecialty field of interest, cardiopulmonary transplantation and mechanical circulatory support. Most reference guides were large, cumbersome, and already outdated by the time they were published. Henceforth, I felt the need to embark on this handbook project. I was further encouraged and supported by my mentors Dr Carmelo Milano, MD, Duke University Medical Center, USA, and Mr Edward 'Ted' Brackenbury, FRCS C/Th, Royal Infirmary of Edinburgh, UK. Furthermore, Duke University Heart Center generously supported the project financially.

Cardiopulmonary Transplantation and Mechanical Circulatory Support is a comprehensive yet succinct and readily available pocket guide of the most up-to-date developments in the field of heart and lung transplantation and mechanical circulatory support. The most prominent and globally respected experts in Europe and North America were selected as editors and authors for this handbook and the content, for the most part, reflects their personal experience, hints, and tips for practitioners on the front line. The handbook is accompanied by informative text and high-resolution practical illustrations making it relevant to all tiers of healthcare professionals such as nurses, advanced care practitioners, surgical, medical, and critical care residents and fellows, as well as junior attending/consultant physicians and surgeons looking after such critically ill patients. This handbook will be readily available both as a hard copy and online. I strive to continuously update it with the most recent evidence-based practice.

Maziar Khorsandi, FRCS C/Th
Assistant Professor of Surgery
Attending Cardiothoracic Surgeon
Division of Cardiothoracic Surgery
University of Washington Medical Center
Seattle, WA, USA

Acknowledgements

We would like to gratefully acknowledge the generous donation by Duke University Heart Center in funding the illustrations for this handbook.

Contents

Contributors *xix*

Abbreviations *xxvii*

Section 1 **Heart failure**

1 Medical and minimally invasive aspects of heart
failure management 3
Marc D. Samsky and Joseph G. Rogers

2 Myocarditis: diagnosis and treatment 15
Stuart D. Russell

3 Cardiac amyloidosis and other restrictive
myopathies: diagnosis and treatment 27
Rahul Loungani and Chetan Patel

Section 2 **Mechanical circulatory support**

4 Indications for ventricular assist devices 41
Antonios Kourliouros

5 Surgical techniques for left ventricular assist device
implantation and associated procedures 49
Igor Gosev and Scott Silvestry

6 Clinical trials with durable left ventricular
assist devices 61
Yuting P. Chiang and Mani A. Daneshmand

7 Diagnosis and management of ventricular assist
device complications 69
*Maziar Khorsandi, Philip Curry, Sukumaran Nair, and
Nawwar Al-Attar*

8 Extracorporeal membrane oxygenation 79
Jeffrey Javidfar, Maziar Khorsandi, and Mani A. Daneshmand

9 Percutaneous mechanical circulatory support 97
Dominick Megna Jr, Maziar Khorsandi, and Danny Ramzy

Contributors

Ahmed S. Al-Adhami, FRCS C/Th
Specialty Registrar
Department of Cardiothoracic Surgery
Golden Jubilee National Hospital
Glasgow, UK
Chapter 13

Nawwar Al-Attar, FRCS C/Th, PhD
Director of Heart Transplantation and Consultant Cardiac and Transplant Surgeon Department of Cardiothoracic Surgery
Golden Jubilee National Hospital
Glasgow, UK
Chapters 7,11,13

Barbara D. Alexander, MD
Professor of Medicine and Pathology
Division of Infectious Diseases
Duke University Medical Center
NC, USA
Chapter 21

Jason Ali, MRCS, PhD
Speciality Registrar in Cardiothoracic Surgery
Department of Cardiothoracic Surgery
Royal Papworth Hospital
Cambridge, UK
Chapter 33

Anders Andreasson, FRCS C/Th, PhD
Speciality Registrar in Cardiothoracic Surgery
Department of Cardiothoracic Surgery
Freeman Hospital
Newcastle, UK
Chapter 27

Francisco Arabia, MD
Professor of Surgery
Division Chief of Cardiothoracic Surgery
University of Arizona College of Medicine
AZ, USA
Chapter 10

Abbas Ardehali, MD
Director of UCLA Heart and Lung Transplantation Program
Professor of Surgery and William E Conner Chair of Cardiopulmonary Transplantation Division of Cardiothoracic Surgery
Ronald Reagan UCLA Medical Center
CA, USA
Chapter 27

Sana Arif, MBBS
Assistant Professor of Medicine
Division of Infectious Diseases
Duke University Medical Center
NC, USA
Chapter 21

Yaron Barac, MD, PhD
Associate Professor of Surgery and Cardiovascular Physiology
Director
Heart and Lung Transplant and Mechanical Circulatory Support Program
Rabin Medical Center
Sackler Faculty of Medicine
Tel Aviv, Israel
Chapters 14,16,34

Andrew S. Barbas, MD
Assistant Professor of Surgery
Division of Abdominal Transplant Surgery
Duke University Medical Center
NC, USA
Chapter 34

Anna K. Barton, MSc, MRCP
Clinical Research Fellow and
Honorary Cardiology Registrar
Centre for Cardiovascular Science
The University of Edinburgh
Edinburgh, UK
Chapter 18

Marius Berman, FRCS C/Th
Consultant Cardiac and Transplant
Surgeon
Department of Cardiothoracic
Surgery
Royal Papworth Hospital
Cambridge, UK
Chapter 15

Desiree Bonadonna, MPS
Director of Extra-Corporeal Life
Support
Duke University Medical Center
NC, USA
Chapters 8, 19

Karen Booth, FRCS C/Th
Consultant Cardiac and Transplant
Surgeon
Department of Cardiothoracic
Surgery
Freeman Hospital
Newcastle, UK
Chapters 27, 32

Brandi Bottiger, MD
Associate Professor of Anesthesia
Division of Cardiothoracic
Anesthesia and Critical Care
Duke University Medical Center
NC, USA
Chapter 37

Benjamin Bryner, MD
Co-Director of Duke ECMO
Program and Assistant Professor
of Surgery
Division of Cardiothoracic Surgery
Duke University Medical Center
NC, USA
Chapter 12

Anthony Castleberry, MD
Assistant Professor of Surgery
Division of Cardiothoracic Surgery
University of Nebraska Medical
Center
NE, USA
Chapter 14

Pedro Catarino, FRCS C/Th
Director of Heart and Lung
Transplantation and Mechanical
Circulatory Support and Consultant
Cardiac and Transplant Surgeon
Royal Papworth Hospital
Cambridge, UK
Chapter 28

Yuting P. Chiang, MD
Resident in Cardiothoracic Surgery
Columbia University Medical Center
NY, USA
Chapter 6

Stephen C. Clark, FRCS C/Th
Director of Heart and Lung
Transplantation and Professor
of Cardiothoracic Surgery and
Cardiopulmonary Transplantation
Department of Cardiothoracic
Surgery
Freeman Hospital and Newcastle
University
Newcastle, UK
Chapter 25

Sylvia Costa, MD
Adjunct Assistant Professor of
Medicine
Division of Infectious Diseases
Duke University Medical Center
NC, USA
Chapter 21

Philip Curry, FRCS C/Th, PhD
Clinical Director of Cardiothoracic
Surgery and Consultant Cardiac and
Transplant Surgeon
Department of Cardiothoracic
Surgery
Golden Jubilee National Hospital
Glasgow, UK
Chapters 7, 11, 13

Jonathan R. Dalzell, FRCP
Consultant Heart Failure
Cardiologist
Scottish National Advanced Heart
Failure Services
Golden Jubilee National Hospital
Glasgow, UK
Chapters 17,18

Mani A. Daneshmand, MD
Director of Heart and Lung
Transplantation and MCS Programs
and Associate Professor of Surgery
Division of Cardiothoracic Surgery
Emory University School of
Medicine
GA, USA
Chapter 6

John Dark, FRCS
Professor of Cardiothoracic
Surgery and Cardiopulmonary
Transplantation
Past President of ISHLT
Newcastle University
Newcastle, UK
Chapter 27

Adam D. DeVore, MD
Assistant Professor of Medicine
Division of Cardiology
Duke University Medical Center
NC, USA
Chapter 20

Julie Doberne, MD, PhD
Resident in Cardiothoracic Surgery
Duke University Medical Center
NC, USA
Chapters 12,26

Hari Doshi, FRCS C/Th
Consultant Cardiac and Transplant
Surgeon
Department of Cardiothoracic
Surgery
Golden Jubilee National Hospital
Glasgow, UK
Chapter 13

Kamrouz Ghadimi, MD
Associate Professor of
Anesthesiology
Division of Cardiothoracic
Anesthesia and Critical Care
Duke University Medical Center
NC, USA
Chapter 35

Igor Gosev, MD, PhD
Assistant Professor
Division of Cardiothoracic Surgery
University of Rochester Medical
Center
NY, USA
Chapter 5

John Haney, MD
Surgical Director of Lung
Transplantation and Assistant
Professor of Surgery
Division of Cardiothoracic Surgery
Duke University Medical Center
NC, USA
Chapter 28

Matthew Hartwig, MD
Associate Professor of Surgery
Division of Cardiothoracic Surgery
Duke University Medical Center
NC, USA
Chapters 26,29

Asif Hasan, FRCS C/Th
Consultant Congenital Cardiac and
Transplant Surgeon
Children's Heart Unit
Freeman Hospital
Newcastle, UK
Chapters 22.1,22.2,23

Nazish Hashmi, MD
Assistant Professor of Anesthesia
Division of Cardiothoracic
Anesthesia and Critical Care
Duke University Medical Center
NC, USA
Chapter 37

Jeffrey Javidfar, MD
Assistant Professor of Surgery and
Assistant Surgical Director of the
Lung Transplantation Program
Division of Cardiothoracic Surgery
Emory University School of Medicine
GA, USA
Chapter 8

Louise Kenny, FRCS C/Th
Specialist Registrar in Congenital
Cardiac Surgery
Children's Heart Unit
Freeman Hospital
Newcastle, UK
Chapters 22.2, 23

Maziar Khorsandi, FRCS C/Th
(Managing editor)
Assistant Professor of Surgery
Division of Cardiothoracic Surgery
University of Washington Medical
Center
WA, USA
Chapters 7,8,9,11

Alan J. Kirk, FRCS
Honorary Professor of Surgery
Consultant Thoracic Surgeon
Golden Jubilee National Hospital
and University of Glasgow
Glasgow, UK
Chapter 18

Jacob Klapper, MD
Assistant Professor of Surgery
Division of Cardiothoracic Surgery
Duke University Medical Center
NC, USA
Chapter 26

**Antonios Kourliouros, FRCS
C/Th, PhD**
Consultant Cardiac Surgeon
Oxford Heart Centre
John Radcliffe Hospital
Oxford, UK
Chapter 4

Stephen Large, FRCS C/Th
Consultant Cardiac and Transplant
Surgeon
Department of Cardiothoracic
Surgery
Royal Papworth Hospital
Cambridge, UK
Chapter 15

Rahul Loungani, MD
Cardiology Fellow
Division of Cardiology
Duke University Medical Center
NC, USA
Chapter 3

**Michael W. Manning,
MD, PhD**
Associate Professor of Anesthesia
Division of Cardiothoracic
Anesthesia and Critical Care
Duke University Medical Center
NC, USA
Chapter 35

Philip McCall, FRCA
Fellow in Cardiothoracic
Anaesthesia and Critical Care
Golden Jubilee National Hospital
Glasgow, UK
Chapter 36

Lynn McGugan, ACNP
Critical Care Nurse Practitioner
Duke University Medical Center
NC, USA
Chapter 19

Dominick Megna Jr, MD
Assistant Professor of Surgery
Surgical Director of Lung
Transplantation Program
Division of Cardiothoracic Surgery
Cedar Sinai Medical Center
CA, USA
Chapters 9,10

Simon Messer, MRCS, PhD
Registrar in Cardiothoracic Surgery
Department of Cardiothoracic
Surgery
Royal Papworth Hospital
Cambridge, UK
Chapter 15

Carmelo Milano, MD
Professor of Surgery
Chief Section of Adult Cardiac
Surgery
Division of Cardiothoracic Surgery
Duke University Medical Center
NC, USA
Chapter 36

Michael Mulvihill, MD
Resident in Cardiothoracic Surgery
Duke University Medical Center
NC, USA
Chapter 29

Jagan Murugachandran, MRCP
Registrar in Internal and Respiratory
Medicine
Specialty Registrar in Respiratory
Critical Care and General Internal
Medicine
Royal Papworth Hospital
Cambridge, UK
Chapter 31

Arun Nair, FRCP
Consultant in Respiratory Medicine
and Lung Transplantation
Department of Respiratory
Medicine and Lung Transplantation
Freeman Hospital
Newcastle, UK
Chapter 30

Sukumaran Nair, FRCS C/Th
Consultant Cardiac and Transplant
Surgeon
Golden Jubilee National Hospital
Glasgow, UK
Chapters 7,11,17

Basil Nasir, FRCSC
Assistant Professor of Surgery
Division of Thoracic Surgery
Centre Hospitalier de l'Université
de Montréal
Montreal, Canada
Chapters 24,28

Mohamed Nassar, FRCS C/Th
Consultant Congenital Cardiac and
Transplant Surgeon
Freeman Hospital
Newcastle, UK
Chapter 22.1

Alina Nicoara, MD
Associate Professor of Anesthesia
Division of Cardiothoracic
Anesthesia and Critical Care
Duke University Medical Center
NC, USA
Chapter 36

Yejide Odedina, MRCP
Specialty Registrar in Respiratory
and General Internal Medicine
Department of Respiratory and
Internal Medicine
Royal Papworth Hospital
Cambridge, UK
Chapter 31

Jasvir Parmar, FRCP, PhD
Consultant in Respiratory Medicine
Department of Lung
Transplantation
Royal Papworth Hospital
Cambridge, UK
Chapters 31,33

Chetan Patel, MD
Associate Professor of Medicine
Division of Cardiology
Duke University Medical Center
NC, USA
Chapters 3,12

Ed Peng, FRCS C/Th
Consultant Cardiac Surgeon, Royal
Hospital
Children Glasgow and Golden
Jubilee National Hospital
Scotland, UK
Chapters 22.2, 22.3

Mihai Podgoreanu, MD
Chief of Division of Cardiothoracic
Anesthesia and Critical Care and
Associate Professor of Anesthesia
Duke University Medical Center
NC, USA
Chapter 37

Danny Ramzy, MD, PhD
Associate Professor of Surgery
Division of Cardiothoracic Surgery
Cedar Sinai Medical Center
CA, USA
Chapter 9

John M. Reynolds, MD
Medical Director of Lung
Transplantation and Associate
Professor of Medicine
Division of Lung Transplantation,
Pulmonary and Critical Care
Duke University Medical Center
NC, USA
Chapter 24

Joseph G. Rogers, MD
Chief Medical Officer and Professor
of Medicine
Division of Cardiology
Duke University Medical Center
NC, USA
Chapter 1

Sebastian V. Rojas, MD
Co-Director of Cardiac
Transplantation
Department of Cardiothoracic,
Transplantation and Vascular
Surgery
Hannover Medical School
Hannover, Germany
Chapter 14

Stuart D. Russell, MD
Director of Heart Failure and
Professor of Medicine
Division of Cardiology
Duke University Medical Center
NC, USA
Chapter 2

Marc D. Samsky, MD
Cardiology Fellow
Division of Cardiology
Duke University Medical Center
NC, USA
Chapter 1

Julie R. Samuel, FRCPath
Clinical Director of the Department
of Clinical Microbiology and
Consultant Clinical Microbiologist
Freeman Hospital
Newcastle, UK
Chapter 32

Jacob Schroder, MD
Director of Heart Transplantation
Program and Assistant Professor
of Surgery
Division of Cardiothoracic Surgery
Duke University Medical Center
NC, USA
Chapters 14,16,34

Sounok Sen, MD
Cardiology Fellow
Division of Cardiology
Duke University Medical Center
NC, USA
Chapter 20

Jigesh A. Shah, DO
Fellow in Abdominal Organ
Transplantation
Division of Abdominal
Transplantation
Duke University Medical Center
NC, USA
Chapter 34

Scott Silvestry, MD
Surgical Director of Thoracic
Transplantation and Associate
Professor of Surgery
Division of Cardiothoracic Surgery
Florida Hospital Transplant Institute
FL, USA
Chapter 5

Andrew Sinclair, FRCA
Director of Mechanical Circulatory
Support and Consultant in
Anaesthesia and Critical Care
Golden Jubilee National Hospital
Glasgow, UK
Chapters 17,36

Sanjeet A. Singh, MRCS, PhD
Clinical Fellow in Heart
Transplantation
Department of Cardiothoracic
Surgery
Golden Jubilee National Hospital
Glasgow, UK
Chapter 17

Alison I. Smyth, MRCP
Clinical Fellow in Heart Failure
Cardiology
Scottish National Advanced Heart
Failure Services
Golden Jubilee National Hospital
Glasgow, UK
Chapter 18

Steven Tsui, FRCS C/Th
Clinical Director of Transplant
Services and Director of Mechanical
Circulatory Support
Consultant Cardiac and Transplant
Surgeon
Royal Papworth Hospital
Cambridge, UK
Chapters 15,33

Nathan Waldron, MD
Assistant Professor in Anaesthesia
and Critical Care
University of Colorado Health
Memorial Hospital Central
CO, USA
Chapter 29

Evelyn Watson, RN
Specialist Charge Nurse
Regional Transplant Unit
Freeman Hospital and Newcastle
University
Newcastle, UK
Chapter 19

Christopher White, FRCSC, PhD
Heart Failure Surgeon
Assistant Professor of Surgery
Dalhousie University
New Brunswick Heart Center
NB, Canada
Chapter 16

Lorenzo Zaffiri, MD
Assistant Professor of Medicine
Division of Lung Transplantation,
Pulmonary and Critical Care
Duke University Medical Center
NC, USA
Chapter 30

Abbreviations

ABOi	AABO incompatible	CNS	central nervous system
ACC	American College of Cardiology	COPD	chronic obstructive pulmonary disease
ACE	angiotensin-converting enzyme	CPB	cardiopulmonary bypass
ACEi	angiotensin-converting enzyme inhibitor	CPR	cardiopulmonary resuscitation
		CPX	cardiopulmonary exercise
ACHD	adult congenital heart disease	CRT	cardiac resynchronization therapy
ACT	activated clotting time		
ADHERE	Acute Decompensated Heart Failure National Registry	CSF	cerebrospinal fluid
		CVP	central venous pressure
AHA	American Heart Association	CXR	chest X-ray
AL	amyloid light chain	DBD	donation after brain death
AMR	antibody-mediated rejection	DC	direct current
Ao	aorta	DCD	donation after circulatory death
aPTT	activated partial thromboplastin time		
		DCM	dilated cardiomyopathy
ARB	angiotensin II receptor blocker	DLCO	diffusion capacity of the lung for carbon monoxide
ARDS	acute respiratory distress syndrome	DPC	distal perfusion cannula
		DSA	donor-specific antibody
ASD	atrial septal defect	EACTS	European Association for Cardio-Thoracic Surgery
ATG	anti-thymocyte globulin		
ATTR-CM	transthyretin amyloid cardiomyopathy	EBV	Epstein–Barr virus
		ECG	electrocardiogram
AV	atrioventricular	ECLS	extracorporeal life support
BAL	bronchoalveolar lavage	ECMO	extracorporeal membrane oxygenation
BB	beta blocker		
BiVAD	biventricular assist device	E-CPR	extracorporeal cardiopulmonary resuscitation
BMI	body mass index		
BNP	B-type natriuretic peptide	EF	ejection fraction
BOS	bronchiolitis obliterans syndrome	eGFR	estimated glomerular filtration rate
BSA	body surface area	ELSO	Extracorporeal Life Support Organization
BSD	brainstem death		
BTT	bridge to transplantation	ESR	erythrocyte sedimentation rate
CAD	coronary artery disease	EVLP	ex vivo lung perfusion
CAV	cardiac allograft vasculopathy	FDA	Food and Drug Administration
CDAD	Clostridium difficile-associated diarrhoea	FEV1	forced expiratory volume in 1 second
		FiO$_2$	fraction of inspired oxygen
CF	cystic fibrosis	FVC	forced vital capacity
CI	cardiac index	GFR	glomerular filtration rate
CLAD	chronic lung allograft dysfunction	GI	gastrointestinal
		GTN	glycerol trinitrate
CMV	cytomegalovirus	HB	hepatitis B
CNI	calcineurin inhibitor		

HBV	hepatitis B virus	LVEDP	left ventricular end-diastolic pressure
HCV	hepatitis C virus	LVEF	left ventricular ejection fraction
HF	heart failure	LVH	left ventricular hypertrophy
HFpEF	heart failure with preserved ejection fraction	MAP	mean arterial pressure
HFrEF	heart failure with reduced ejection fraction	MCS	mechanical circulatory support
		MELD	Model for End-Stage Liver Disease
HFSS	Heart Failure Survival Score	MFI	mean fluorescent intensity
HHV	herpesvirus	MMF	mycophenolate mofetil
HIT	heparin-induced thrombocytopenia	MR	mitral regurgitation
		MRA	mineralocorticoid receptor antagonist
HIV	human immunodeficiency virus	MRI	magnetic resonance imaging
HKTx	heart–kidney transplantation	MRSA	methicillin-resistant Staphylococcus aureus
HLA	human leucocyte antigen		
HLTx	heart–lung transplantation	mTOR	mechanistic target of rapamycin
HM	HeartMate		
HSV	herpes simplex virus	MV	mitral valve
hTTR	hereditary transthyretin	NAAT	nucleic acid amplification testing
HZ	herpes zoster		
IA	invasive aspergillosis	NICM	non-ischaemic cardiomyopathy
IABP	intra-aortic balloon pump/ counterpulsation	NO	nitric oxide
		NODAT	new-onset diabetes after transplantation
ICD	implantable cardioverter defibrillator		
		NRAD	neutrophilic reversible allograft dysfunction
ICU	intensive care unit		
Ig	immunoglobulin	NTM	non-tuberculous mycobacteria
IJ	internal jugular	NT-proBNP	N-terminal pro-B type natriuretic peptide
IL-2	interleukin-2		
IL2R	interleukin-2 receptor	NYHA	New York Heart Association
IL2RA	interleukin-2 receptor antagonist	OHT	orthotopic heart transplantation
ILD	interstitial lung disease	PA	pulmonary artery
INR	international normalized ratio	PAC	pulmonary artery catheter
INTERMACS	Interagency Registry for Mechanically Assisted Circulatory Support	PaCO$_2$	partial arterial pressure of carbon dioxide
		PaO$_2$	partial arterial pressure of oxygen
ISHLT	International Society for Heart and Lung Transplant	PCCS	post-cardiotomy cardiogenic shock
IV	intravenous		
IVIG	intravenous immunoglobulin	PCO$_2$	partial pressure of carbon dioxide
LA	left atrial/atrium		
LAA	left atrial appendage	PCR	polymerase chain reaction
LAS	lung allocation score	PCWP	pulmonary capillary wedge pressure
LKTx	lung–kidney transplantation		
LLTx	lung–liver transplantation	PEEP	positive end-expiratory pressure
LV	left ventricular/ventricle		
LVAD	left ventricular assist device	PFO	patent foramen ovale
LVEDD	left ventricular end-diastolic diameter	PFT	pulmonary function testing
		PGD	primary graft dysfunction

PH	pulmonary hypertension		SVR	systemic vascular resistance
PJP	*Pneumocystis jirovecii* pneumonia		TAH	total artificial heart
PLE	protein-losing enteropathy		TAVR	transcatheter aortic valve replacement
PO	*per os* (orally)		TBBX	transbronchial biopsy
PO_2	partial pressure of oxygen		TEG	thromboelastography
PRA	panel-reactive antibody		TLC	total lung capacity
PT	physical therapy		TMP–SMX	trimethoprim–sulfamethoxazole
PTLD	post-transplant lymphoproliferative disorder		TOE	transoesophageal echocardiography/echocardiogram
PVR	pulmonary vascular resistance			
RA	right atrial/atrium		TR	tricuspid regurgitation
RAA	right atrial appendage		TTE	transthoracic echocardiography
RAAS	renin–angiotensin–aldosterone system		TTR	transthyretin
RAS	restrictive allograft syndrome		UFH	unfractionated heparin
rATG	rabbit anti-thymocyte globulin		UNOS	United Network for Organ Sharing
RCM	restrictive cardiomyopathy		V/Q	ventilation/perfusion
rpm	revolutions per minute		VA	venoarterial
RV	right ventricular/ventricle		VAD	ventricular assist device
RVAD	right ventricular assist device		VAV	venoarteriovenous
RVEDP	right ventricular end-diastolic pressure		VO_2max	maximal oxygen consumption
RVEF	right ventricular ejection fraction		VSD	ventricular septal defect
SHFM	Seattle Heart Failure Model		VV	venovenous
SOT	solid organ transplant		VZV	varicella zoster virus
SVC	superior vena cava		WHO	World Health Organization
SvO_2	mixed venous oxygen saturation		wtTTR	wild-type transthyretin

Heart failure

Medical and minimally invasive aspects of heart failure management

Epidemiology of chronic heart failure

Heart failure (HF) is a major public health concern affecting >6 million Americans. The care of patients with HF places a significant burden on the US healthcare system in terms of morbidity, mortality, and cost. In 2012, there were nearly 2 million clinic visits, 500,000 emergency room visits, and >1 million hospital discharges (~25% of discharged patients are readmitted within 30 days) for HF-related care with an associated total cost of $30 billion. Projections estimate $70 billion in total HF-related spending by 2030, with approximately 80% of costs coming directly from hospital admissions.

Clinical assessment of heart failure

HF is characterized by functional limitations resulting from sequelae of increased intracardiac filling pressures or low cardiac output. Clinical assessment including a detailed history and physical examination is imperative to differentiate patients with HF from a variety of alternative diagnoses. Worsening dyspnoea, orthopnoea, paroxysmal nocturnal dyspnoea, peripheral oedema, and elevated jugular venous pulsations are all common signs and symptoms of HF patients and are suggestive of increased left- and right-sided filling pressures. Patients with low cardiac output may complain of fatigue and poor exercise tolerance though cool/mottled extremities, resting tachycardia, and a narrow pulse pressure are findings more specific of a low output state. Pertinent items from the patient history, common signs and symptoms, and important physical examination findings for HF are listed in Box 1.1.

After confirmation of a HF diagnosis, further stratification should be based on disease severity and/or functional limitation. The American College of Cardiology (ACC) and American Heart Association (AHA) developed a staging system focused on disease progression whereas the New York Heart Association (NYHA) classification is based upon functional limitation (Table 1.1). Both classification systems provide unique and complementary schemas that facilitate an understanding of the clinical condition and prognosis of individuals and cohorts of patients.

Aetiologies of heart failure

Development of primary cardiomyopathy can result from impaired structure/functioning of the myocardium, cardiac valves, or conduction system. Cardiomyopathy can also occur secondary to disordered functioning of another organ, such as cor pulmonale, where chronic lung disease leads to pulmonary hypertension (PH) and subsequent right HF.

Meta-analyses suggest that underlying coronary artery disease (CAD) is the most common aetiology of heart failure with reduced ejection fraction (HFrEF), and is responsible for at least 65% of the diagnoses. Chronic hypertension and diabetes are also important risk factors for development of HFrEF. In fact, CAD, hypertension, and diabetes act synergistically to augment the risk of development of HFrEF. As such, an emphasis on HFrEF prevention has become an important mission of the ACC and AHA.

Box 1.1 Common findings in heart failure

Pertinent items from patient history suggestive of heart failure
- Previous history of HF.
- Other cardiovascular comorbidities (CAD, congenital heart disease, valvular disease, left bundle branch block).
- Previous myocardial infarction.
- Risk factors for heart failure (diabetes, hypertension, obesity).
- Systemic illnesses with cardiac involvement (amyloidosis, sarcoidosis, Chagas, rheumatic, glycogen storage disease).
- Chronic human immunodeficiency virus (HIV) infection or acquired immune deficiency syndrome (AIDS).
- Recent viral-like illness.
- Toxic exposures.
- Substance abuse (e.g. alcohol).
- Current malignancy or previous exposure to chemotherapy.

Signs and symptoms of heart failure
- Shortness of breath.
- Dyspnoea on exertion.
- Peripheral oedema.
- Orthopnoea/paroxysmal nocturnal dyspnoea.
- Increasing abdominal girth/bloating.
- Early satiety.
- Fatigue.
- Altered mental status.
- Dizziness/presyncope/syncope.
- Bendopnea (shortness of breath when bending over).

Physical examination findings suggestive of heart failure
- Tachycardia.
- Narrow pulse pressure or thready pulse.
- Tachypnoea.
- Elevated jugular venous pressure.
- Rales or diminished breath sounds.
- Point of maximal cardiac impulse laterally displaced.
- S3 or S4 heart sounds.
- Hepatomegaly with or without pulsatile liver.
- Ascites.
- Peripheral oedema with or without chronic skin changes.
- Cheyne-Stokes breathing (Oscillatory breathing pattern).

Non-ischaemic cardiomyopathies (NICMs) are also an important group of diagnoses that should always be considered when evaluating patients with HF. Valvular heart disease (rheumatic and non-rheumatic), electrical conduction system disorders (incessant/inappropriate tachycardia or chronic left bundle branch block chronic right ventricular pacing), toxin and chemotherapy exposure, excessive alcohol consumption, infiltrative systemic diseases, viral infections, Chagas disease, and other NICMs constitute approximately 25% of cases of HFrEF. Genetic cardiomyopathies are also an important aetiology of NICM and have been reported to be responsible

Table 1.1 Heart failure staging and functional classification

ACC/AHA staging		NYHA functional classification	
At high risk of HF but without structural abnormalities or symptoms	A	None	
Structural heart disease present but without symptoms of HF	B	I	No limitation; ordinary physical exertion does not cause HF symptoms
Structural heart disease present, with previous or current symptoms of HF	C	I	No limitation; ordinary physical exertion does not cause HF symptoms
		II	Slight limitation; no resting symptoms; ordinary physical exertion causes HF symptoms
		III	Marked limitation; no resting symptoms; less than ordinary activity causes HF symptoms
Refractory HF requiring specialized interventions	D	IV	Significant limitation; symptoms of HF present at rest or with minimal exertion

for up to 50% of idiopathic dilated cardiomyopathies. It is important to evaluate for these exposures, even in the presence of risk factors for ischaemic cardiomyopathy, as many of them can be at least partially treated, resulting in improvement of native cardiac function. Importantly, a substantial number of patients have an idiopathic cardiomyopathy, which usually

---

Box 1.2 Aetiologies of heart failure
- CAD (acute myocardial infarction and chronic ischaemia).
- Chronic hypertension.
- Valvular heart disease (stenotic and regurgitant lesions).
- Intra- or extracardiac shunting.
- Familial/genetic.
- Toxins.
- Medications (anthracycline chemotherapies, taxane chemotherapies, tumour necrosis factor alpha inhibitors, neuropsychiatric stimulants, etc.).
- Infiltrative diseases (sarcoidosis, amyloidosis).
- Metabolic disorders (e.g. thyrotoxicosis, beriberi, glycogen storage disease).
- Myocarditis.
- Chronic tachyarrhythmias.
- Chronic bradyarrhythmias.
  - Left bundle branch block
  - Chronic RV pacing
- Cor pulmonale.

presents as dilated NICM. Aetiologies of cardiomyopathy and HF are listed in Box 1.2.

Evaluation for patients with heart failure with reduced ejection fraction

Transthoracic echocardiography

Non-invasive cardiac imaging plays a vital role in the assessment of patients with HF. Transthoracic echocardiography (TTE) can be performed at the bedside without risk to the patient and without associated radiation exposure. TTE can be used to help determine the aetiology of HF via assessment of structural abnormalities, electromechanical dyssynchrony, valvular pathology, and pericardial disease. Routine assessment includes quantitatively measuring systolic function, wall thickness, chamber sizes and volumes. These measurements can be particularly helpful in considering HF aetiology, chronicity, and potential for recovery. Furthermore, TTE can be used to measure intracardiac filling pressures and flow across valves.

TTE is also commonly used to assess right-sided filling pressures, which can be helpful in guiding diuretic therapy. Right atrial (RA) pressure can be estimated by measuring inferior vena cava (IVC) diameter and relative change in size with inspiration. Normal IVC size with inspiratory collapse of >50% is associated with normal RA pressure. An enlarged IVC or smaller inspiratory collapse is associated with increased RA pressures.

Heart catheterization

Determining the presence of significant concomitant CAD in HFrEF has important therapeutic and prognostic implications. Cardiac catheterization via invasive coronary arteriography is considered the 'gold standard' for assessing the presence and severity of CAD and its contribution to HF. Based on results from the Surgical Treatment for Ischemic Heart Failure (STICH) and associated STICH Extension Study (STICHES), patients with CAD and HF with reduced systolic dysfunction benefit from coronary artery bypass grafting.

Direct measurement of intracardiac pressures and cardiac output via right heart catheterization can be useful when there is uncertainty regarding aetiology of symptoms or when precise measurements are required for determining candidacy of surgical HF therapies (transplantation or durable mechanical circulatory support). Furthermore, right heart catheterization can be helpful when dynamic changes in intracardiac pressure and volume need to be measured. A common example is an exercise right heart catheterization to determine the severity of mitral regurgitation (MR) or diastolic dysfunction. Right heart catheterization with concomitant pulmonary vasodilator administration may be performed to determine the aetiology of PH, candidacy for medications, and response to treatment.

Functional testing

Reduced exercise tolerance is a common complaint in patients with even mild HF, and can be exacerbated by common comorbidities. The 6-minute walk test is a valuable tool that can be safely administered to quantify submaximal functional capacity in patients with HF. Furthermore, it can be measured serially and has been shown to predict outcomes. Cardiopulmonary exercise (CPX) testing is typically used to more completely quantify and characterize exercise capacity in patients with HF. CPX testing distinguishes between aetiologies of functional limitation including poor effort, pulmonary disease, or lack of cardiovascular reserve. Peak oxygen consumption, commonly referred to as 'VO$_2$max', is measured during CPX testing and provides the most objective assessment of functional capacity. Peak oxygen consumption is a foundational component in the determination of patients likely to benefit from surgical HF therapies including transplantation or durable mechanical circulatory support.

Pharmacotherapies for heart failure with reduced ejection fraction

Chronic HF is characterized by a compensatory activation of the sympathetic nervous system and the renin–angiotensin–aldosterone system (RAAS) as a result of decreased cardiac output, reduced stimulation of arterial baroreceptors, and renal hypoperfusion. Activation of the RAAS system ultimately results in the conversion of angiotensin I to the biologically active molecule angiotensin II via angiotensin-converting enzyme (ACE). Angiotensin II has several negative effects in chronic HF including vasoconstriction, sodium retention, stimulation of aldosterone release causing myocardial fibrosis, and co-stimulation of the sympathetic nervous system leading to increased levels of plasma catecholamines. Thus, the pharmacological foundation for chronic HF is centred around reducing sympathetic nervous system activation and RAAS signalling.

Beta blockers

Long-term treatment of chronic HF with beta blockers (BBs) reduces symptom burden, improves functional status, halts or reverses disease progression, and reduces hospitalization and mortality. Beta antagonists inhibit circulating catecholamine stimulation of adrenergic receptors by competitive binding to reduce the compensatory sympathetic overdrive of patients with chronic HF.

Patients with symptomatic HF and a left ventricular ejection fraction (LVEF) of ≤40% should be treated with a BB. Three BBs have evidence supporting their use in patients with chronic HF: bisoprolol, metoprolol succinate, and carvedilol. Beta antagonists are a complex class of drugs with a variety of pharmacological effects. BBs may inhibit only the β_1 receptor, both β_1 and β_2 receptors, or β_1, β_2, and alpha receptors. In addition, some of the BBs have intrinsic sympathomimetic properties that mimic the effects of epinephrine and norepinephrine increasing both heart rate and blood pressure. Improved outcomes from BB use in patients with chronic HF is not a class effect. Bucindolol and metoprolol tartrate (short acting) have not been shown to be as effective, especially in select subgroups of patients. One of the three guideline-directed BBs should be prescribed to all patients with stable HF unless there is a contraindication or there has been previous intolerance. In general, it is recommended that patients be on stable doses of diuretic (if needed) prior to initiation of BB as there is a well-documented transient increase in risk of fluid retention with initiation or increase in BB dose.

Renin–angiotensin–aldosterone system antagonists

Inhibition of the RAAS is a key component of treatment for chronic HF. Increased RAAS signalling as a result of relative renal hypoperfusion increases circulating levels of angiotensin II. Until recently, use of either an angiotensin converting enzyme inhibitor (ACEi), or angiotensin II receptor blocker (ARB), in addition to a BB was considered cornerstone therapy for patients with symptomatic HF and an LVEF of ≤40%. Treatment of patients with chronic HF with an ACEi or ARB (in patients with ACEi intolerance) has been repeatedly shown to reduce mortality, reduce HF hospitalization, and improve functional status.

A new class of drugs that inhibit the angiotensin receptor and neutral endopeptidase (neprilysin) have been shown to be superior to an ACEi for reducing mortality and HF hospitalization in patients with symptomatic HF. The Prospective Comparison of ARNI [angiotensin receptor–neprilysin inhibitor] with ACEI to Determine Impact on Global Mortality and Morbidity in Heart Failure (PARADIGM-HF) trial was a randomized double-blind trial comparing sacubitril–valsartan with enalapril in patients with class II–IV HFrEF. The trial was stopped prematurely given the benefit of treatment with sacubitril–valsartan. Sacubitril–valsartan was associated with an absolute risk reduction of nearly 5% in the combined endpoint of cardiovascular death or HF hospitalization, and 3% for cardiovascular death alone. Given the positive data for use of sacubitril–valsartan, the ACC and AHA have published updates to the HF management guidelines to assist physicians and other providers with initiation and dosing. Criteria for initiation include elevated serum natriuretic peptide levels, a systolic blood pressure of >100 mmHg, and a glomerular filtration rate (GFR) of at least 30 mL/min/1.73 m^2. As with all other HF therapies, dose adjustments should be titrated to systolic blood pressure or evidence of intolerance such as renal dysfunction or angioedema.

Mineralocorticoid receptor antagonists

Mineralocorticoid receptor antagonists (MRAs) such as spironolactone and eplerenone also block the effects of RAAS activation and have been shown to improve outcomes in patients with chronic HF treated with maximally tolerated doses of BB and ACEi/ARB. Mechanistically, MRAs inhibit the deleterious effects of aldosterone, which acts directly on the heart by promoting development of cardiac fibrosis. Mineralocorticoid receptors are overexpressed in diseased hearts in proportion to the degree of cardiac dysfunction. Aldosterone binding to the mineralocorticoid receptor in the diseased heart creates a cycle of production of angiotensin II and thus a propagating cycle of RAAS activation and worsening left ventricular (LV) dysfunction and symptomatic HF.

Sodium Glucose Co-transporter 2 Inhibitors

Sodium Glucose Co-transporter 2 Inhibitors (SGLT2i) are a class of medications that inhibit glucose reabsorption in the proximal convoluted tubule of the nephron. These medications have been repeatedly shown to reduce all-cause mortality, cardiovascular mortality, and HF hospitalizations in patients with HF regardless of diabetes status. The mechanism of action related to improving cardiovascular outcomes in patients with HF is not yet understood.

Ivabradine

Ivabradine is a selective sinus node inhibitor which acts specifically on the hyperpolarization-activated cyclic nucleotide-gated channels within the sinoatrial node. Thus, ivabradine slows depolarization within the sinus node to lower resting heart rate without affecting myocardial contractility or relaxation. Further, ivabradine has no impact on blood pressure. The Systolic Heart Failure Treatment with the IF Inhibitor Ivabradine Trial (SHIFT) randomized patients already on maximally tolerated HF medications and a resting sinus heart rate of at least 70 beats per minute to ivabradine or placebo. Patients randomized to ivabradine experienced an improvement in the primary combined endpoint of cardiovascular death or hospital admission for worsening HF. Ivabradine is therefore recommended for patients with chronic HF with an LVEF of ≤35% and are in sinus rhythm with a resting heart rate of at least 70 beats per minute despite maximal BB dosage and RAAS inhibition. Importantly, ivabradine should not be used as a full or partial substitute for BB.

Hydralazine and isosorbide dinitrate

Fixed-dose combination hydralazine plus isosorbide dinitrate for treatment of chronic HF is reserved for selected patient populations. Specifically, for patients intolerant of RAAS blocking agents due to angioedema, or for black patients with persistent symptoms of HF despite optimally titrated BB plus ACEi/ARB and MRA. The African-American Heart Failure Trial (A-HeFT) was terminated early due to significant improvement in the combined endpoint of death, HF hospitalization, and quality of life in patients treated with fixed-dose combination hydralazine plus isosorbide dinitrate compared to placebo (6.2% vs 10.2%, p = 0.02). While not directly assessed in clinical trials, the relative benefits of sacubitril–valsartan are sufficiently pronounced such that it should take priority over the use of hydralazine–nitrates.

Loop diuretics

Despite a glaring absence of evidence to support their use, loop diuretics are among the most frequently used pharmacotherapies for HF. Loop diuretics including furosemide, torsemide, and bumetanide work on the apical surface of the thick ascending loop of Henle to directly inhibit transport of sodium, potassium, and chloride ions. Inhibition of ion reabsorption in this location effectively leads to the natriuretic effect of loop diuretics. Administration of loop diuretics intravenously can also have a vasodilatory effect via action on ion transporters located in vascular smooth muscle cells.

Each loop diuretic has a different bioavailability when administered orally. Furosemide has the greatest variability, with a mean of 50% and ranges from 10% to 90%. Furosemide absorption can be delayed with food intake as well as in patients with significant gut oedema or low duodenal blood flow. This in turn leads to reduced peak plasma concentration and can contribute to diuretic resistance.

Torsemide and bumetanide have higher and more predictable oral bio-availability (>90%) with associated pharmacokinetics not limited by absorption. Of the loop diuretics, torsemide has the longest half-life (6 hours vs 2.7 hours for furosemide vs 1.3 hours for bumetanide). There are limited data comparing loop diuretics in patients with HF. The ongoing Torsemide Comparison with Furosemide for Management of Heart Failure (TRANSFORM-HF) trial will determine if treatment with torsemide improves 12-month all-cause mortality for patients with HF.

When dosing loop diuretics, it is important to remember that they all have steep dose–response curves or 'threshold effect'. Increasing or escalating doses of medication will not increase the natriuretic effect, but may act to prolong the time of serum drug concentration above the required threshold to achieve desired effect. It is important to account for this concept and relative bioavailability when choosing and dosing diuretics for patients with HF.

Inotropes

Positive inotropic agents cause an increase in cardiac output via a variety of pharmacological targets including inhibition of phosphodiesterase-3 (milrinone), beta-adrenergic receptor agonism (dobutamine), calcium sensitization (levosimendan), and increased intracellular calcium via inhibition of cell membrane ion exchange (digoxin). Though these medications may temporarily improve haemodynamics via their ability to augment cardiac contractility and/or reduce pulmonary and systemic vascular resistance (SVR), the use of intravenous inotropes for management of acute or chronic HF lacks evidence.

Digoxin can be administered either orally or intravenously and has been studied prospectively for patients with chronic HF. The Digitalis Investigation Group (DIG) study randomized patients receiving ACEi and diuretic to either placebo or oral digoxin. Patients in the treatment arm experienced a reduced rate of overall hospitalization and HF hospitalization. There was no difference in all-cause mortality. The results of the DIG trial, in combination with use of other evidence-based guideline-directed medical therapy for HF, has dramatically reduced the use of oral digoxin for patients with chronic HF. Interestingly, findings from the Randomized Assessment of the Effect of Digoxin on Inhibitors of the Angiotensin Converting Enzyme (RADIANCE) and Prospective Randomized Study of Ventricular Failure and the Efficacy of Digoxin (PROVED) trials suggest that discontinuation of digoxin increases the risk of adverse outcomes in ambulatory patients with HFrEF. Similar findings have been found in patients who are hospitalized for HF and have digoxin discontinued during admission.

Prevention of sudden cardiac death

Ventricular arrhythmias are common in patients with chronic HF. Sustained ventricular arrhythmias and sudden cardiac death are responsible for as much as two-thirds of HF-related mortality. As such, implantation of primary and secondary prevention cardioverter defibrillators is considered a class I recommendation with a strong level of evidence. Clinical practice guidelines recommend placement of an implantable cardioverter defibrillator (ICD) in patients with NYHA class II–III symptoms and an LVEF of ≤35% who are on maximally tolerated guideline-directed medical therapies for HF. For patients with ischaemic heart disease, clinical trials and guidelines recommend waiting at least 40 days post myocardial infarction and at least 3 months following revascularization for ICD implantation (if applicable). Placement of a secondary prevention ICD should be done following an event of sudden cardiac death if obviously reversible causes of ventricular arrhythmias have been excluded such as acute myocardial ischaemia/infarction, electrolyte abnormalities, and toxic exposures including medication exposures that are proarrhythmic.

Cardiac resynchronization therapy

Observational studies suggest that electrical and mechanical dyssynchrony induced by a left bundle branch block on electrocardiogram (ECG) can lead to cardiac remodelling with subsequent cardiomyopathy, chronic HF with exacerbation of functional MR, and increased mortality. Cardiac resynchronization therapy (CRT) involves implantation of a permanent transvenous pacing system that provides concomitant pacing of the left and right ventricles. This promotes electrical and mechanical ventricular synchrony. Randomized trials have shown benefit in patients with a QRS of at least 150 milliseconds with a left bundle branch block morphology, symptomatic HF, on maximally tolerated evidence-based pharmacotherapies, and an LVEF of ≤35%. Similar to ICD therapy, implantation should be at least 40 days following an episode of myocardial ischaemia or an acute myocardial infarction. Reversible causes of cardiomyopathy and HF should also be addressed prior to referral for CRT. Importantly, there is no evidence of benefit in patients with right bundle branch block or incomplete/partial left bundle branch block. For patients with an LVEF of >35% but <50%, if a high burden of ventricular pacing is needed for another indication, it is also reasonable to pursue CRT placement.

Transcatheter valvular therapies for heart failure

Transcatheter mitral repair for secondary mitral regurgitation

MR can occur as a result of primary pathology of the mitral valve (MV) leaflets or secondary to pathology of the structure and function of the heart. For secondary MR due to LV dilation and secondary distortion of the MV annulus, transcatheter MV repair has been recently shown to be a viable therapy. The MitraClip, based on the Alfieri edge-to-edge leaflet repair, is the only US Food and Drug Administration-approved device for percutaneous repair of MR.

The Cardiovascular Outcomes Assessment of the MitraClip Percutaneous Therapy for Heart Failure Patients with Functional Mitral Regurgitation (COAPT) and Percutaneous Repair with the MitraClip Device for Severe Functional/Secondary Mitral Regurgitation (MITRA-FR) trials provide the only evidence to guide percutaneous repair of secondary MR. The COAPT trial enrolled >600 patients with moderate to severe or severe secondary

MR with associated LVEF of 20–50% and at least NYHA class II HF symptoms despite maximal tolerated doses of HF pharmacotherapies. Patients were randomized to continue medical therapies plus transcatheter MV repair (MitraClip) or medical therapy alone. Patients treated with MitraClip had a significant reduction in mortality and HF hospitalization (evident within 30 days of therapy) compared to the medical therapy arm. Furthermore, patient-reported outcomes related to functional capacity and quality of life were improved after receiving transcatheter MV repair compared to medical therapy alone.

In MITRA-FR, 304 patients with at least moderate secondary MR, with associated LVEF of 15–40% and symptomatic HF, were randomized to either medical therapy plus transcatheter MV repair or medical therapy alone. The results of MITRA-FR were negative for the primary outcome of all-cause mortality at 12 months or in the rate of unplanned HF hospitalization.

The discrepant results of these trials are not entirely obvious but important differences include a larger study population, longer duration of follow-up, and a higher severity of MR in COAPT. Taken in aggregate, the data from COAPT and MITRA-FR suggest that in appropriately selected patients, transcatheter MV repair is a reasonable strategy to improve important clinical outcomes, functional capacity, and quality of life.

Transcatheter aortic valve replacement for heart failure

Transcatheter aortic valve replacement (TAVR) is an alternative to surgical valve replacement in patients with severe aortic stenosis, especially those at increased risk of death from surgery. Aortic stenosis and HF are common diagnoses in older patients (>75 years old) and likely synergistically lead to worsened outcomes. Unfortunately, evidence-based HF medications have no effect on the valvular component of afterload in aortic stenosis and associated outcomes. Thus, the Transcatheter Aortic Valve Replacement to Unload the Left Ventricle in Patients with Advanced Heart Failure (TAVR UNLOAD) trial (NCT02661451) was designed to test the hypothesis that TAVR on top of optimal medical therapy improves outcomes in patients with moderate aortic stenosis and HFrEF.

Prognostication for heart failure

Risk scores

In addition to assessment of ACC/AHA staging and NYHA functional classification, routine assessment of the potential for adverse outcome is an important part of the evaluation and management of patients with HF. Validated scores for risk stratification in patients with chronic and acute HF exist. The Seattle Heart Failure Model (SHFM) is the most robust and commonly used risk score to predict timing and mode of death in ambulatory patients with chronic HF. The SHFM can be accessed online (https://depts.washington.edu/shfm) and incorporates multiple clinical variables including demographics, LVEF, vital signs, medications, and various laboratory values to accurately predict 1-, 2-, and 3-year survival. Importantly, the SHFM model has been validated repeatedly in multiple contexts.

For patients admitted with acutely decompensated HF, a model developed from the Acute Decompensated Heart Failure National Registry (ADHERE) can be used readily at the bedside to predict in-hospital mortality. Importantly, the ADHERE score for acute HF involves only three routinely measured clinical variables: systolic blood pressure, blood urea nitrogen, and serum creatinine.

Referral to advanced heart failure specialists

Patients with chronic HF who progress to develop persistent and severe symptoms despite optimal medical therapy should be referred to an advanced HF team. Further manifestations of worsening HF or development of end-stage disease include intolerance of evidence-based medical therapies due to hypotension, NYHA class IV symptoms, refractory volume overload requiring frequent hospitalization, cardiac cachexia with associated unintentional weight loss not otherwise explainable, or requirement of intravenous inotropes to assist with diuresis or for management of hypotension. Ultimately, earlier referral allows for trained specialists to evaluate a patient for surgical HF therapies before becoming too unstable to tolerate life-sustaining treatments.

Chapter 2

15

Myocarditis: diagnosis and treatment

Introduction

Myocarditis is an inflammatory disease of the myocardium caused by a number of infectious and non-infectious problems and the subsequent inflammatory response to the initial insult. It can present either acutely or subacutely and result in a spectrum of clinical manifestations ranging from mild cardiac damage (normal ejection fraction (EF) and mild symptoms) to fulminant myocarditis associated with either cardiogenic shock or sudden death. In this chapter, the aetiologies, clinical presentation, diagnostic modalities, therapies, and prognosis will be reviewed.

Definition

Myocarditis is defined as inflammation of the heart muscle related to either a cellular or humoral immune process and is established by either histological, immunological, or immunohistochemical criteria. It may either occur in the setting of a systemic immune-mediated disorder or in isolation to just the heart. It should also be distinguished from dilated cardiomyopathy (DCM) which is a clinical diagnosis with dilation and reduced contraction of the left and/or both ventricles not related to another cause (CAD, valvular heart disease, inflammation).

Epidemiology

The true incidence of myocarditis is undefined due to many cases being relatively asymptomatic. A study using the International Classification of Diseases estimated a prevalence of about 22 cases per 100,000 patients annually. In young competitive athletes, studies rank myocarditis as the third leading cause of sudden death. Studies have also shown that between 1% and 5% of patients testing positive for acute viral infections exhibit a form of myocarditis. A large study evaluating causes of cardiomyopathy in 1230 patients performed endomyocardial biopsies and found that 9% had myocarditis. Similarly, in the Myocarditis Treatment Trial, evidence of myocarditis was found in 10% of the patients who underwent endomyocardial biopsy (214/2233 patients) for presumed myocarditis based on a history of HF and an appropriate clinical syndrome. Based on the low prevalence in patients presenting with NICM, one must remember that there are many other reasons for cardiomyopathy and have an increased suspicion for myocarditis in those with an acute presentation, a viral prodrome, and elevated biomarkers.

Aetiology

Although this chapter focuses on viral myocarditis, the causes of myocarditis are extensive and include both infectious and non-infectious agents as outlined in Box 2.1. The most common cause of myocarditis are viral infections including adenovirus, cytomegalovirus (CMV), enterovirus including coxsackie virus A and B, hepatitis C virus, human immunodeficiency virus, human herpesvirus 6, influenza virus, and parvovirus B19. Although exact mechanisms are unclear, based on animal data from coxsackie B virus studies, the currently accepted mechanism is that the virus enters the cardiomyocyte via specific receptors on the cell surface. An immunological response consisting of T lymphocytes and macrophages leads to the elimination of the virus. In some patients, this immune response persists for weeks to months after viral elimination resulting in DCM. Additionally, this damage may result in the formation of autoantibodies to various cardiac epitopes resulting in further damage to the myocardium. This response is more likely to occur in patients with a genetic predisposition, leading to the hypothesis that there might be a genetic relationship to the development of myocarditis. The inability to eliminate the virus or turn off the immune response results in chronic myocarditis.

The European Society of Cardiology Working Group on Myocardial and Pericardial Disease has developed a model with three phases. In phase 1, direct microbial or toxin damage results in myocyte death, release of chemokines and cytokines, and activation of the immune system resulting in active myocarditis. Phase 2 is the elimination of the agent and either resolution of the inflammation (healed myocarditis) or continued infection or inflammation or both (chronic myocarditis). Phase 3 is split up into four groups. Chronic microbial myocarditis occurs when the offending agent is present with ongoing inflammation and destruction. Chronic microbial and immune myocarditis occurs when both the microbial agent is present and autoantibodies are present with ongoing inflammation and destruction. Chronic autoreactive myocarditis occurs when there are autoantibodies but no microbial agent. Finally, DCM occurs when there is no active inflammation but either the microbial agent or autoantibodies or both are present with ongoing destruction.

Box 2.1 Causes of myocarditis

Infectious
- Viruses—most common.
- Bacteria.
- Fungi.
- Parasites.
- Protozoa.
- Rickettsiae.
- Spirochetes.
- Helminths.

Non-infectious
- Autoimmune.
- Sarcoidosis.
- Giant cells.
- Systemic disorders
- Hypersensitivity reactions.
- Radiation.
- Antibiotics.
- Psychiatric medications.
- Cardiotoxins.
- Checkpoint inhibitor drugs.
- Illicit drugs.

In addition to viral and other infectious agents, a similar process can occur via the non-infectious mechanisms including drugs, toxins, and many of the rheumatological disorders. After the initial insult to the heart, the immune system responds in a similar manner as described above, resulting in an inflammatory state.

Giant cell myocarditis is an autoimmune process characterized by a mixed inflammatory process with T lymphocytes and multinucleated giant cells plus extensive necrosis. Patients tend to present with fulminant myocarditis with rapidly progressive HF, ventricular arrhythmias, and heart block. It is a particularly aggressive form of myocarditis with the median survival being 3 months without immunosuppressive therapy. Treatment with aggressive immunosuppression with two or three different agents similar to early after heart transplantation has been shown to improve survival with a 5-year transplant-free survival rate of >50%. One of the primary reasons to perform a biopsy is looking for giant cell myocarditis since it is responsive to immunosuppressive therapy.

Clinical features (symptoms/diagnosis)

The clinical presentation of myocarditis is quite varied and can range from mild dyspnoea and chest pain with a normal EF to cardiogenic shock. The 'classic' presentation is of a patient experiencing a viral illness which is often fairly benign prior to developing acute HF symptoms including exertional dyspnoea followed by oedema, orthopnoea, and paroxysmal nocturnal dyspnoea. Many patients also have conduction disturbances or arrhythmias resulting in complaints of tachycardia and palpitations. Others will present with chest pain and an acute coronary syndrome-type presentation. Unfortunately, some patients present in cardiogenic shock or after sudden death.

Although classically myocarditis is thought of as a common reason for HF, many patients will present with a normal EF. An Italian registry of patients with myocarditis recently reported its findings on clinical presentation. Of 443 patients either under the age of 50 or under the age of 70 with a negative cardiac catheterization, the diagnosis of myocarditis was confirmed by either positive endomyocardial biopsy or the combination of a positive troponin plus peripheral oedema plus late gadolinium enhancement on cardiac magnetic resonance imaging (MRI). It was found that only 26.6% of the patients presented with either an EF of <50% or ventricular arrhythmias or a low cardiac output syndrome. Additionally, there were differences in the presentation between the two groups with the complicated group having a higher incidence of dyspnoea (55.7% vs 6.2%), syncope (16.5% vs 2.5%), and a history of autoimmune disorder (15.4% vs 4.2%). Patients with a normal EF were more apt to have chest pain (59.1% vs 96.6%) and ST segment elevation with a normal catheterization as their presenting symptom. Of note, there was no difference in the number of patients presenting with a flu-like syndrome between the two groups with 64.5% having fever, 80.5% having flu prodromal symptoms, and 36.8% having sore throat.

The diagnosis of myocarditis begins with a high clinical suspicion. These patients are often young and present with dyspnoea and including cardiac problems in the differential diagnosis often doesn't occur. Patients usually present with either signs and/or symptoms of HF, chest pain, or arrhythmias. About half of the patients will have a history of a recent upper respiratory illness. The ECG will often demonstrate sinus tachycardia but might also show signs of myocardial inflammation including repolarization abnormalities and QRS prolongation. Heart block is often suggestive (but not required) of either cardiac sarcoidosis or giant cell myocarditis. The ECG might also only be suggestive of pericarditis with PR segment depression and non-specific ST, T-wave changes instead of elevation.

Laboratory findings will include an elevated B-type natriuretic peptide (BNP) reflective of HF and usually elevated troponin I or T. Studies have shown though that patients with biopsy-proven myocarditis can have normal troponin levels so the absence of a troponin elevation does not rule out myocarditis. An elevated erythrocyte sedimentation rate (ESR) is also frequently found. A complete blood count with differential should always be performed to evaluate for peripheral eosinophilia. The European Society of Cardiology guidelines suggest monitoring of serum troponin, ESR, and C-reactive protein. Routine viral serologies have not been proven to be helpful and are no longer recommended as part of the evaluation.

The chest X-ray (CXR) can be suggestive of HF with pulmonary vascular congestion or an enlarged heart. However, the absence of these findings does not rule out myocarditis and, in general, the CXR should be used to rule out other aetiologies of dyspnoea or chest pain such as a pneumonia.

The echocardiogram is quite helpful in the diagnosis. Patients will often present with diffuse hypokinesis and possibly ventricular dilation. An increase in LV wall thickness can be a sign of myocardial oedema and might correlate with reduced voltage on ECG. A surrounding pericardial effusion can often be present. If the LV is dilated, that is usually a sign of less acute presentation and tends to correlate with a reduced incidence of recovery of LV function. Additionally, the echocardiogram should be used to rule out other possible causes of HF including valvular heart disease and focal wall motion abnormalities suggestive of CAD. A normal EF does not rule out myocarditis as many patients will have a normal EF.

Cardiac MRI is now quite frequently used in the diagnosis of myocarditis. A consensus conference resulted in the Lake Louise Criteria for the diagnosis of myocarditis by MRI which are outlined in Box 2.2.

For patients who present with acute cardiogenic shock or heart block or arrhythmias, a cardiac MRI often cannot be performed due to safety issues and one should consider an endomyocardial biopsy. The ACC issued a consensus statement on the indications for biopsy and gave recommendations for endomyocardial biopsy for the following patients:
- New-onset HF of <2 weeks and haemodynamic compromise.
- New-onset HF of 2 weeks to 3 months associated with a dilated LV and either new ventricular arrhythmias or second- or third-degree heart block or failure to respond to usual medical therapy.
- HF for >3 months with a dilated LV and either new ventricular arrhythmias or second- or third-degree heart block or failure to respond to usual medical therapy.
- HF and a suspected allergic reaction.

Not included in the guidelines but a new consideration is to perform endomyocardial biopsy in patients who have recently received checkpoint inhibitors and have new HF due to the increased incidence of myocarditis.

Box 2.2 Cardiac MRI criteria for the diagnosis of myocarditis

Requires the setting of clinically suspected myocarditis. Need at least two criteria for the diagnosis:

1. Regional or global increased signal intensity of T2-weighted images suggesting oedema.
2. Increased global early gadolinium enhancement ratio between myocardium and skeletal muscle on gadolinium-enhanced T1-weighted images suggestive of capillary leakage.
3. Late gadolinium enhancement defined as at least one focal lesion in a non-coronary distribution typically involving the myocardium or subepicardium.

A repeat study is suggested if none of the above are present but symptoms are recent and there is a strong clinical suspicion of myocarditis or only one of the criteria is present.

The presence of LV dysfunction or pericardial effusion is supportive evidence for myocarditis.

Reproduced from Friedrich MG, Sechtem U, Schulz-Menger J, et al; International Consensus Group on Cardiovascular Magnetic Resonance in Myocarditis. Cardiovascular magnetic resonance in myocarditis: A JACC White Paper. J Am Coll Cardiol. 2009 Apr 28;53(17):1475–87. doi: 10.1016/j.jacc.2009.02.007 with permission from Elsevier.

To improve diagnostic accuracy, one should take at least six pieces of tissue. In addition to the routine pathological evaluation, it is ideal to perform immunohistochemistry and polymerase chain reaction (PCR) to look for a viral genome. One should simultaneously study the peripheral blood to rule out an acute systemic infection and possible contamination of the myocardial samples. As outlined in the section on therapy (see p. 22), aggressive immunosuppression for patients with 'virus-negative' myocarditis has been shown to improve outcomes in small trials. The Dallas criteria were developed to define myocarditis in biopsy specimens (Box 2.3). The definition of active myocarditis required both an inflammatory infiltrate of the myocardium with necrosis and/or degeneration of adjacent myocytes not typical of damage associated with CAD (Fig. 2.1). Additionally, occasionally the cause of myocarditis can be found for patients with Chagas disease, Lyme carditis, and CMV. The diagnostic criteria for clinically suspected myocarditis as outlined by the European Society of Cardiology are outlined in Box 2.4.

Finally, for patients at high suspicion of CAD, cardiac catheterization should be performed to rule out CAD.

Box 2.3 Dallas criteria for the diagnosis of myocarditis

First biopsy
- Myocarditis with or without fibrosis.
- Borderline myocarditis.
- No myocarditis.

Subsequent biopsy
- Ongoing (persistent) myocarditis with or without fibrosis.
- Resolving (healing) myocarditis with or without fibrosis.
- Resolved (healed) myocarditis with or without fibrosis.

Box 2.4 Diagnostic criteria for clinically suspected myocarditis

Clinical presentation

- Chest pain.
- New-onset or worsening dyspnoea (<3 months).
- Subacute/chronic or worsening dyspnoea (>3 months).
- Palpitations or other arrhythmia symptoms.
- Unexplained cardiogenic shock.

Diagnostic criteria

- ECG: new second- or third-degree heart block, bundle branch block, ST/T wave changes, ventricular tachycardia or fibrillation, frequent atrial or ventricular ectopy.
- Elevated troponin.
- Imaging abnormalities (echocardiography/MRI/angiography): LV dysfunction, ± effusion, increased wall thickness, thrombi.
- MRI: tissue oedema of late gadolinium enhancement pattern. Suspect if >1 clinical and >1 diagnostic criteria are present.

Reproduced from Caforio AL, Pankuweit S, Arbustini E, et al; European Society of Cardiology Working Group on Myocardial and Pericardial Diseases. Current state of knowledge on aetiology, diagnosis, management, and therapy of myocarditis: a position statement of the European Society of Cardiology Working Group on Myocardial and Pericardial Diseases. Eur Heart J. 2013 Sep;34(33):2636–48, 2648a–2648d. doi: 10.1093/eurheartj/eht210 with permission from Oxford University Press.

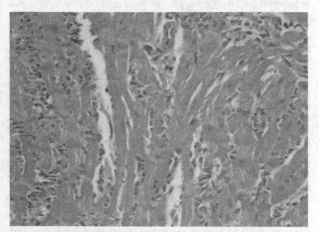

Fig. 2.1 Haematoxylin–eosin staining of an endomyocardial biopsy sample showing an inflammatory infiltrate with associated cellular necrosis consistent with acute myocarditis. See plate section.

Therapy

The initial management of patients with myocarditis and HF should focus on the usual therapy for patients with HF as outlined in Chapter 1. If patients are haemodynamically unstable, one should use caution with beta blocker therapy due to the acute, negative inotropic properties of those agents. Other agents used to control tachycardia should be used carefully as the increased heart rate may be compensatory for a low stroke volume. The treatment of arrhythmias should be as per usual protocol. Because many of these patients recover function, ICD therapy should be performed as well as per the usual guidelines.

For patients who present in cardiogenic shock, the initial management should focus on haemodynamic support of the patient with inotropes and vasopressors. Additionally, early transfer to a centre equipped with the ability to perform specialized diagnostic studies (MRI, endomyocardial biopsy) and mechanical support should be consider as patients can quickly decompensate. There are no randomized studies on the acute management of shock with myocarditis. In patients with shock after an acute myocardial infarction, norepinephrine has a lower incidence of arrhythmias and improved survival compared to dopamine. If an endomyocardial biopsy is performed, consideration should be given to also perform a right heart catheterization and leave it in place to help with management, although the use of right heart catheterization has not been associated with improved outcomes in this group. As outlined later in this chapter, some patients will be found to have a specific diagnosis on biopsy and in addition to supportive care, directed therapy towards that diagnosis should be performed. Finally, since complete recovery from myocarditis occurs so frequently, one should use aggressive temporary support including percutaneous assist devices or extracorporeal membrane oxygenation (ECMO) acutely in patients who are unresponsive to vasopressor therapy.

Left ventricular assist devices (LVADs) should be considered in patients who require temporary mechanical support and are not improving. In deciding whether or not to place permanent mechanical support, one should consider signs of irreversibility as outlined in Box 2.5. Even in that setting, over a period of a few months many patients will recover and can potentially have their device removed. In a study of 24 patients with a ventricular assist device (VAD) placed for fulminant myocarditis, the best predictor of recovery was an onset of symptoms within 1 week of presentation and female sex. A report from the Intervention in Myocarditis and Acute Cardiomyopathy 2 (IMAC2) study found that patients who did not recover after the VAD had a larger LV (left ventricular end-diastolic diameter (LVEDD) 7.0 cm vs 5.3 cm), less inflammation (0% vs 75%), and more fibrosis (100% vs 25%).

Finally, in patients who don't recover after placement of their VAD, consideration should be given to cardiac transplantation if appropriate. Early case reports of patients transplanted for lymphocytic myocarditis showed an increased rate of rejection and reduced survival. A larger study from the United Network for Organ Sharing (UNOS) database showed no differences in outcomes between patients with myocarditis versus other aetiologies. Finally, Columbia University reported the results of 32 patients transplanted with lymphocytic myocarditis and found similar survival and

> **Box 2.5 Factors associated with reduced incidence of recovery in acute myocarditis**
> • Lower EF (<40%).
> • Ventricular arrhythmias.
> • Low cardiac output requiring inotropes or MCS.
> • Cardiac-specific autoantibodies.
> • Syncope.
> • Biventricular dysfunction.
> • Persistence of viral genome.
> • Presence of fibrosis.
> • LVEDD >7.0 cm.

rejection rates to patients transplanted with idiopathic cardiomyopathy. At this time, one might consider heightened surveillance for rejection in these patients, but the presence of myocarditis before transplantation should not be a contraindication for transplantation.

Therapies for specific forms of myocarditis

Lymphocytic myocarditis is defined as the presence of a cellular infiltrate and LV dysfunction. A number of clinical trials have been performed to evaluate the benefits of immunosuppressive therapy in patients with biopsy-proven myocarditis. The first large trial was the Myocarditis Treatment Trial which evaluated the use of ciclosporin and steroids versus placebo. Over 2000 patients were screened to find the 111 with active myocarditis. There was no significant different in the endpoint of improvement in EF between the two arms. Based on data showing improvement in children with myocarditis, intravenous immunoglobulin (IVIG) has been studied as well. In two randomized studies, one showed no improvement in EF and the other, which included the use of plasmapheresis followed by IVIG, showed a small change in EF of 6% and improved NYHA functional class in 25 patients.

More recently, a number of studies have been performed in patients who are virus negative but have inflammation on biopsy. The largest trial was a randomized, placebo-controlled trial of 85 patients with half receiving steroids and azathioprine versus placebo. Of those receiving immunosuppressive therapy, 88% had an improvement in EF of at least 10% versus none in the placebo arm. Other retrospective trials have shown similar results. At this time, if treating a virus-negative patient with active inflammation, consideration of immunosuppressive therapy is reasonable but a definitive approach requires more prospective data.

Randomized trials of antiviral therapy have not been performed in patients with virus-positive myocarditis. Small studies have shown improvement in EF with the use of interferon beta for patients with enterovirus or adenovirus genomes. A follow-up randomized trial of 143 patients included those with parvovirus B19 and showed improvement in quality of life and clearance of virus, but no change in EF when compared to placebo. It should be noted that these patients had the presence of virus on biopsy, but not acute, active myocarditis.

Patients with giant cell myocarditis have been shown to be responsive to immunosuppressive therapy. In a trial of 11 patients with biopsy-proven myocarditis, all received ciclosporin and prednisone and nine of the 11 received muromonab-CD3. Two patients underwent early heart transplantation and one patient died of respiratory complications, but the others survived past a year which is much improved from historical data. This is in contrast to an earlier study of 63 patients with giant cell myocarditis who had a rate of death or cardiac transplant of 89% with a median survival of 5.5 months. In patients who do progress to require an assist device, one should strongly consider the placement of biventricular support since these patients will often progress to biventricular standstill. Finally, there are reports of recurrence of giant cell myocarditis after transplantation that has usually been shown to be responsive to enhanced immunosuppressive therapy.

Eosinophilic myocarditis is characterized by an eosinophilic infiltrate that may be caused by hypersensitivity to a drug or toxin, parasite, or hypereosinophilic syndrome. It usually presents as an acute myocarditis associated with a peripheral eosinophilia and has been shown to be responsive to aggressive steroid therapy. Additionally, one should ensure that the offending agent is discontinued or removed.

Outcomes

The vast majority of patients with myocarditis have normal LV function and seem to do well in comparison to patients who are more symptomatic and have biopsy-proven myocarditis. The Myocarditis Treatment Trial showed that all patients improved their EF from a baseline of 25% to 34% by 28 weeks. Twenty per cent of the patients were dead at 1 year and 56% were dead at 4.3 years. Patients with less severe disease tended to do better. Slightly better outcomes were reported by a group from Germany in patients with myocarditis and positive virus with 19.2% mortality at 4.7 years. Similar data were reported in an Italian registry of 174 patients with myocarditis with a rate of 13% at 2 years of death or transplantation. They found that patients with signs or symptoms of persistent left or right HF had the largest association with need for transplantation or death.

Patients with fulminant myocarditis defined as LV dysfunction and low cardiac output requiring inotropes or MCS have had varying outcomes depending on the study. A retrospective analysis of 147 patients with biopsy-proven myocarditis reported that the 15 patients with fulminant myocarditis had a 93% transplant-free survival rate at 11 years after biopsy compared to only 45% of those with acute myocarditis. A recent report of 187 consecutive patients with clinical myocarditis between 2001 and 2016 provides more recent data on outcomes of patients with advanced, fulminant myocarditis with symptoms for <1 month. One hundred and thirty of the patients presented with a viral prodrome but endomyocardial biopsies looking for positive virus were not performed. The authors defined fulminant myocarditis as patients with LV dysfunction and low cardiac output requiring inotropes or MCS. Thirty five of the 55 patients with fulminant myocarditis required MCS which was usually a balloon pump. Mortality in the fulminant myocarditis group was 18.2% (10/55), four had an early heart transplant, and one received an LVAD. There were no events in the non-fulminant group of patients. It should be noted that most of these patients received immunosuppressive therapy.

Myocarditis is a difficult disease process because of varying clinical presentations, aetiologies, and outcomes. One should have a heightened suspicion for diagnosis, especially in children and young adults who rarely present with cardiac issues. Aggressive diagnosis and therapy including referral to institutions equipped with therapeutic modalities is required.

Cardiac amyloidosis and other restrictive myopathies: diagnosis and treatment

Introduction

Restrictive cardiomyopathies (RCMs) are a heterogeneous group of diseases characterized haemodynamically by impaired ventricular filling and abnormal diastolic function. These can be characterized pathophysiologically as infiltrative diseases, metabolic storage diseases (less commonly diagnosed in the adult population), sarcomeric protein disorders, endomyocardial diseases, or idiopathic. A simplified list of aetiologies is presented in Table 3.1.

Table 3.1 Aetiology of restrictive cardiomyopathy by pathophysiology

Pathophysiological classification of RCM	Specific diseases
Infiltrative	Amyloidosis
	Sarcoidosis
Metabolic storage disease	Fabry disease
	Gaucher disease
	Haemochromatosis
	Glycogen storage disease
	Niemann–Pick disease
Sarcomeric protein disorders	Spectrum of hypertrophic cardiomyopathy
Endomyocardial disease	Endomyocardial fibrosis
	Radiation induced

Each of these disorders leads to alteration of normal myocardial or endocardial tissue, resulting in progressive ventricular dysfunction in diastole where efficient cardiac relaxation and filling are critical. Impaired ventricular filling leads to elevated intracardiac pressures with resultant symptoms of congestive HF. Ultimately, this progresses to low stroke volume with poor cardiac output in the advanced stages. Each of these diseases has specific nuance to its diagnosis and treatment. This chapter will focus on presentation, management, and indications for referral to advanced therapies for RCMs. Due to its increasing recognition, amyloid cardiomyopathy will be discussed in greater detail.

Clinical presentation and diagnosis

RCM should always be suspected when a patient presents with clinical signs of congestion in the setting of preserved EF. Many types of RCM affect both ventricles, thus patients can often manifest right HF symptoms (ascites, anasarca, and lower extremity oedema) in addition to left-sided HF symptoms (dyspnoea, fatigue, exercise intolerance, and pulmonary oedema).

A mainstay of diagnosis is echocardiography. RCM can present with increased wall thickness in infiltrative disorders (amyloidosis) or normal wall thickness in non-infiltrative disorders (radiation, endomyocardial fibrosis). Chronic pressure overload often leads to impressive biatrial enlargement which can predispose to atrial tachyarrhythmias and affiliated embolic complications. Systolic function is often preserved until the later stages of disease, and echocardiographic signs of diastolic dysfunction are a *sine qua non*. These include elevated early diastolic filling velocity (E wave) with decreased late diastolic filling velocity (A wave), often with an E/A ratio of >2; and decreased tissue Doppler velocity of the lateral mitral annulus (e') with an elevated E/e', often >14 (Fig. 3.1). Chronic left-sided pressure overload eventually leads to postcapillary PH, thus many patients develop significant tricuspid regurgitation (TR) in later disease stages as a result of right ventricular (RV) remodelling. Invasive haemodynamics can be used to support non-invasive diagnostic studies. Findings on right heart catheterization include elevated right- and left-sided filling pressures, PH, and the classic 'square-root sign' indicating early and rapid ventricular filling with subsequent plateau phase.

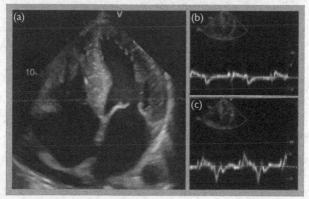

Fig. 3.1 Still image of infiltrative RCM highlighting normal LV size, thickened ventricular walls, enlarged RV, and biatrial enlargement indicative of late-stage disease (a). Figure on right reveals low tissue Doppler velocities at medial (b) and lateral (c) mitral annulus. See plate section.

Echocardiography and haemodynamics can also help distinguish between RCM and constrictive pericardial disease, which can often have a similar clinical presentation. As mentioned, RCM presents with low mitral annular tissue Doppler velocities (e') whereas constriction presents with normal e' and 'annulus reversus' (medial > lateral e'). An invasive haemodynamic study can further help this distinction; RCM is characterized by ventricular concordance during respiration, elevated pulmonary pressures, and LV > RV diastolic pressures. Constriction demonstrates ventricular discordance during respiration, equalization of ventricular diastolic pressures, and often absent PH (Table 3.2). If diagnosis is still uncertain, cardiac computed tomography (CT) and MRI can enrich diagnostic yield by providing anatomic features of the pericardium, including thickness, calcification, or inflammation.

Table 3.2 Constellation of findings associated with restrictive cardiomyopathy

Evaluation	Findings
History and physical	• Right side: lower extremity oedema, elevated JVP, Kussmaul's sign, anasarca
	• Left side: dyspnoea, fatigue, pulmonary oedema
Echocardiogram	• ↑ E/e' (>14)
	• ↑ E/A (>2)
	• ↓ e' velocity (<10 cm/s)
	• Lateral > medial e' velocity
Haemodynamics	• Ventricular concordance with respiration
	• 'Square-root sign'
	• ↑ pulmonary artery pressures
	• LVEDP > RVEDP

A, late atrial filling velocity; E, early transmitral filling velocity; e', tissue Doppler velocity at mitral annulus; JVP, jugular venous pressure; LVEDP, left ventricular end-diastolic pressure; RVEDP, right ventricular end-diastolic pressure.

Once RCM is suspected, diagnosis of the specific aetiology often relies on a constellation of findings including family history, imaging findings, and endomyocardial biopsy. Histopathology can diagnose amyloidosis, sarcoidosis, endomyocardial fibrosis, Fabry disease, Danon disease, and hypertrophic cardiomyopathy. A retrospective study from the Johns Hopkins Hospital revealed that endomyocardial biopsy conducted for unexplained RCM was diagnostic in 29% of cases, changed patient management in 25% of cases, and most commonly revealed amyloidosis. Prognosis often depends on the specific condition that is diagnosed, but is generally considered to be poor if aetiology is felt to be idiopathic.

Management of RCM revolves around treatment of the underlying condition (if such treatment exists) in addition to management of HF. Targeted therapies are available for specific cardiomyopathies. Fabry disease can be treated with enzyme replacement therapy with agalsidase beta; haemochromatosis can be treated with iron chelation therapy; endomyocardial fibrosis can sometimes be surgically managed with endocardiectomy; and sarcoidosis can be treated with immunosuppression. Treatment for light-chain and transthyretin (TTR) cardiac amyloidosis will be discussed further in the next section (see Amyloid cardiomyopathy, p. 31).

Unlike dilated cardiomyopathies with depressed ventricular function, there are no specific guideline-directed medical therapies for RCM. In fact, as the disease progresses, many therapies used in HF with reduced EF can actually be detrimental. In advanced RCM, stroke volume becomes markedly reduced, and cardiac output is dependent on heart rate, limiting the use of beta blockade. Hypotension and renal dysfunction often limit the use of renin-angiotensin inhibitors. Thus, these therapies are frequently not tolerated and have resulted in no mortality benefit in RCM. The mainstay of therapy revolves around management of the patient's volume status (which can be tenuous due to the steep LV diastolic pressure–volume relationship in RCM) and control of atrial arrhythmias (with concomitant thromboembolism risk) which are frequent in this population. There may, however, be a role for mineralocorticoid antagonism to augment diuresis and potentially improve outcomes. Referral for durable mechanical circulatory support (MCS) or heart transplantation is indicated when patients have severe functional impairment (NYHA class III or greater HF). Pacemakers may be needed for progressive conduction disease, and defibrillators have varying indications dependent on specific RCM and prognosis at the time of disease identification; indications for cardiac implantable electronic devices are discussed in detail elsewhere.

Amyloid cardiomyopathy

An increasingly recognized aetiology of RCM is amyloid cardiomyopathy, a condition characterized by extracellular deposition of misfolded proteins. While there are many known amyloidogenic proteins, two primarily affect the heart: immunoglobulin light-chains or misfolded TTR. Light-chain amyloidosis (AL amyloid) is a result of abnormal production of immunoglobulin light chains from a plasma cell dyscrasia.

TTR is a molecule produced primarily by the liver to carry retinol-binding protein and thyroxine. It exists normally as a stable tetramer; disassociation of the tetramer into monomeric intermediates leads to formation of amyloid fibrils which can subsequently deposit in tissue. Instability of TTR is either the result of pathogenic mutations inherited in an autosomal dominant fashion with variable penetrance (resulting in hereditary transthyretin (hTTR) amyloidosis) or age-related deposition of the wild-type TTR protein (wtTTR or senile TTR).

Interstitial deposition of amyloid fibrils results in ventricular wall thickening, decreased ventricular compliance, diastolic dysfunction, and subsequent RCM. Microvascular deposition can lead to coronary flow abnormalities and micro-ischaemia to the conduction system. Deposition in atria can lead to decreased compliance, atrial pressure overload, and can contribute to atrial arrhythmias. hTTR can also present with polyneuropathy with symptoms including tendinopathy, carpal tunnel syndrome, and autonomic dysfunction. The degree of neurological and cardiac involvement is mutation dependent. AL amyloidosis can result in protein deposition anywhere in the body, including the gastrointestinal (GI) tract, kidneys, and skin.

Prevalence

Recent studies have demonstrated that amyloid cardiomyopathy, in particular transthyretin amyloid cardiomyopathy (ATTR-CM), is far more prevalent than previously recognized. In a Finnish autopsy study of 256 patients aged >85 years, nearly 25% were found to have myocardial TTR amyloid deposition via immunohistochemistry, although the clinical significance was undefined. In patients with heart failure with preserved ejection fraction (HFpEF) and left ventricular hypertrophy (LVH), 13% above the age of 60 years were found to have ATTR-CM; this number increased to 30% when the age of 75 years was used as a cut-off. Finally, in patients undergoing TAVR at one centre, 17% were found to have ATTR-CM. Mutations leading to hTTR have geographic variation; the Val122Ile mutation is present in 3–4% of African Americans in the USA, and the Thr60Ala mutation is present in 1% of the Northern Ireland population. Overall, there must be a high clinical suspicion for this disorder when patients present with RCM.

Diagnosis

Diagnosis of amyloid cardiomyopathy involves integration of a constellation of clinical symptoms, imaging characteristics, and laboratory findings. Histopathology can also be used for diagnostic confirmation. Initial, heightened clinical sensitivity to the various manifestations of amyloid cardiomyopathy as mentioned previously (autonomic dysfunction, carpal tunnel syndrome, atrial arrhythmias, conduction disease) is paramount to diagnosis. ECG may reveal low voltages despite increased ventricular wall thickness, though this is more common in AL amyloidosis and has poor sensitivity for ATTR-CM. Echocardiography may reveal typical features of RCM highlighted in Table 3.2 (see p. 30). In addition, speckle tracking echocardiography can be used to define longitudinal myocardial strain. Characteristic findings in amyloid cardiomyopathy include impaired global longitudinal strain despite normal EF, but with relative preservation of regional longitudinal strain at the apex, translating to a 'cherry-on-top' or 'bullseye' pattern during strain imaging. Finally, MRI will reveal diffuse late gadolinium enhancement in a subendocardial pattern and is specific for diagnosis of cardiac amyloidosis. Imaging findings representative of cardiac amyloidosis are highlighted in Fig. 3.2.

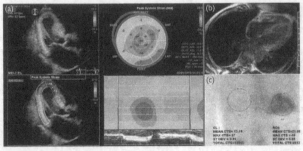

Fig. 3.2 Characteristic imaging findings of cardiac amyloidosis. (a) Typical findings of longitudinal strain imaging with characteristic 'bullseye' pattern. (b) MRI with diffuse subendocardial late gadolinium enhancement. (c) Pyrophosphate (PYP) scan with heart/contralateral (H/Cl) ratio >1.5. See plate section.

Definitive diagnosis of a subtype of amyloidosis requires further serological testing, nuclear imaging and, in many cases, biopsy. Our institution's algorithm is shown in Fig. 3.3. First, serological testing to exclude AL amyloid must be performed via measurement of serum free light chains, serum protein electrophoresis, and urine protein electrophoresis with immunofixation. If all three of these are negative, this effectively rules out the presence of AL amyloidosis. Concurrently, nuclear imaging should be performed. Two molecules, pyrophosphate (PYP) and 3,3-diphosphono-1,2-propanodiacarboxylic acid (DPD), previously used as bone tracers, were found to have avidity to TTR deposits in the myocardium. These

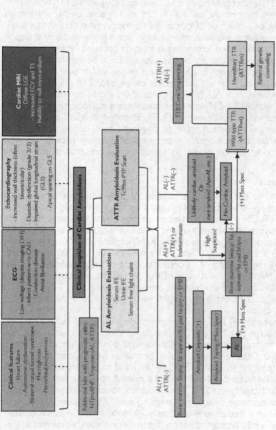

Fig. 3.3 Duke University approach to diagnosis of cardiac amyloidosis. CAD, coronary artery disease; ECV, extracellular volume; EMB, endomyocardial biopsy; IFE, immunofixation; LVH, left ventricular hypertrophy; NTproBNP, N-terminal pro-B-type natriuretic peptide; Tc99m, technetium 99m.

Courtesy of Dr Michel Khouri.

are tagged to technetium allowing quantification of TTR deposits via nuclear scintigraphy. Absolute counts and mean counts are measured over the heart and on the contralateral (control) side of the chest. A heart/contralateral ratio of mean counts ≥1.5 was found to have a 97% sensitivity and 100% specificity for diagnosing TTR amyloid. Once diagnosed as ATTR-CM, further genotyping is required to distinguish wtTTR from hTTR. If pathways for both AL and ATTR-CM are negative, cardiac amyloidosis is unlikely, or a rare type of cardiac amyloidosis is present. If clinical suspicion for cardiac amyloidosis remains high, tissue biopsy is the next step. If both are positive, then further tissue must be obtained for histopathology. We favour endomyocardial biopsy, which should be subsequently typed via mass spectrometry, to definitively diagnose which type of amyloid is affecting the heart. Fat pad aspirate has low yield for TTR (15–40%) but has higher sensitivity for AL (80%). Importantly, it should be noted that many patients with ATTR-CM may have concomitant monoclonal gammopathy of undetermined significance (MGUS), identified in >20% in one series, which can be a common cause of diagnostic confusion. Consultation of a haematologist/oncologist is recommended, as these patients may also require bone marrow biopsy to assess for the presence of plasma cell dyscrasia.

Prognosis

Prognosis for this condition is variable. AL amyloidosis typically presents more acutely, progresses rapidly, and thus has a prognosis that is worse than ATTR-CM and is dependent on degree of cardiac involvement. The Mayo Clinic has developed a staging system utilizing cardiac biomarkers: N-terminal pro-B type natriuretic peptide (NT-proBNP) ≥1800 ng/dL, cardiac troponin T ≥0.025 mcg/L, and difference in serum light-chain concentrations ≥18 mg/dL. Prognosis worsens as more of these biomarkers are abnormal. Median survival if none of the biomarkers are above threshold is 55 months, but if all are elevated, median survival is only 5 months. This improves to 22 months in patients who are able to undergo stem cell transplantation.

Prognosis for ATTR-CM is dependent on a variety of factors, including age, genotype (if hTTR), NYHA functional class, serum biomarkers, and imaging findings, but overall median survival is in the order of 3–5 years. The Mayo Clinic derived a similar biomarker-based prognostic scoring system using NTproBNP (>3000 pg/mL) and cardiac troponin T (>0.05 ng/mL) and found that 4-year overall survival if no biomarkers were above threshold (stage I) was 57%, one biomarker abnormal (stage II) was 42%, and both biomarkers abnormal (stage III) was 18%. Notably, patients with stage III had a median survival of only 20 months. NYHA functional class also plays a role in prognostication (higher NYHA class, worse median survival) and identifies patients who better respond to treatment (discussed in following treatment section). Finally, for hTTR amyloid, the Val122Ile mutation present in many African Americans in the USA confers a worse prognosis than other genotypes. Fig. 3.4 highlights various prognostic features that have been identified in the literature. Prognosis is particularly important because patients early in the course of disease may derive benefit from TTR-targeted therapeutics, whereas those later in the course of disease may require transplantation or only be eligible for a more palliative approach to disease management.

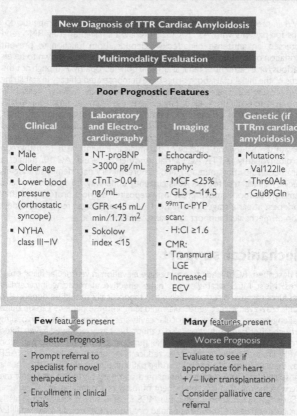

Fig. 3.4 Prognostic variables in ATTR-CM with guidance for future therapy. CMR, cardiac magnetic resonance; cTnT, cardiac troponin T; ECV, extracellular volume; GFR, glomerular filtration rate; GLS, global longitudinal strain; H/Cl, heart/contralateral; LGE, late gadolinium enhancement; MCF, myocardial contraction fraction; NTproBNP, N-terminal pro B-type natriuretic peptide; NYHA, New York Heart Association; TTR, transthyretin; TTRm, mutant TTR.

Treatment

For both AL cardiomyopathy and ATTR-CM, therapy is focused on (1) management of HF, treated similarly as other RCM, and (2) treatment of the underlying condition. For AL cardiomyopathy, this requires chemotherapy directed at the underlying plasma cell dyscrasia and necessitates consultation of a haematologist/oncologist. Regimens are generally comprised of an alkylating agent (cyclophosphamide), proteasome inhibitor (bortezomib), and dexamethasone, along with novel CD38 inhibitors (daratumamab).

While previously considered untreatable, there are now therapeutic options for patients with ATTR-CM. Patisiran, a small-interfering RNA, and inotersen, an antisense oligodeoxynucleotide, both function to prevent translation of TTR mRNA into TTR protein and have been shown to be efficacious for treatment of familial amyloid polyneuropathy. Although not the focus of the initial trials, both drugs have demonstrated efficacy in stabilizing or improving surrogate cardiac endpoints such as LV wall thickness, NT-proBNP, and 6-minute walk distance. Recently, tafamidis, a molecule which causes stabilization of the TTR tetramer and prevents monomerization, was approved for use for both hTTR and wtTTR cardiomyopathy based on reductions in all-cause mortality and cardiovascular-related hospitalizations in the Safety and Efficacy of Tafamidis in Patients with Transthyretin Cardiomyopathy (ATTR-ACT) trial. Another molecule, AG-10, mimics a tetrameric stabilizing mutation, and has preliminary data demonstrating efficacy. A clinical trial for AG-10 is currently underway. Of note, tetrameric stabilizers do not remove previously deposited amyloid protein, and thus work best at early stages of disease. Later disease stages require consideration of mechanical support and transplantation.

Mechanical support

As described, RCM leads to progressive elevation in ventricular filling pressures. Most MCS strategies are quite effective at reducing intracardiac pressures through direct unloading and theoretically should be beneficial in RCM. However, direct ventricular unloading in these patients can be quite challenging owing to small ventricular cavity size. Augmentation of unloading through afterload reduction also cannot be easily achieved given fixed stroke volume, making strategies like intra-aortic balloon counterpulsation (IABP) limited in their capacity to reduce filling pressures. However, IABP may be used in specific cases to bridge patients to durable support or heart transplantation, and through augmented coronary perfusion, can limit the micro-ischaemia that is a component of many of the infiltrative RCMs.

Surgical implantation of durable MCS faces a similar challenge. This is particularly true for isolated left-sided circulatory support devices. Small LV size can cause mechanical obstruction of a LVAD inflow cannula. Abutment of the inflow cannula to the myocardium can result in obstruction, risk suction events, and lead to dangerous ventricular arrhythmias. Restrictive haemodynamics often lead to chronic RV pressure overload and resultant RV failure, a major source of morbidity and mortality post LVAD. In patients with DCM and biventricular dysfunction, post-implantation RV failure can occur in 20–30% of patients. These patients require longer inotropic support, longer intensive care unit (ICU) stays, and longer hospitalizations. In many patients with DCM, RV performance eventually improves such that they can be discharged from the hospital without significant HF symptoms. However, development of late or recurrent right HF results in a higher 1- and 2-year mortality. In RCM treated with LVAD, this risk of RV dysfunction is further increased due to the underlying structural and haemodynamic changes of the RV which are less likely to respond to LV unloading.

The Mayo Clinic has reported their experience of LVAD implantation in 28 patients with RCM. The most common indications for implant were amyloidosis, hypertrophic cardiomyopathy, and sarcoidosis, and most patients had Interagency Registry for Mechanically Assisted Circulatory Support (INTERMACS) profiles I and II, indicating true end-stage RCM. As expected, the vast majority had evidence of RV dysfunction and elevated right-sided pressures prior to implantation, and 54% of patients underwent concurrent tricuspid valve intervention. A LVAD was implanted as a bridge to transplantation (BTT) in 61% of patients and destination therapy (DT) in the rest.

Thirty-nine per cent of patients experienced postoperative RV failure requiring inotropic support, 25% experienced postoperative renal failure, and in-hospital mortality was 14%. Overall 1-year survival in the entire cohort was 64%, far lower than the 85% 1-year event-free survival in patients with DCM treated with newest generation centrifugal pumps. The authors also compared LVAD outcomes by aetiology of RCM and found no difference in mean survival time between amyloid and non-amyloid aetiologies. Finally, the authors found that increased LV diameter in systole and diastole were both significantly associated with greater survival. An LVEDD of ≤46 mm was significantly associated with mortality.

In registry analysis from 2008 to 2014, only 1% of all LVAD implants were for RCM and another 0.9% were for hypertrophic cardiomyopathy. The most common aetiologies of RCM were amyloidosis, sarcoidosis, and idiopathic disease. Interestingly, those who received LVAD in this cohort had some features of 'burned-out' disease and shared a phenotype with DCM: only approximately 5% had LVEF ≥40% and over half had an LVEDD ≥6.0 cm. In the context of this mixed phenotype, the authors saw no significant difference in 1-year survival between RCM (74%) and DCM (81%). However, they also identified small LVEDD (50 mm in their study) as being significantly associated with higher overall mortality (1-year survival estimated at only 30%).

Our group infrequently uses MCS as a long-term solution for patients with end-stage restrictive disease. However, the data previously described indicate that, in the appropriately selected patient, it may improve short-term survival until transplantation can be achieved. Further, there are also data indicating that MCS may reduce reactive PH, which can be a contraindication to transplantation. We recommend using LVAD in RCM only when ventricular geometry is favourable (LVEDD ≥50 mm) and in patients without significant clinical RV failure. These suggestions are in keeping with those issued by the International Society for Heart and Lung Transplant (ISHLT), which state that MCS with LVAD cannot be routinely recommended, but can be considered in highly select cases at specialized centres (IIb recommendation). Alternative strategies of MCS in RCM include biventricular mechanical support (total artificial heart) or ECMO. Specifically for cardiac amyloidosis, an approach providing biventricular support via total artificial hearts has demonstrated reasonable long-term outcomes in a small cohort of patients.

Transplantation

Referral for orthotopic heart transplantation (OHT) is considered a class I indication in RCM patients with NYHA class III and IV symptoms, and is often the only therapy that can improve prognosis in these patients.

Patients with RCM often develop reactive PH in response to chronically elevated left-sided pressures, resulting in a phenotype of combined pre- and postcapillary PH. Elevated pulmonary pressures often preclude these patients from transplantation listing; thus, timely referral is critical.

The number of OHTs performed for RCM is increasing over time, from 1.4% in the period from 1987 to 2010 to 3.4% in the period from 2009 to 2016. In a cohort evaluated from 2000 to 2013, approximately 7.4% of RCM patients are bridged to transplantation using LVAD support. At our centre, we often list these patients with inotropic support with or without haemodynamic monitoring. As mentioned, MCS in these patients can be technically challenging, and IABP is less helpful. Unfortunately, per the revised UNOS allocation system, these patients often get relegated to status 3 or 4, despite the severity of their illness. Indeed, data indicate that patients with RCM have a higher risk of death while awaiting OHT as compared to other forms of cardiomyopathy, though these data were obtained prior to changes to the UNOS classification and likely reflect the overall poor prognosis of this group of diseases. Outcomes after OHT for RCM appear to be similar to those for the combined group of 'non-RCM' patients but worse when compared to DCM directly.

Given the various aetiologies of RCM, there are special treatment considerations that need to be recognized prior to transplantation in this group of patients. For example, patients with underlying sarcoidosis should be concomitantly treated with disease-specific immunosuppression; those with haemochromatosis should continue to receive iron-reduction therapy; and those with Fabry disease should continue to receive enzyme replacement therapy.

Specifically for amyloidosis, thorough evaluation for extracardiac manifestations should be performed, as these can lead to worsening morbidity and mortality after transplantation. In particular, evaluation for renal involvement (proteinuria), neuropathy (peripheral neuropathy, autonomic dysfunction), and GI involvement (elevated alkaline phosphatase, malabsorption) should be undertaken. Severe manifestations of the above may serve as contraindications to transplantation. For AL amyloidosis in particular, light-chain reductive chemotherapy should be given both before and after OHT (as soon as it is deemed safe).

Wild-type amyloidosis requires only OHT, but these patients are often older and have additional comorbidities, which may preclude them from being optimal candidates. For hTTR, strategies include combined heart-liver transplant versus isolated heart transplant followed by ongoing TTR-directed therapies. Recent data suggest outcomes for both isolated OHT and combined heart–liver transplantation in cardiac amyloid patients are approaching those of OHT in other patients.

In conclusion, RCMs represent a minority of HF patients, but with growing recognition of cardiac amyloidosis, will be increasingly encountered. Mainstay of therapy involves management of volume status and utilization of disease-specific therapies when they exist. MCS can be technically challenging, but utilized in the appropriate patients. If patients are safely bridged to transplantation, they often do well compared to their non-RCM counterparts.

Mechanical circulatory support

Indications for ventricular assist devices

Short-term VAD therapy

Extracorporeal right VAD (RVAD)

Patients requiring short-term mechanical support of the right heart can receive a temporary RVAD which is an extracorporeal bypass configuration of the RV obtaining drainage from the RA or the RV with blood returning into the main pulmonary artery (PA). This can be done as an open surgical procedure or percutaneously. Illustration of an open RVAD is seen in Fig. 4.1.

The main indications for extracorporeal RVAD are:
- RV failure post myocardial infarction or severe pulmonary hypertension.
- Post-cardiotomy isolated RV failure not responsive to inotropic support.
- RV failure post heart transplantation.
- RV failure following durable LVAD implantation.

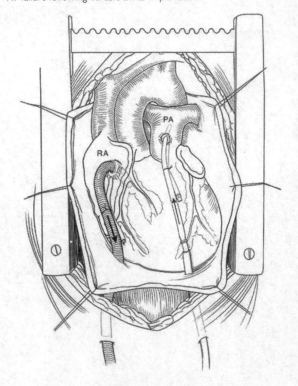

Fig. 4.1 Open extracorporeal RVAD.

Careful assessment of the function of the LV is required so that the increased preload provided by the RVAD can be accommodated by the contractile function of the LV. In those cases, in which the acute RV failure requiring mechanical support is accompanied by respiratory failure, an oxygenator can be attached to the RVAD circuit (oxy-RVAD).

Extracorporeal LVAD

Selective bypass of the left heart can be accomplished with an open-chest drainage of the left atrium (LA) (via the right superior pulmonary vein) or the apex of the LV and return to the ascending aorta with the use of an extracorporeal centrifugal pump (Fig. 4.2). Devices implanted percutaneously, or via surgical cutdown of a peripheral artery, in the form of microaxial pumps (Impella, Abiomed, Danvers, MA, USA) are also gaining popularity. The main indications for temporary LVAD support are:

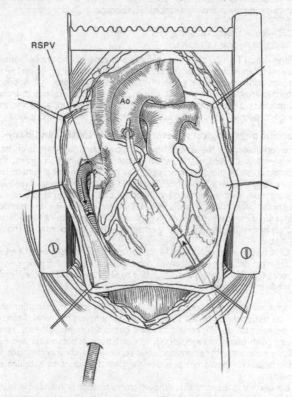

Fig. 4.2 Extracorporeal LVAD. Ao, aorta; RSPV, right superior pulmonary vein.

- Cardiogenic shock post myocardial infarction.
- Cardiomyopathies affecting mainly the LV.
- Post cardiotomy.
- Acute viral myocarditis.
- Acute decompensation of transplant candidate—BTT.

Durable LVADs

LVAD systems for long-term use comprise a pump, which for most modern devices is centrifugal and intrapericardial, with an inflow component attached to the LV apex and an outflow graft attached to the ascending aorta.

Developments in technology and perioperative management have improved outcomes of patients on durable LVAD support, which has led to an expansion in their current indications. The principal indications are:

- BTT.
- DT—lifelong support.
- Bridge to myocardial recovery.

Within the BTT group there are a subgroup of patients who are potentially transplant candidates but remain satisfied with their quality of life on LVAD support and may willingly come off the transplant waiting list. Another subgroup are those who present with transient contraindications to transplantation or are too sick until a donor could be identified, and form the bridge-to-decision cohort, representing almost 40% of LVAD recipients.

Specific physiological criteria for durable LVAD candidacy

Decision-making for the listing of the heart transplant candidate takes into consideration the prognostic benefit of heart transplantation against the natural course of the disease process. Risk prediction models such as the Heart Failure Survival Score (HFSS) and the SHFM have been utilized for this purpose. With recent survival outcome data in LVAD patients, these scores can inform decision-making for LVAD candidacy as well. In countries where LVAD therapy is reserved for those who are transplant candidates, such as in the UK, the ISHLT listing criteria for heart transplantation should be met:

- CPX testing with peak VO$_2$ ≤14 mL/kg/min (if not on BB) or ≤12 mL/kg/min if receiving BB, in conjunction with unfavourable HF prognosis score (<80% 1-year survival calculated by SHFM or a HFSS in the high/medium risk range).

The following negative criteria suggest unsuitability for transplantation and can be extrapolated to the LVAD candidates: irreversible renal, hepatic, or neurological disease remain absolute contraindications. Obesity, renal failure (with potential reversibility), cancer history, tobacco use, and significant pulmonary hypertension, albeit conventional contraindications to transplantation, should not preclude mechanical support as a bridge to candidacy.

It is becoming apparent that although transplantation is intended in many LVAD recipients, only a small percentage will eventually receive an organ. Hence, the distinction between BTT and DT is less pertinent in the modern era and the aforementioned guidance for transplant listing can only be informative for the LVAD candidate.

With a changing landscape in organ availability, heart transplant waiting lists, evolving technology, and the available evidence from transplant and VAD studies, it is methodologically challenging to produce stringent guidelines for durable LVAD therapies. For these reasons, the European Association for Cardio-Thoracic Surgery (EACTS) published an expert consensus statement (rather than guidelines) on long-term MCS highlighting the main indications for durable LVADs:

- Functional limitations with NYHA class IIIb or IV *and*
- EF ≤25% *and*
- At least one of the following criteria:
  - INTERMACS levels 2–4.
  - Inotrope dependence.
  - Progressive end-organ dysfunction.
  - CPX testing with peak VO$_2$ ≤12 mL/kg/min.
  - Temporary MCS dependence.

Specific considerations of the LVAD candidate:
- Chronic biventricular failure poses a challenge to durable LVAD support and temporary extracorporeal or implantable RVAD support should be considered.
- Unlike transplantation, age is not a contraindication to durable LVADs as long as age-associated comorbidities and frailty are carefully assessed.
- Similarly, in patients with poor glycaemic control and end-organ complications, durable LVADs may still be considered.

It is essential that before any definitive conclusions are made with regard to organ dysfunction reversibility, cardiac output and filling status are optimized. That applies to renal but more importantly to liver function, as irreversible liver damage poses a contraindication to LVAD therapies.

Other patient groups where durable LVADs are generally contraindicated

- Patients with intractable ventricular tachycardia are not isolated LVAD candidates.
- Patients with restrictive cardiomyopathy are not LVAD candidates due to small LV cavities which would preclude effective LV apical drainage.
- Ventricular septal defect not amenable to repair.
- Infective endocarditis.
- Proven malignancy with expected survival <1 year.

Risk stratification and timing of implantation of durable LVADs

Risk stratification models have been developed to identify those who would benefit the most from durable LVADs and help to inform timing for implantation. It is recognized that a deterioration of the general medical condition as evidenced by low albumin, and derangement of liver and kidney function tests exponentiates the risk associated with LVAD implantation. The Lietz–Miller stratification score, which was based on outcomes of older-generation devices, yielded strong concordance between those with high-risk profile and mortality after LVAD implantation. The Model for End-Stage Liver Disease (MELD) was originally a risk stratification tool for patients with cirrhosis undergoing portosystemic shunts, but it has been shown to also predict transfusion requirements and mortality following

LVAD implantation. The formula variables of bilirubin, creatinine, and the international normalized ratio (INR) provide a surrogate of end-organ function, that could influence timing of LVAD surgery. The above-mentioned risk stratification tools, in addition to the Destination Therapy Risk Score (DTRS), were predominantly based on pulsatile flow LVADs and their discriminatory ability for continuous flow devices is limited. A more relevant risk stratification model for the modern era, the Heart Mate II Risk Score, was superior to both the DTRS and MELD in predicting 90-day mortality. Age, albumin, creatinine, INR, and low LVAD volume cardiac surgical units were the independent variables used to calculate the risk profiles of LVAD candidates. While these models offer some prognostication, a multidisciplinary approach with a dedicated advanced HF team is recommended to guide the most appropriate treatment strategy.

Myocardial recovery following durable LVAD implantation

Although reverse remodelling of the failing ventricle supported with a durable LVAD tends to occur within the first 6 months from implantation, only a small proportion of these patients (~1%) will meet criteria for separation from mechanical support within the first year. Durable mechanical support that leads to recovery of the failing LV and to explant is termed bridge to recovery and has an incidence of approximately 3% at 3 years. Patient-related parameters such as younger age, shorter duration of HF, and absence of pulmonary hypertension or significant LV dilatation (LVEDD <6.5 cm) are positive prognostic factors for myocardial recovery. Likewise, myocarditis and postpartum cardiomyopathy patients are more likely to recover compared to those with an ischaemic cause. Targeted pharmacological interventions may enhance reverse remodelling, the likelihood of myocardial recovery, and ultimately LVAD explantation in select patient groups. There are no universally accepted LVAD explantation protocols, but different groups have proposed the following parameters as indicators of appropriate recovery prior to explant:

At low LVAD speed, 'off-pump' testing:

- LVEDD <60 mm.
- LV end-systolic diameter <50 mm.
- EF >45%.
- LV end-diastolic pressure <12 mmHg.
- Resting cardiac index (CI) >2.8 L/min/m^2.
- VO$_2$ >16 mL/kg/min.

Are durable LVADs alternatives to heart transplantation?

While heart transplantation is the standard of care for those who have favourable characteristics to qualify and timely receive an organ, there is an increased number of HF patients who do not meet the criteria for listing. It is now well established that durable LVADs offer improved survival and quality of life versus optimal medical management. With improved safety characteristics of the newer devices, the US FDA has given approval for their use as DT. But for those ambulatory patients who are also eligible for transplantation, is durable LVAD implantation a suitable option?

For LVAD therapies to be true alternatives to transplantation the following conditions should be met:

- Symptom relief. Optimization of pump speed based on central venous and pulmonary capillary wedge pressure (PCWP) reading and echocardiographic indices can improve filling pressures and ventricular unloading and translate to better symptom control.
- Reduction in adverse events. Pump thrombosis and stroke are the main complications associated with LVADs; however, modern pump engineering and blood pressure and anticoagulation protocols have led to a modest reduction of these events. VAD-related infections and sepsis are still prevalent in part due to the need for exteriorization of the driveline and are associated with high morbidity and mortality.
- Ease of implantation. Modern LVADs allowing for a fully intrapericardial implantation through median sternotomy or less invasive techniques are associated with low operative mortality and reproducibility.

In the absence of randomized trials examining mid- and long-term survival and quality of life between LVADs and heart transplantation, we can only extrapolate data from observational studies, which demonstrated equipoise at 1 year. However, the shortage of donor organs, which may impact especially patients with certain group types, size, and antibody profile, mandates the use of LVADs even if in their current state they are unlikely to match the excellent long-term results of a successful heart transplant. Where LVADs may be a true alternative to transplantation is in the 'high-risk' recipients—those who fail to meet standard criteria for transplantation—receiving marginal organs, where median survival is approximately 5 years. Finally, for those who achieve myocardial recovery with their durable LVAD leading to explant, not receiving a transplant may be advantageous.

Surgical techniques for left ventricular assist device implantation and associated procedures

Operative planning

A preoperative plan is determined after a full patient evaluation is completed, reviewing all relevant haemodynamic data, echocardiography, and radiographic imaging. The need for concomitant procedures is assessed preoperatively and confirmed in the operating room after review of the intraoperative haemodynamic status and the transoesophageal echocardiography (TOE). The TOE is reviewed to establish overall function, the integrity of the interatrial septum, aortic valve competency, and the presence of other valvular lesions and LV thrombus. An operative time out reviewing not only patient information but operative plan and conduct is a practice that high-performance teams have developed and maintain.

Sternotomy approach

Implanting an LVAD through a median sternotomy utilizing cardiopulmonary bypass (CPB) is the most common implantation technique. Most LVADs are recommended to be implanted using this approach in their FDA-approved instructions for use. Specific operative steps may relate to size, outflow location, driveline exit site, and positioning of the implanted LVAD.

The patient is brought into the operating room and placed in a supine position. General anaesthesia is induced and maintained. Monitoring lines are placed typically including arterial line, pulmonary artery catheter (PAC), and a TOE probe. In case of previous cardiac surgery with the associated risks of sternal re-entry, vascular access is typically established as per team preference ranging from arterial and venous wires and/or lines, to anticipatory exposure of the femoral or axillary arteries to facilitate emergent initiation of CPB. A midline incision is made and a full sternotomy is performed. The diaphragm is mobilized and divided to a varying extent to allow placing the pump body or outflow graft when dictated by pump size and configuration. The pocket must be large enough to prevent pump displacement or compromise in the final, closed chest pump position. The pericardium is opened liberally towards the apex. A pericardial cradle is created with consideration for an asymmetric vertical opening to allow the pericardium to be re-approximated at the conclusion of the implantation. For LVADs that require a true pocket, the diaphragm is divided with a linear stapler and a preperitoneal pocket is created anterior to the posterior rectus sheet. Adequate spacing requires a pocket that is wide enough to allow full sub-diaphragmatic pump body placement with the pump parallel to the axial plane. The HeartMate (HM) 3 (Abbott, Abbott Park, IL, USA) intrapericardial placement as well as extended extrapericardial placement by augmentation of the pericardium with prosthetic material. Most LVAD implantation can be completed with most or all of the left pleura intact.

Driveline

After establishing a pump pocket, consideration is given to tunnelling the driveline prior to giving heparin. The driveline is tunnelled exiting on either side of the abdomen in the midclavicular line below the costal margin but above the belt line. The ideal exit site is marked prior to surgery, with the patient sitting or standing, and wearing typical clothes. The exit site is selected and a small skin incision is made and dissected to the rectus fascia. The driveline is tunnelled internally engaging the rectus sheath within the chest, maintaining the initial depth to avoid compression from the costal margin. The driveline is ideally placed within the rectus sheath until immediately below the chosen exit site where it traverses the fascia perpendicular with minimal subcutaneous distance (Fig. 5.1). All velour should remain within the fascia with no visible velour at the skin interface to decrease risk of driveline infection. An anchoring suture is placed approximately 5 cm from the exit site to stabilize the driveline in the event of sudden driveline traction until the driveline is healed. Alternative driveline techniques employ an initial lateral path to a temporary exit on the flank, with a second medial pass of the trocar to the final exit site to create a longer tunnel in an attempt to decrease the risk of driveline infection.

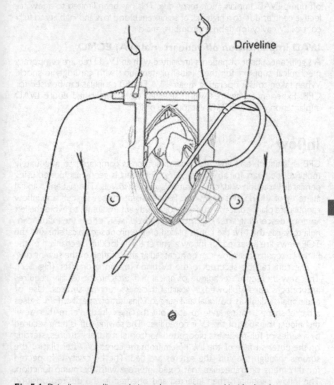

Fig.5.1 Driveline tunnelling technique: the trocar is passed inside the chest, engaging the posterior fascia to a pre-marked exit site, remaining extraperitoneal, within the rectus sheath until exiting through the subcutaneous fascia.

Cardiopulmonary bypass

Cannulation is performed according to the surgeon's preference with consideration to avoid excess tissue dissection in patients with anticipated future operations. In patients with pre-existing MCS, utilizing previously placed cannulas and/or other components can be accomplished in many cases.

Before initiating CPB, the intraoperative TOE findings should be reviewed for significant valvular lesions, atrial septal defect (ASD), or thrombus in LV or left atrial appendage (LAA). The tissue quality of the LV and apex should be assessed for apical calcifications with consideration for alternative implantation techniques in the setting of a hostile apex.

Off-pump implantation

Concern for the body's pathophysiological response to CPB has led to some specific pump designs that would facilitate off-pump procedures and off-pump LVAD implantation technique. This has been limited to a few selective centres due to a high risk of significant blood loss and inability to fully control LV cavity for debris, thrombus, and air.

LVAD implantation off venoarterial (VA) ECMO

A significant subset of patients implanted with an LVAD require temporary mechanical support for their initial presentation with cardiogenic shock. When taken to the operating theatre, VA ECMO cannulas can be used for CPB. Experienced centres will in selected cases performed entire LVAD implantation off VA ECMO without use of CPB.

Inflow

CPB is initiated, and any additional dissection is completed to adequately mobilize the heart for apical exposure. The heart is gently positioned using pericardial traction and/or operative sponges/towels. The patient's apical anatomy of the heart is examined. Positioning of the sewing cuff and inflow cannula are planned at the true apex or slightly anterolateral, to avoid the left anterior descending artery. In order to appropriately orient the inflow cannula towards the MV, the cuff is placed on the proposed apical site and the TOE views are assessed for inflow alignment. The locking mechanism of the HM 3 to secure the inflow can be accessed at any rotation of the sewing ring.

The cuff can be secured to the LV prior to coring or after (Fig. 5.2). The 'sew-then-core' technique of apical cuff attachment usually requires anchoring sutures followed by partial-thickness running sutures. Use of additional sealants is optional and surgeon/institution specific. HM 3 uses a barrel-shaped coring knife to core out the apex. In the 'core-then-sew' technique, the apex of the LV is cored first. The sewing cuff is then secured by a series of full-thickness pledgetted horizontal mattress sutures, starting on the outer surface of the LV, 1.5 cm from the cored LV. After placing the sutures through the cuff, the sutures are tied. The LV cavity is inspected for thrombus or trabeculae that could interfere with the pump function. The inflow cannula is then inserted and oriented in the desired position and secured. In the Multicenter Study of MagLev Technology in Patients Undergoing Mechanical Circulatory Support Therapy with HeartMate 3 (MOMENTUM 3) study, the 'core-then-sew' technique required longer CPB duration but the two techniques yielded similar outcomes.

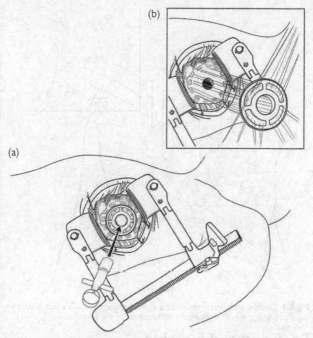

Fig.5.2 (a) 'Sew-then-core' technique for apical sewing cuff. (b) 'Cut-then-sew' technique showing pledgetted mattress sutures placed after the LV apex is cored.

The heart is returned into the pericardium, and the pump position is assessed for stability and orientation on the TOE. Adjustments to the orientation and angulation can be made at this point.

Outflow

At this point, the outflow graft is attached to the pump and clamped. The HM 3 outflow graft clip is then placed in order to prevent outflow graft twists and in HM II and HM 3 bend relief is attached to the pump.

The outflow graft is bevelled for an acute angle of 45–75° and placed on the lateral aspect of the ascending aorta distal to the sinotubular junction (Fig. 5.3). A partial occluding clamp is applied to the aorta and the 14 mm HM 3 graft is anastomosed to the aorta after confirming occlusion and sizing the aortotomy. The anastomosis is performed with a 4-0 or 5-0 continuous polypropylene suture. Just before tying the anastomotic suture, the outflow graft clamp is released, the heart is filled, and lung ventilation is initiated to de-air the graft. The graft is then clamped and the partial aortic cross-clamp is removed.

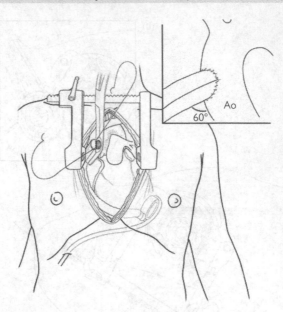

Fig.5.3 Outflow graft anastomosis to the ascending aorta (Ao). The graft is cut on a bevel to create a 40–60° angle on the lateral aspect of the aorta.

De-airing and weaning from cardiopulmonary bypass

Embolism of air into the coronary circulation may contribute to RV failure whereas air embolism to the cerebral circulation may result in transient neurological dysfunction or a stroke. Multiple de-airing strategies can be used to decrease the risk of significant air embolism. Using CO_2 to flood the surgical field decreases the air entrained in the heart as does continuing low-rate and tidal volume ventilation throughout the procedure. At the end of the procedure, a de-airing vent can be placed in the ascending aorta distal to outflow graft anastomosis or directly through the hood of the graft into the aortic root. Additional manoeuvres include using a small-bore needle at the highest level of the outflow graft.

Ventilation is restarted and preparations are made in anticipation of weaning from CPB. Separation from CPB requires normothermia, a satisfactory cardiac rhythm with appropriate respiratory dynamics, the absence of surgical bleeding, and mean arterial pressure (MAP) of at least 70 mmHg. TOE is used to assess RV function, residual air, the presence of an interatrial shunt, septal position, as well as new aortic insufficiency. Inotropes and inhaled pulmonary vasodilators are used as per institutional protocols primarily to support the RV. Once the left-sided cardiac chambers are sufficiently filled, the LVAD is turned on at its lowest speed and slowly ramped up while the CPB flow is decreased. The position of the intraventricular septum, MR and TR, and aortic valve opening are closely monitored as CPB is weaned. After successful separation from CPB, CPB cannulas are removed and anticoagulation is reversed. The inflow and outflow anastomoses are examined for bleeding. Chest tubes are placed into the mediastinum and pleural spaces. Using prosthetic material to cover the LVAD components to enable easier re-entry is done as per surgeon practice. The sternum and soft tissue are closed as per surgeon routine.

Thoracotomy approach

Smaller sized LVADs and the availability of instruments designed for minimally invasive cardiac surgery have enabled increased adoption of less invasive approaches for LVAD implantation as a strategy to improve perioperative outcomes. Less invasive implants may be accomplished with a small left anterior thoracotomy in conjunction with an upper hemi-sternotomy or a right anterior mini-thoracotomy (Fig. 5.4).

The patient is positioned in a modified supine position with a slight bump or inflatable support under the left chest to enhance apical exposure. Defibrillator pads are placed laterally to avoid planned left-sided incisions and/or right-sided pericardial sutures. The sterile field is extended to the side of the bed on the left. This set-up enhances the ability of two surgeons working in tandem, one performing the upper hemi-sternotomy or right anterior mini-thoracotomy while the other is focused on the left anterolateral thoracotomy.

To help plan for the left thoracotomy incision, a CT scan or a TTE is used to locate the LV apex. The specific intercostal space is planned to optimally access the apex, which is typically the fifth space. A 6–8 cm skin incision is made directly over the LV apex and the intercostal muscle is divided laterally to the midaxillary line in order to facilitate exposure. Alternatively, a portion of the rib overlying the LV apex can be divided to provide the space to accommodate the device and avoid inadvertently fracturing a rib. A soft tissue retractor is placed followed by an intercostal retractor. The pericardium is opened anterior to the phrenic nerve and several stay sutures are placed to improve exposure of the LV apex. To improve exposure, a stay suture may be placed in the fibrous portion of the diaphragm and brought out through a stab wound in the lower chest wall for retraction.

The decision to perform an upper hemi-sternotomy or right anterior mini-thoracotomy depends on surgeon preference, prior cardiac surgery, and the position of the aorta relative to the sternum. The right anterior thoracotomy is performed using a 4–5 cm skin incision at the second intercostal space. The third rib is disarticulated and a soft tissue retractor inserted into the wound. The upper hemi-sternotomy is performed through a 4–6 cm upper midline incision. The sternotomy can be extended into the right second intercostal space or teed off into both sides with sternal plate fixation later. A retractor is then placed and the pericardium is opened, exposing the ascending aorta. Pericardial retraction sutures are placed to pull the aorta rightward, improving exposure in primary surgery patients. A slightly larger incision may be considered in reoperative cases.

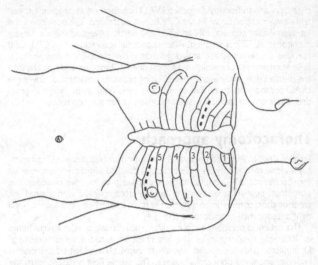

Fig.5.4 Less invasive exposure for LVAD implantation. Small bilateral thoracotomy.

Anticoagulation is given as per protocol and the aorta is cannulated directly while venous cannulation is performed percutaneously to the femoral vein into the SVC. The sewing cuff can be affixed to the apex prior to bypass according to surgeon preference, or bypass can be initiated for enhanced exposure for sewing cuff placement. The patient is placed in the steep Trendelenburg position for apical coring and the cuff attached in the sequence as per surgeon preference.

The LVAD pump is connected to the outflow graft and assembled if not previously completed. The driveline and outflow graft are then tunnelled. In primary sternotomy patients the outflow graft is tunnelled intrapericardially while in re-do patients the outflow graft is tunnelled beneath the sternum after dissecting a tunnel into the right pleural space. In some reoperative cases, a small sub-xiphoid incision is made to assist in outflow graft positioning and for additional exposure when necessary.

The pump is then inserted in the incision and secured to the apical sewing ring. The graft is initially de-aired by allowing the outflow graft to fill before it is clamped. After tunnelling the outflow graft to the upper incision and checking the path and length, the outflow graft is cut and bevelled. A partial occlusion clamp is applied to the ascending aorta and anastomosis is performed. Upon completion, the heart and VAD are de-aired in antegrade and retrograde fashion and the patient is weaned off CPB.

Prior to thoracotomy closure, chest tubes are placed, one in the right chest and two from the left chest, one in the pericardium, and one in a pleural space. The pericardium is closed around the device with pericardial membrane to minimize adhesions between the pump body and the lung.

Descending aorta and axillary artery outflow

In patients with multiple prior sternotomies or a hostile ascending aorta due to calcifications or previous surgeries, the descending aorta and axillary artery may be considered for alternative outflow graft sites.

Access to the intrathoracic descending aorta is achieved by dividing the left inferior pulmonary ligament to the level of the inferior pulmonary vein. The diaphragm is retracted with a stitch in the fibrous portion brought out through the chest wall. A partial clamp is then applied and anastomosis performed.

For axillary artery outflow, standard exposure of the left axillary artery is performed with care not to injure the brachial plexus. A right and left radial arterial line is placed to monitor outflow. The outflow graft is tunnelled through the first interspace and the anastomosis performed on the inferior aspect of the artery. A distal restricting band may be placed around the axillary artery to limit left arm overflow. With restriction and full LVAD flow, the arterial pressure in the left radial should be 75% of that in the right radial arterial line.

Pump speed is adjusted in both alternative outflow positions to allow aortic valve opening in order to prevent aortic root thrombosis and possible embolic stroke.

Concomitant procedures

The surgical management of associated valvular disease in patients undergoing LVAD implantation remains controversial. There is evidence (class 1, level of evidence C) of benefit from repairing or replacing an aortic valve with more than mild to moderate insufficiency, but the benefit in intervening on the MV and tricuspid valve is unclear. Closure of a sizeable patent foramen ovale (PFO) is recommended in order to prevent hypoxia associated with significant right-to-left shunt after LVAD implantation. There is growing evidence from retrospective studies that concomitant LAA occlusion may decrease subsequent thromboembolic events.

Aortic valves with moderate insufficiency can be repaired, replaced with a bioprosthetic valve, or oversewn. Aortic valve repair using a central stitch to coapt the leaflets (Park's stitch) will, if placed appropriately, reduce central aortic insufficiency while allowing flow through the aortic valve and washing of the aortic root. A pledgetted 4-0 or 5-0 polypropylene suture is placed centrally halfway into all three aortic cusps and tied. This manoeuvre can be performed through the aortotomy for the outflow graft or through a separate aortotomy. If the aortic cusps are damaged or not coapting, replacement with a bioprosthetic aortic valve or oversewing the valve can be performed. These manoeuvres require cross-clamping the aorta but the aortic valve can be addressed through a right mini-thoracotomy or upper hemi-sternotomy as well as a full sternotomy.

Concomitant MV repair for severe functional MR remains controversial. Repair can be performed through full and upper mini-sternotomy incisions. The valve is exposed through the interatrial groove after the sewing cuff is attached and coring has been performed. The patient is placed in the steep Trendelenburg position to avoid entrapping air. Aortic cross-clamping is not necessary to perform mitral repair in this setting. Alternatively, an Alfieri stitch can be placed through the core of the LV and effectively decreases MR.

The tricuspid valve can also be repaired through both sternotomy and thoracotomy approaches with bicaval cannulation. TR is often secondary due to left-sided failure, with a higher afterload in the RV and subsequent tricuspid annulus dilatation. Consideration should be given for repairing a tricuspid valve with more than moderate regurgitation and reversal of flow in the hepatic veins demonstrated on intraoperative echocardiography, in the absence of an increase in the RV short/long axis ratio. Repair is performed through the RA without aortic cross-clamping with an annuloplasty ring placed prior to VAD implantation. In less invasive approaches, a right thoracotomy can be performed through the third interspace to allow tricuspid valve exposure in addition to the ascending aorta.

Occlusion of the LAA has been suggested to decrease thromboembolic events in patients with and without atrial fibrillation with LVAD. Multiple techniques exist and occlusion can be safely performed through most incisions on CPB with occlusion devices or standard ligation. Prior to occlusion, the presence of clot is excluded with TOE and post occlusion, the LAA is assessed to confirm closure.

Exchange

The need for pump exchange due to thrombosis, infection, or driveline/pump failure created new surgical challenges. Most commonly, exchanges performed offer an opportunity to upgrade pump selection to newer devices (e.g. from HM II or HVAD [withdrawn from the market] to HM 3). Depending on the indication for pump exchange, the option for less invasive and possibly off-pump exchange of the LVAD body alone is possible in many circumstances.

HM II to HM II pump body exchange can be performed through either sternotomy or subcostal access, on or off pump. Subcostal access via an 8–10 cm subcostal incision with dissection down to the pocket is performed. The inflow, outflow elbow, and proximal outflow graft are exposed. The driveline is controlled from the incision if infection is not present. Once the pump is explanted, the new pump is implanted and the new driveline is usually tunnelled to the opposite side from the previous driveline position. When CPB is used, femoral cannulation is employed. Anticoagulation is administered after exposure of the pump and the femoral vessels are cannulated for CPB. The bend relief is disconnected and the pump is stopped. The outflow graft is clamped and disconnected. In off-pump exchange, the inflow may be clamped or occluded with a balloon catheter. De-airing is performed with a small-bore needle, and maintaining LV filling to prevent air from being entrapped. CO_2 is used to flood the field.

Exchange of HM II or HVAD to HM 3 is a more extensive procedure than a subcostal exchange. The assessment of patient candidacy for this exchange includes preoperative TOE and right heart catheterization to assess for valvular abnormalities, an assessment of RV function, and CT of the chest to exclude outflow graft obstruction/thrombus.

HM II to HM 3 exchange can be performed through a re-sternotomy or through a subcostal incision. In the latter approach, the HM II pump body and outflow graft elbow is exposed through the main subcostal incision, while a small left thoracotomy is made to access the apex of the heart and the prior inflow cannula (Fig. 5.5). In most cases, the HM II sewing cuff can be trimmed to 12–15 mm and the HM 3 implanted through this cuff, securing the pump with cable ties. Alternatively, a HM 3 specific cuff can be sewn after excising the HM II cuff on CPB. HVAD to HM 3 exchange is performed through a median sternotomy or a left thoracotomy. The thoracotomy exchange is performed on CPB with femoral cannulation. The HVAD apical cuff is excised and the HM 3-specific apical cuff in secured in standard fashion.

Upon removal of the prior HM II, and after securing the HM 3, the new outflow graft can be tunnelled into the subcostal incision and an end-to-end bevelled anastomosis performed to the original HM II outflow graft.

Due to outflow graft size discrepancies, when exchanging a HVAD (10 mm outflow graft) to HM 3 (14 mm outflow graft), the outflow graft-to-graft anastomosis needs to be carefully sized and tapered, and bend relief length may need to be trimmed for appropriate visualization. Deairing is performed by the use of a vent placed in the outflow graft or with a small-bore needle.

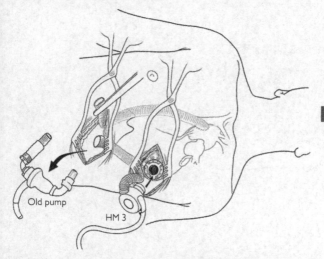

Old pump

HM 3

Fig. 5.5 HM II to HM 3 exchange through subcostal and thoracotomy approach.

Chapter 6

Clinical trials with durable left ventricular assist devices

Pre-trial era

The first human implantation of a total artificial heart as a BTT occurred in 1969. Over the next two decades, several LVADs—all volume displacement pumps—were developed, including the HeartMate implantable pneumatic left ventricular assist system (IP LVAS), the Thoratec Pierce–Donachy VAD, and the Novacor LVAS. However, data about these devices were limited to case reports and series, and adoption remained limited to a handful of centres. In the late 1980s, the US FDA granted investigational device exemption approval to these first-generation devices, paving the way for large-scale trials.

Early trials in first-generation devices

Issues facing early trials

Double-blind, randomized, placebo-controlled trials are the gold standard of clinical evidence. However, implementation of this design in surgery can be impractical and even at times unethical. Challenges include the incorporation of blinding and placebo controls (e.g. sham procedures), the difficulties of standardizing complex surgeries, and the learning curve associated with novel procedures.

The small population of BTT patients was a key challenge facing early LVAD trials. The Novacor LVAS trial, which started in 1996, enrolled 'cardiac transplant candidates in imminent danger of death'. In that year, heart transplant waiting list candidates numbered 2,436 in the USA; only a small fraction would qualify. Eliminating the randomized control arm could reduce the sample size and shorten recruitment time, potentially leading to more rapid approval. However, this would be at the cost of study validity. This trade-off was accepted by all of the early trials, which used either a single-arm design or incorporated non-randomized controls: historical controls or contemporaneous controls who either declined the device or for whom the device was unavailable.

Results of early trials

These early trials convincingly demonstrated improved survival until transplant for deteriorating waiting list patients. The HeartMate IP was implanted in 75 patients at 17 centres between August 1985 and September 1993. Compared to 33 non-randomized controls, HeartMate IP patients had greater survival until transplantation (71% vs 36%, p = 0.001). The Novacor LVAS trial, which recruited 129 patients at 22 centres between March 1996 and June 1998 as well as 35 non-randomized controls, also demonstrated improved survival until transplantation: 75% versus 37% (p <0.001). Similarly, in a single-arm trial, 63% of 186 BTT patients at 41 centres who received a Pierce–Donachy VAD (also known as the PVAD) survived until transplantation. These results led to FDA approval of all three devices for BTT.

An important secondary finding of these trials was significant end-organ function improvement. Additionally, the major complications following LVAD implantation were characterized. Among HeartMate IP patients, complications included bleeding (41%), infection (41%), thromboembolism

(4%), and right HF (15%) during a mean follow-up of 76 days. Novacor LVAS patients experienced similar adverse events (with a notably higher risk of stroke): bleeding (39%), infection (30% systemic, 12% pocket, and 10% driveline), central nervous system (CNS) thromboembolism (25%), and RV dysfunction (9%). Thoratec PVAD patients, during a mean support of 24 days, also experienced bleeding (26%), infection (55%), and thromboembolism (6%). Adverse event data from these trials served as benchmarks for future trials investigating upgraded devices.

These early trials lacked many features now commonly accepted as obligatory: protocols were not published, primary endpoints were not specified, sample size calculations were not reported, and adverse event definitions were not described. However, they successfully demonstrated the potential of LVAD therapy. Together, these trials gave LVAD therapy a solid foothold within the armamentarium of HF therapies and motivated the development of upgraded, implantable devices that allowed BTT patients to leave the hospital and paved the way for DT.

Expansion to destination therapy

Bethesda Conference

In 1995, the Bethesda Conference, attended by clinicians, scientists, industry, and the FDA, met to create guidelines for DT trials, including a general definition of the DT population and the endpoints that would define success in this setting. Additionally, future trials would be expected to determine pre-specified sample sizes based on statistical power and to use standardized adverse event definitions.

REMATCH trial

The Randomized Evaluation of Mechanical Assistance for the Treatment of Congestive Heart Failure (REMATCH) was the first DT trial. This was the first LVAD trial to publish a detailed protocol and the first to employ a randomized control arm. Between May 1998 and July 2001, 129 patients with chronic end-stage HF ineligible for heart transplantation were randomly assigned to HeartMate XVE implantation (N = 68) or optimal medical management (N = 61). Survival at 1 year was 52% in device recipients and 25% in the controls (p = 0.002). Adverse events remained common, in particular bleeding and sepsis, and device failure at 24 months was 35%. Based on these data, the HeartMate XVE became the first LVAD to receive FDA approval for DT.

INTrEPID trial

Enrolment in the REMATCH trial was slower than expected. This was attributed to a lack of equipoise among patients and clinicians, given the successful BTT trials. In view of this concern and the anticipation of high rates of control arm dropout, the Investigation of Nontransplant-Eligible Patients who are Inotrope Dependent (INTrEPID) DT trial with the Novacor LVAS used non-randomized controls. INTrEPID enrolled 37 patients between March 2000 and May 2003 and followed 18 non-randomized controls. While Novacor LVAS patients had superior 1-year survival compared to controls (27% vs 11%, p = 0.02), these results appeared inferior to the

REMATCH device group. Additionally, Novacor LVAS patients had a high 1-year stroke risk (62%), a concerning finding consistent with the Novacor LVAS BTT trial. The investigators hypothesized these differences might have been due to patient selection, smaller trial sample size resulting in less accumulation of clinical experience, or inherent device differences. Ultimately, this device did not receive DT approval.

Second-generation devices

Continuous flow devices

First-generation volume displacement devices had many disadvantages: their large size limited application to female and paediatric patients, the multitude of moving parts limited durability, and the large drivelines promoted infection. Second-generation, continuous flow LVADs were much smaller, had a single moving part (the rotor), and required a slimmer driveline. Examples include the Thoratec HeartMate II, the MicroMed DeBakey VAD, and the Jarvik 2000 Heart. However, many feared their minimal pulsatility was incompatible with normal physiology. Additionally, aortic root thrombus was a concern. Definitive demonstration of safety and efficacy required trial data.

Updated FDA guidance

Second-generation devices also raised questions about trial design—specifically, whether control arms should include contemporaneous subjects randomized to first-generation devices or whether historical controls should be used instead. Again, major stakeholders convened to discuss strategies, and in 2006 the FDA published separate design guidelines for BTT and DT trials. Given the large DT patient population, DT trials would include randomized controls. Additionally, given the permanent nature of DT, high-quality data demonstrating improved durability and safety were desired. In contrast, the BTT population remained small. Therefore, these trials could continue using single-arm designs, with the following caveats: in lieu of controls, investigators would use objective performance criteria as benchmarks for success (e.g. pre-specifying a threshold proportion of patients meeting the primary endpoint); additionally, post-marketing studies including contemporaneous controls were mandated. This was enabled by the creation of the INTERMACS registry in 2005, which could facilitate comparison of first- and second-generation devices while controlling for baseline comorbidities (uniformly collected using standardized definitions).

HeartMate II BTT trial

The HeartMate II BTT trial was a single-arm, prospective, multicentre study. The primary endpoint was the proportion of patients who were transplanted, weaned off LVAD support, or alive on the heart transplant waiting list at 180 days. To demonstrate success, a pre-specified objective performance criteria was defined as the lower end of the 95% confidence interval for the primary endpoint exceeding 65%. Between March 2005 and May 2006, 133 patients at 26 centres were enrolled. In addition to similar inclusion and exclusion criteria as prior BTT trials, this trial excluded patients with mechanical aortic valves and aortic aneurysms. At 180 days,

75% of patients achieved the primary endpoint. Additionally, compared to historical data from the HeartMate XVE BTT trial, reductions in bleeding, infection, and right HF were demonstrated. After receiving BTT approval in April 2008, a post-marketing study using the INTERMACS registry was performed, corroborating the trial results.

HeartMate II DT trial

The HeartMate II DT trial included a randomized control arm. Given the focus on reducing device complications in DT patients, the primary endpoint was a composite endpoint: survival free from disabling stroke and reoperation at 2 years. Between March 2005 and May 2007, 200 patients were enrolled and randomly assigned 2:1 to either the HeartMate II (N = 134) or HeartMate XVE (N = 66). At 2 years, 46% of HeartMate II patients and 11% of controls achieved the primary endpoint (hazard ratio 0.38; 95% confidence interval 0.27–0.54; p <0001). Again, significant reductions in device-related infection and right HF were demonstrated. The HeartMate II received DT approval in January 2010.

Assessment of second-generation LVAD trials

The results of the HeartMate II trials and other trials investigating second-generation devices represented another leap forward in device performance as well as trial design. These trials demonstrated how collaboration between academia, industry, and the FDA could result in creative solutions to complex challenges that balanced timely approval of life saving devices with patient safety. However, LVAD patients continued to be plagued by complications such as pump thrombosis and stroke, and further improvements of LVADs were required to offer this therapy to more patients.

Third-generation devices

The focus on reducing pump thrombosis and thromboembolism motivated the development of third-generation devices. The shearing of blood and heat generation at bearing contact points were thought to promote thrombosis. Thus, third-generation devices, such as the HeartWare Ventricular Assist Device (HVAD)-now withdrawn from production and the HeartMate 3 (currently the only FDA approved third generation LVAD on the market) are characterized by a 'bearingless' rotor held in place by magnetic and/or hydrodynamic forces. Additionally, these miniaturized devices could be implanted completely within the thorax, thus eliminating the need for an abdominal pump pocket. Trial design continued to evolve: innovations included use of contemporaneous registry-based controls, adaptive trial designs, and a paradigm shift in the concept of LVAD indications. Additionally, while these upgraded devices were anticipated to reduce adverse events, short- and long-term survival were not expected to significantly improve; trials during this era therefore typically performed non-inferiority comparisons of the primary endpoint. Although the HVAD has been removed from production, we have made the decision to include some pertinent trials, since there currently are many patients around the world who are still supported with this device for both DT and BTT, implanted prior to the device withdrawal.

ADVANCE trial

The ADVANCE trial, investigating the HeartWare HVAD for BTT, was the first to include a contemporaneous, registry-based, control arm. Demonstrating that these arms were comparable at baseline was critical. To accomplish this, the investigators enrolled contemporaneous INTERMACS registry BTT patients who met identical inclusion and exclusion criteria. Next, they used baseline data to calculate for each subject a propensity score predicting likelihood of being in the treatment arm. Subjects were then stratified into propensity score quartiles, and comparability was assessed by confirming that each arm contained five subjects per quartile. The primary endpoint was survival until transplantation or recovery or continued survival on the waiting list at 180 days. The two arms were then compared by calculating the weighted average of quartile-specific differences in the proportions of patients achieving this endpoint. Between August 2008 and February 2010, 140 patients were enrolled in the treatment arm; 499 INTERMACS control patients were identified. Overall, 92.0% of HVAD patients met the primary endpoint compared to 90.1% of controls, and the HVAD was found to be non-inferior.

Although the ADVANCE trial successfully resulted in BTT approval for the HVAD in November 2012, this experience demonstrated the challenges of using registry-based controls. Although the pre-specified comparability criteria were satisfied, a significantly larger proportion of control patients were within INTERMACS profiles 1 and 2. Additionally, differences in adverse events definitions and reporting precluded direct comparison.

ENDURANCE trial

The HVAD was next evaluated for DT in the ENDURANCE trial, a prospective, randomized, multicentre trial. Subjects were randomly assigned 2:1 to receive the HVAD or HeartMate II. A novel feature of this trial was the adaptive design for sample size determination, allowing for early trial termination: after 300 patients reached 2 years of follow-up, an interim analysis would determine the proportion of control patients meeting the primary endpoint (survival free from disabling stroke or reoperation). If this proportion exceeded 55%, the trial would be terminated (under these conditions the study would still achieve 90% power to establish non-inferiority); otherwise, 450 subjects would be enrolled. From August 2010 through May 2012, 446 patients received either the HVAD (N = 297) or HeartMate II (N = 148). The HVAD was shown to be non-inferior to the HeartMate II (55.4% vs 59.1%, p = 0.01). While similar rates of major bleeding and infections were found, a higher stroke risk was demonstrated in HVAD recipients (29.7% vs 12.1%, p <0.001). The HVAD received DT approval in 2017.

MOMENTUM 3 trial

During this period, the traditional dichotomy of BTT versus DT began to be challenged. Rather than seeing these patients as clustering statically within two distinct populations, some argued that the whole LVAD population represented a dynamic continuum of transplant eligibility, given that LVAD support frequently reversed major barriers to eligibility (e.g. renal dysfunction or PH). According to INTERMACS data, 20% of DT patients ultimately underwent heart transplantation. Calls emerged instead for a single LVAD indication and the investigation of short-term and long-term endpoints in a single trial, with the added benefits of reducing device development time and trial-related costs.

The MOMENTUM 3 trial, a prospective, multicentre, randomized trial comparing the HeartMate 3 with the HeartMate II, was the first to implement a single set of inclusion and exclusion criteria including both BTT and DT patients. Subjects were organized into a short-term cohort (consisting of the first 294 patients, in whom 6-month outcomes would be analysed) and a long-term cohort (consisting of the first 366 patients, in whom 2-year outcomes would be analysed). The primary endpoint was survival free from disabling stroke or pump exchange at both time points. At 6 months, the primary endpoint occurred in 86.2% of HeartMate 3 patients and 76.8% of HeartMate II patients ($p < 0.001$ for non-inferiority). At 2 years, the primary endpoint occurred in 79.5% of HeartMate 3 patients and 60.2% of HeartMate 2 patients, meeting significance for not only non-inferiority but also superiority. Need for pump exchange and stroke risk were also significantly lower in the new device. FDA approvals for BTT and DT were granted for HeartMate 3 in August 2017 and October 2018 respectively.

Conclusion

Clinical trials have played a central role in the development and adoption of LVAD devices. The specific challenges raised by investigating these devices were met by innovations in trial design and aided by cooperation between clinicians, scientists, industry, and the FDA. Together, these investigators successfully paved the way for a promising new era in the treatment of HF patients.

Diagnosis and management of ventricular assist device complications

Introduction

Over the past two decades, there have been major advancements in the management of patients with end-stage HF. Patients with VADs are no longer bed-bound and are encouraged to ambulate to mitigate the risks of physical and psychological deconditioning. Newer generation centrifugal durable VADs confer superior flow dynamics and significantly improved event-free recovery and survival. In this chapter we will focus on the most common complications pertaining to surgical and percutaneous VADs. In the surgical VAD category, the term 'durable VAD' refers to long-term, surgically implantable LVADs (most commonly the HeartMate (HM) 3 (Abbott, Abbott Park, IL, USA) or HVAD (Medtronic, Minneapolis, MN, USA)-now withdrawn from production, no approved implantable, durable RVAD currently exists), and the term 'extracorporeal VAD' denotes central cannulation for purposes of shorter-term and temporary LVAD, RVAD, or biventricular assist device (BiVAD) support, connected extracorporeally to a centrifugal pump. While these two broad surgical VAD categories are separate entities, they serve the same purpose. Hence, there are some complications that are common between the two modes of surgical VAD support and there are some complications unique to each. We shall also touch upon the complications of the most commonly utilized percutaneous VADs. Although the HVAD has been removed from production, we have made the decision to include some pertinent trials, since there currently are many patients around the world who are still supported with this device for both DT and BTT, implanted prior to the device withdrawal.

Surgical VADs

The 'extracorporeal VADs' are inserted via direct central cannulation most commonly through median sternotomy. LVADs are instituted via direct cannulation of the LA or the LV apex as an inflow connection to the pump and a cannula directly inserted into the ascending aorta as an outflow connection. RVADs are instituted through venous cannulation of the RA as an inflow connection to the pump and a main PA cannulation as outflow connection. A combination of both would constitute a BiVAD system. A membrane oxygenator can be spliced into either of these two circuits if there is impaired oxygenation or ventilation (see Chapter 5).

The 'durable' LVADs are inserted for the purposes of BTT or for DT. Eligible patients by definition should have worsening end-stage LV failure (INTERMACS level 3 or lower) while being on intravenous (IV) inotropic support and/or IABP with sub-normal cardiac indices and/or high PVR, or as an outpatient with worsening symptomatic HF (NYHA class IV) and EF <25% on maximal medical therapy (see Chapter 4). Over the past two decades there has been enormous development in LVAD technology from pulsatile devices (HM XVE) to axial continuous flow (HM II) to centrifugal pumps (HM 3 and HVAD) with more superior flow dynamics.

Complications of surgical VADs

Mortality rate (durable VAD)

The reported 2-year 'event-free' (freedom from disabling stroke, need for device exchange or removal) survival rate according to the MOMENTUM 3 trial (see Chapter 6) was 77.9% for the centrifugal flow HM 3 device versus 56.4% for the axial flow HM II device, hence there has been a significant paradigm shift towards this newer technology.

Major mediastinal/cannulation site bleeding (durable and extracorporeal VAD)

Bleeding is the most commonly encountered complication of surgical VADs and can occur in as many as 50–80% of patients. A significant proportion will require blood product transfusion. As many as 30% of patients would require re-exploration in the operating room. Major bleeding occurs because of coagulopathy, inadequate surgical haemostasis, or a combination of both, hence checking coagulation screen and thromboelastography (TEG) and correction of any coagulopathy should take place as a matter of priority. Frequently the patients may have been on another form of MCS, for example, IABP and/or VA ECMO with heparinization for a prolonged period of time, increasing the risk of bleeding from coagulopathy or platelet dysfunction (e.g. acquired von Willebrand disorder). Some may have had previous median sternotomies requiring sternal re-entry and extensive adhesiolysis. Hence, there should be meticulous attention to haemostasis during VAD implantation surgery. Temporary VAD cannulation sites are particularly prone to bleeding. We recommend that the cannulation sites in the aorta, the LV apex (in cases of LVAD support), the RA, and the PA (in cases of RVAD support) should utilize double purse strings with pledgets. The lines should be tunnelled with care. Wide-bore chest drains should be placed in the pericardium and the mediastinum. These typically stay until after full heparinization is commenced and the desired activated partial thromboplastin time (aPTT) has been achieved. Unless excessive bleeding is encountered, the sternum is commonly closed with sternal wires in a routine fashion. Attention should be paid to wire puncture sites prior to chest closure as these frequently bleed. Some practices elect to leave the chest open routinely until all coagulation has been corrected and mediastinal drainage has subsided in order to mitigate the risk of cardiac tamponade and bleeding. Anticoagulation with unfractionated heparin is typically held for the day of operation and recommenced the following day. The aPTT range for the extracorporeal VADs should be set at 40–50 seconds and increased incrementally to 60–70 seconds with careful attention to chest drain output. However, for the durable VADs such as the HM 3 with low risk of thrombosis, aPTT can kept at a lower range (40–50 seconds). In case of bleeding, there should be a low threshold for returning to the operating room for re-exploration. Human leucocyte antigen (HLA) allosensitization in BTT patients and transfusion-related lung injury are two major adverse effects of blood product transfusion. In cases of excessive bleeding and TEG prolongation of 'R time', coagulation factor transfusion is indicated. Antifibrinolytics such as tranexamic acid are good adjuncts for perioperative haemostasis. A low-dose recombinant factor VII can be administered with extreme caution in a select number of cases. Desmopressin (e.g. DDAVP) can be used in patients with suspected acquired von Willebrand disorder.

Gastrointestinal tract bleeding (durable and extracorporeal VADs)

This complication can occur in both durable and extracorporeal VADs. Durable VAD GI bleeding has an incidence of around 10% per patient year. The bleeding sites are commonly from the stomach, the duodenum, or from colonic angiodysplasias. Any GI bleeding should trigger cessation of anticoagulation, correction of coagulopathy and thrombocytopenia and administration of antifibrinolytics (e.g. tranexamic acid). Upper and lower GI endoscopy with or without angiography and embolization are indicated. Emergent surgical intervention should be reserved for massive life-threatening haemorrhage. Careful planning and attention to the path of the durable LVAD driveline as it traverses the anterior abdominal wall should be made prior to embarking on an exploratory laparotomy as there is a risk of iatrogenic damage to the driveline.

Driveline infection (durable VADs)

Surgical site infection is a common complication and the rate of driveline infection can be as high as 30% per patient year. Any evidence of purulent discharge, erythema, heat, pain, and swelling at the driveline tract or exit site (with or without systemic manifestations) should alert the surgical team of the possibility of deep-seated driveline infection. The most commonly implicated microorganisms include *Staphylococcus aureus*, *Pseudomonas* species, and enteric Gram-negative bacteria. Blood cultures should be drawn and followed by commencement of empirical broad-spectrum IV antimicrobial agents and CT scanning. The CT scan should demonstrate any evidence of abscess formation or subcutaneous gas, warranting surgical exploration and debridement. A tractotomy is performed along the path of the driveline and the driveline is relocated from the site of infection. At the operation, all infected and necrotic tissue should be removed and irrigated down to the bleeding and healthy tissues. Vacuum-assisted closure application can aid wound healing after debridement; however, in the short term it can potentially accentuate bleeding from the surgical site especially following recommencement of anticoagulation. If the infection has extended near the LVAD device, exchange is indicated in a selected group of patients. The diagnosis of driveline infection prioritizes patients on the heart transplant list in the USA, highlighting the importance of this diagnosis.

Stroke (durable and extracorporeal VADs)

This is one of the most devastating complications of LVAD implantation. All patients should be anticoagulated following VAD implantation. Stroke in VAD patients can be haemorrhagic or embolic. Hence, meticulous attention to coagulation studies should be paid by both clinicians and the patients themselves. Embolic strokes occur twice as commonly than haemorrhagic strokes in VAD patients. The rate of stroke in VAD patients can be as high as 10% for the HM 3 vs 20% for the axial flow HM II device (2-year outcomes of MOMENTUM 3 trial, see Chapter 6). The highest risk of stroke nevertheless appears to be in patients supported with the HVAD even compared to the axial flow HM II device and careful anticoagulation monitoring and blood pressure control of patients receiving this device is advised (ENDURANCE trial, see Chapter 6). Cerebral CT scanning should be performed urgently, and neurology and neurosurgical opinion should be sought following a suspected stroke to consider surgical/interventional therapy if possible. However, prognosis remains poor in VAD patients sustaining large strokes, and the BTT patients may be removed from the heart transplant list with only a minority reconsidered for transplantation upon recovery.

Arrhythmias (durable and extracorporeal VADs)

Atrial or ventricular arrhythmias can be a cause of RV dysfunction, reducing LVAD preload and causing low cardiac output states. In stable patients, atrial arrhythmias can be terminated with class III antiarrhythmics (e.g. amiodarone or sotalol) and with correction of electrolytes (e.g. K^+ and Mg^{2+}). Haemodynamically unstable or symptomatic patients should receive direct current (DC) cardioversion. Ventricular arrhythmias, on the other hand, can cause more acute deterioration of haemodynamics and should be treated more promptly with electrical cardioversion or defibrillation. Fortunately, most patients who receive durable LVADs will have received a CRT defibrillator or an ICD, which commonly terminate the ventricular tachycardia/ventricular fibrillation rhythms as they occur. Beta-adrenergic agonists and phosphodiesterase inhibitors should be weaned off; common antiarrhythmics such as lidocaine or amiodarone should be initiated. BBs may also be helpful. Less frequently, ventricular arrhythmias are refractory to pharmacological and electrical measures and approaches such as stellate ganglion block or catheter ablation may be necessary.

Cannula displacement (extracorporeal VADs)

There is an increased risk of cannula displacement with patient ambulation. It is imperative that the cannulas are secured with double purse strings and the snares affixed to the cannulas at multiple levels with heavy silk ties. The cannulas should be tunnelled laterally along the costal margin so that they are not in the way of the patient's lower extremities when they ambulate. Externally, the cannulas should be affixed to the skin at multiple levels with heavy braided silk sutures and their tightness should be verified regularly by the nurses and physicians on daily rounds so as to avoid displacement.

Hypoxaemia (durable and extracorporeal VAD)

Hypoxia can be related to the LVAD or RVAD support. Thrombus in an RVAD circuit with pulmonary embolization may manifest as hypoxia. Management consists of increased anticoagulation and replacement of the circuit (see later section). RVAD flows should be adjusted with caution and preferably with echocardiographic guidance; over-setting of RVAD speeds without careful attention to the function of the left heart can lead to supraphysiological pressures in the pulmonary circulation and pulmonary oedema. Where there is intracardiac connection (e.g. PFO), LVADs can significantly accentuate right-to-left shunting, which can lead to significant hypoxaemia. Hence, any intracardiac shunts should be identified by preoperative TOE and closed at the time of LVAD placement. Pre- and postoperatively, percutaneous device closure (e.g. Amplatzer, Abbott, Abbott Park, IL, USA) can be considered if the anatomy of the shunt is suitable. Reverting to VA ECMO support may be a safe salvage strategy if there is a significant decline in the patient's oxygenation or ventilation from any of the above-mentioned causes of respiratory failure.

Right ventricular failure after LVAD (durable and extracorporeal VADs)

This is one of the most dreaded complications of LVADs. It can occur in 9–44% of all durable LVAD implants of which nearly 5% (see Chapter 6 for the MOMENTUM 3 trial) may require RVAD support. The presentation could be sudden (i.e. immediately following LVAD implantation and upon weaning from CPB) or more insidious (i.e. worsening renal and liver function with high right heart filling pressures in the days and weeks following LVAD implantation). The aetiology of this phenomenon is not entirely clear but it is postulated that RV overloading due to increase in venous return as a result of improved cardiac output and leftward displacement of the ventricular septum can lead to RV dysfunction. Preoperative predictive factors of RV failure after durable LVAD implantation include the presence of severe TR, high RA pressures (RA pressure mmHg/PCWP mmHg ratio >0.6) and low (<2.0) PA pulsatility index (= systolic PA pressure – diastolic PA pressure/ RA pressure). Severe TR should be repaired at the time of LVAD implantation. TOE and PA catheters are indispensable tools for the diagnosis of LVAD-induced RV failure. There should be a high index of suspicion with increasing RA pressures (>15 mmHg), low SvO_2, low CI, low PA pressures, reduced pulsatility index, and increased suction events. RV function can be improved through conservative measures (e.g. pacing the RV at higher rates (100–110 bpm), inodilator and inhaled pulmonary vasodilator support). If these measures fail, consideration should be given for reopening the chest to allow more space for the RV and/or placement of extracorporeal or percutaneous RVAD (e.g. ProtekDuo (LivaNova, Pittsburgh, PA, USA)/ Impella RP (Abiomed, Danvers, MA, USA)—see below) implantation before end-organ failure has set-in.

Thrombosis and haemolysis (durable and extracorporeal VADs)

Durable VAD thrombosis is an increasingly rare phenomenon in the context of the newer generation centrifugal HM 3 LVADs as compared to the axial flow devices (e.g. the HM II has a device thrombosis rate of ~10%). It nevertheless remains a more common complication in the context of extracorporeal VADs. The extracorporeal tubing should be examined on a daily basis for fibrin strands and thrombus formation especially around the tubing connectors. If there is significant thrombus formation, the external portion of the tubing should be exchanged to avoid occlusion and/or embolization. Heparin bolus of 5000 units IV should be administered before clamping and dividing any lines. If the patient has a BiVAD and the LVAD tubing requires exchange, the RVAD flows should be weaned and decreased before clamping LVAD lines to avoid pulmonary oedema and haemorrhage. If there is an RVAD that requires exchange, the team should be prepared for significant reduction in LV preload and profound hypotension during the process. Hence, the process of extracorporeal VAD and tubing exchange in any context should be expedient.

As the HM II axial flow device has been almost completely superseded by the centrifugal devices, haemolysis and thrombosis have become exceedingly rare but should be considered as a differential diagnosis with high power consumption, rising lactate dehydrogenase, and plasma free haemoglobin and/or haemoglobinuria. In such instances, the patient should be admitted to a specialized VAD centre as early as possible. CT angiography should be performed to identify large thrombi or kinks in the outflow graft. Unfortunately, a CT angiogram is frequently unable to definitively detect pump thrombosis due to metallic artefact caused by the device. Echocardiography and 'ramp' studies could aid diagnose pump thrombosis as the aetiology of haemolysis if the pump is unable to decompress the LV with incremental echocardiographically guided speed increases. If the aforementioned tests confirm pump thrombosis, consideration should be given for VAD exchange.

Outflow graft obstruction

Due to the flexibility of the outflow graft, obstruction following insertion is possible if the graft is not appropriately sized prior to being sewn (see Chapter 5 for surgical technique). The HM 3 in particular has encountered problems with torsion of the outflow graft, which has since been improved upon (additional lock added to prevent torsion). The clinical manifestation of this complication would depend on the extent of obstruction to the flow. Pump power consumption is typically reduced (in contrast to pump thrombosis, see previous paragraph). The clinical manifestation may range from being asymptomatic to having recurrence of HF or even developing circulatory arrest in extreme cases of obstruction. Diagnosis can be made with a CT angiogram which would identify the obstruction. Following this, the patient should return to the operating room for corrective surgery. To avoid this complication in the first place, the outflow graft should first be connected to the pump and the cardiac apex returned to its natural position before pulling and measuring the graft to reach the right pericardial dimple (pleuro-pericardial junction) and from there pulling and measuring the graft again to reach the suprasternal notch. The excess Dacron should then be removed and the outflow graft sewn to the ascending aorta. We have found that this technique has been very effective to avoid graft length redundancy and subsequent kinking. The lie of the graft should be along the right heart border and away from the sternal edge. Utilization of percutaneous stents to remedy graft obstruction has also been described.

Insertion site infections (extracorporeal VADs)

Such infections are common in extracorporeal VADs as cannulas are frequently in place for protracted periods of time. The dressings around the cannulas should be changed with care and under aseptic conditions. Repeated dressing changes can lead to excoriation and irritation and a silicon, non-stick dressing is preferred. When infection is encountered, the most common offending microorganisms include coagulase-negative staphylococci, *Staphylococcus aureus*, and *Pseudomonas* species. Broad-spectrum antimicrobial therapy, followed by sensitivity-guided, targeted therapy should be commenced. Any concerns about deep-seated infection should prompt CT scanning to delineate pockets of infection and re-exploratory surgery to debride or even relocate the cannulation exit site. Ultimately, the most effective treatment consists of removal of the infected cannula which can occur with ventricular recovery or transplantation.

Air entrainment (durable and extracorporeal VADs)

Air can enter the circuit and lead to embolization and rarely air lock. Most commonly, this occurs when the chest is open and the mechanism consists of reduced intracardiac volume and creation of vacuum with subsequent entrainment of air. Dislodgement of the inflow cannula can also create this problem. As soon as this is identified, the system should be vented to remove air. Pump speed should be reduced to eliminate suction and in many instances the pump may need to be stopped and the outflow clamped. If air has entered the aorta, then venting of the aorta is required.

Percutaneous and minimally invasive VADs

Complications such as bleeding, insertion site infection, hypoxaemia, GI bleeding, thrombosis, and haemolysis and their managements are similar to extracorporeal VADs (described in previous sections in this chapter).

Percutaneous and minimally invasive VADs can be utilized to support the LV, the RV, or both. The percutaneous VADs propel blood forward with an impeller or with centrifugal technology. The most commonly available percutaneous LVAD devices and their characteristics are as follows:

- The Impella 2.5 (9 French (Fr) catheter and 12 Fr pump motor) can flow up to 2.5 L/min. It can be placed using a percutaneous approach and has been used prophylactically in high-risk percutaneous coronary intervention (PCI).
- The Impella CP (9 Fr catheter and 14 Fr pump motor) can flow up to 3.5 L/min. It can also be placed using a percutaneous approach.
- The Impella 5.0 (9 Fr catheter and 21 Fr pump motor) is a 'minimally invasive' VAD requiring surgical cutdown onto the femoral or the axillary artery for insertion. It can flow up to 5 L/min. With similar flow rates to Impella 5.0, the Impella LD (9 Fr catheter and 21 Fr pump motor) can be utilized to support the left heart. However, it is inserted directly into the ascending aorta with a Dacron chimney graft. The Impella 5.0 has been utilized to treat cardiogenic shock for up to 10 days, whereas Impella CP and 2.5 are primarily suited for peri-procedural support during high-risk PCI and for LV venting and decompression in the context of peripheral VA ECMO and poor LV ejection.
- The newer Impella 5.5 (9 Fr catheter and 19 Fr pump motor) is inserted in the same manner as the 5.0. See page 100 for more information.

Percutaneous RVAD devices include the Impella RP (11 Fr catheter and 22 Fr pump motor) and the ProtekDuo dual-lumen catheter connected to the TandemHeart centrifugal pump and are designed as RVAD support. They are both inserted with fluoroscopic guidance. The Impella RP is inserted through the femoral vein. The ProtekDuo catheter is most commonly inserted through the right internal jugular vein and is floated into the main PA.

Anticoagulation with unfractionated heparin with aPTT range of 60–70 seconds is the goal. Serial TTE/TOE assessments should be performed at the time of insertion, following any repositioning, flow adjustments, and following weaning and removal of the devices.

Mortality rate

These data are based on reported observational studies; the 30-day mortality rate while on the Impella device appears to range from 23% to 65%. The reported mortality rate appears to be slightly higher while on the Impella 5.0 than with the narrow-calibre devices.

Major adverse cardiovascular events

The 30-day risk of stroke has been reported to have ranged from 1.7% to 6.3% with the Impella devices. Impella 5.0 appears to convey a higher risk of stroke.

Bleeding

The 30-day observational rate of bleeding requiring an operation for haemostasis has been reported to range from 2.6% to 43.8%, with the Impella 5.0 appearing to have significantly higher bleeding risk as compared to the Impella 2.5 perhaps due to the need for surgical cutdown to place this device.

Haemolysis and thrombosis

These complications are most commonly encountered in narrower calibre percutaneous devices (7.5–10.3% for Impella 2.5 vs 6.3% for Impella 5.0) due to the turbulence caused by the impeller. Following VAD implantation, daily serum lactate dehydrogenase and plasma free haemoglobin should be measured. Rising levels of such parameters with or without haemoglobin-uria should alert the HF team of acute haemolysis. If there is thrombosis, the TTE/TOE can aid the diagnosis by identifying LV dilation or the presence of worsening functional MV regurgitation due to the device's inability to decompress the LV. If untreated, haemolysis can lead to renal failure and the need for dialysis. When haemolysis with or without thrombosis is suspected, the aPTT should be increased to 70–80 seconds and the Impella device should be removed emergently and the patient should be supported with an alternative form of support, such as IABP (if tolerated)/VA ECMO/extracorporeal LVAD.

Catheter migration

The Impella device catheter is positioned with TOE or fluoroscopic guidance, with the inflow placed through the aortic valve and rested in the LV outflow tract and the outflow orifice is positioned in the ascending aorta. Catheter migration can lead to significant haemodynamic compromise and haemolysis. Suspicion of catheter migration can be confirmed with a portable plain radiograph or TTE/TOE. Repositioning also requires TOE or fluoroscopic guidance.

Vascular injury and limb ischaemia

Incidence of major vascular injury can be as high as 17%. Impella catheters can cause limb ischaemia by causing obstruction of blood flow distally leading to limb ischaemia or compartment syndrome. Vascular injury (e.g. arterial dissection) can also occur at the time of introduction or removal of such catheters. Therefore, distal flow should be verified by means of a Doppler ultrasound scan immediately following insertion or removal of the device and documented. Inability to verify Doppler flow should prompt emergent vascular intervention for example, relocation of the catheter, possible angiography, and/or surgical exploration of the site.

Conclusion

VAD complications are numerous and can be debilitating or fatal. Anticipation of such complications and early intervention when complications arise is emphasized and may mitigate deleterious consequences.

Extracorporeal membrane oxygenation

Clinical applications and indications

The basic concept of ECMO is draining the deoxygenated blood from the venous side, using a centrifugal pump to push the blood across a membrane oxygenator, and then returning it to the body via a large-bore cannula. The oxygenated blood is returned to either an artery or a different venous site.

When evaluating patients for extracorporeal support, it is crucial to programmatically develop global inclusion and, more importantly, exclusion criteria. Each patient going on ECMO should have an exit strategy (e.g. BTT, bridge to recovery, etc.) in order to avoid a futile and prolonged ECMO run (i.e. 'bridge to nowhere') which would create an ethical dilemma and eventual withdrawal of support. Although exceptions can be argued for, it is recommended that upper limits for age be established. Additional criteria to consider include prior duration of mechanical ventilation particularly at high inspiratory pressures, body mass index (BMI), and comorbidities, including presence and chronicity of renal failure and incidence of multisystem organ failure. Also, decisions should be made regarding whether or not it should be offered to patients with advanced cancers.

ECMO can provide temporary mechanical support to facilitate surgery on the heart, lung, and airway. Patients can be placed on venoarterial (VA) ECMO to provide haemodynamic support during high-risk catheter interventions. Airway surgeries, such as tracheal resection or airway tumour ablation, can be supported on venovenous (VV) ECMO to obviate the need for cross-table ventilation. VV and VA ECMO can be used to provide intraoperative mechanical support during lung transplantation.

Venovenous ECMO

In terms of respiratory ECMO, inclusion criteria include PaO_2/FiO_2 ratio <60 despite maximum ventilator support. Exclusion criteria can include mechanical ventilation >7–10 days, significant known neurological injury, or profound multiorgan failure.

Before proceeding to ECMO, the critical care team may consider use of inhaled pulmonary vasodilators, pharmacological paralysis, and ventilation in prone positioning. Also, consultation from a high-volume ECMO centre may provide further expertise in ventilator and patient management that may obviate the need for VV ECMO. VV ECMO provides an opportunity to treat patients with refractory hypoxaemic and/or hypercarbic respiratory failure. These are usually single-system or lung-specific aetiologies. Common clinical indications include acute respiratory distress syndrome (ARDS) resulting from viral or bacterial pneumonia, trauma, pulmonary contusions, burn/inhalation injury, reperfusion injury, as well as primary graft dysfunction (PGD) after lung transplantation. Additionally, carefully selected patients with significant gas exchange deficit, or profound hypoxaemia can be supported on VV ECMO as a bridge to lung transplantation.

Configuration

There are three common VV ECMO configurations. Femoro-femoral ('fem-fem', Fig. 8.1), femoro-internal jugular ('fem-IJ', Fig. 8.2), and dual lumen (see Chapter 9). The least technically challenging approach is the standard right IJ-right femoral vein configuration due to the familiarity of most critical care practitioners in central venous line placement. While image guidance is strongly recommended throughout, fluoroscopy at the end is helpful to ensure that the tips of the cannulas are not in close proximity to mitigate against 'recirculation'. In recirculation, the oxygenated blood coming out of the outflow cannula is immediately drained back into the inflow cannula and pushed through the ECMO circuit, reducing the volume of oxygenated blood reaching the patient's vital organs. Benefits of the fem-fem approach include ease of placement and less risk of recirculation, but the IVC can be crowded and it may be more technically challenging to place a left femoral cannula with a right-sided femoral cannula already in place.

The right IJ-right femoral vein configuration can be modified to include the left IJ or left subclavian vein site for outflow, and the left femoral vein for inflow. Each of these represents unique technical challenges and, as such, an experienced cannulator and image guidance with fluoroscopy is helpful.

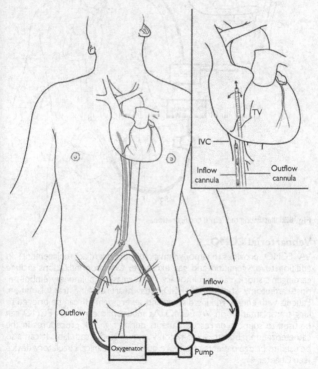

Fig. 8.1 Illustrating the fem-fem VV ECMO configuration. Note the higher position of the outflow cannula (the enlarged image) to minimize 'recirculation'. TV, tricuspid valve.

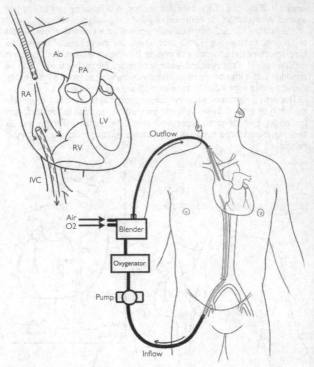

Fig. 8.2 Illustrating the fem-IJ configuration.

Venoarterial ECMO

VA ECMO provides haemodynamic support (cardiac replacement) in addition to oxygenation and gas exchange. Common indications include cardiogenic shock, cardiopulmonary arrest, massive pulmonary embolism, post-cardiotomy shock, and PGD after heart or lung transplantation. Patients with end-stage lung disease and severe right HF can be bridged to lung transplantation on VA ECMO. As mentioned earlier VA ECMO can be used to support or rescue patients during high-risk procedures in the catheterization laboratory (commonly known as the cath lab). It can also be used to bridge patients to a more durable mechanical circulatory device (see Chapter 4).

Configuration

VA ECMO can be configured as central or peripheral (Fig. 8.3). This relates to the location of the cannulas and can offer varying levels of mechanical support and unloading of the LV. Central VA ECMO can be deployed through direct cannulation of the aorta or indirect cannulation via a graft sewn onto the innominate or the subclavian artery, with venous drainage directly from the RA or the vena cava.

Peripheral VA ECMO can be placed percutaneously into the femoral artery and obviates the need for an incision. It can also be deployed into the axillary artery or the femoral artery with the cutdown technique. Venous drainage usually comes from the femoral vein.

A hybrid upper body VA ECMO approach that promotes mobility has been popularized by certain high-volume programmes and is dubbed the 'sport model'. In this approach, the axillary or innominate artery is cannulated and venous drainage is obtained from an upper body site.

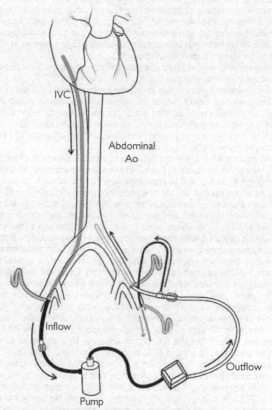

Fig. 8.3 Illustrating the peripheral VA ECMO configuration with a distal perfusion cannula.

VAV ECMO

In patients who are femorally cannulated for VA ECMO, there is a zone of mixing in the thoracic aorta between the oxygenated ECMO blood flowing in retrograde fashion up from the femoral artery and the patient's natural and suboptimally oxygenated (due to impaired lung function, e.g. ARDS/ pulmonary oedema) circulation being ejected from the LV. The blood from the LV perfuses the coronary arteries, and can also supply the innominate artery, left carotid artery, and possibly the left subclavian artery depending on the exact location of mixing. This may initially not be a problem if the LV isn't ejecting and the heart is being rested on VA ECMO or if the LV is ejecting, but the lungs still are functional. However, if the LV starts to recover in the setting of impaired lung function, then patients will experience differential hypoxaemia or North–South syndrome (also known as Harlequin syndrome). It is important that the upper body end-organs and the recovering heart not be subjected to prolonged hypoxaemia as it may lead to permanent dependence upon MCS.

In severe instances of North–South syndrome, the patient's upper body may appear cyanotic despite being on full femoral VA ECMO and having normal lower body saturation or a post-oxygenator PaO_2 >300 mmHg. A simple way to detect suspected differential hypoxaemia would be to check a right radial arterial blood gas or place a pulse oximeter on the right hand. If there is a significant difference between that and lower body saturation, or if the saturation is surprisingly low, then the diagnosis of North–South syndrome should be considered.

The treatment for differential hypoxaemia includes placement of an upper body venous return (outflow) cannula in a venoarteriovenous (VAV) configuration (Fig. 8.4). In this configuration the oxygenated blood is split between the femoral arterial cannula and the new upper body venous return cannula. With this new venous return cannula, oxygenated blood would reach the right-sided circulation and then eventually get pumped across into the ascending aorta. Usually 1–2 L of flow down, aided by a Hoffman clamp and a flow meter, the venous cannula is sufficient. One should avoid excessive outflow from the venous return cannula especially in the context of right heart dysfunction. An alternative treatment strategy for the North–South syndrome would be relocating the femoral arterial cannula centrally to the aorta or to an upper body site such as the axillary, subclavian, or innominate artery. These would all require surgical cannulation of the new vessel or a graft sewn onto the vessel.

An alternative to mitigating differential hypoxaemia includes jugular venous drainage alone as inflow with a femoral arterial cannula as outflow. With this VA configuration, the oxygen-poor blood of the RA/ SVC junction is drained, but the IVC blood, which has been shown to carry an oxygen saturation of around 80%, enters the right heart. This circuit configuration is designed, firstly, to off-set concerns that the new upper body return cannula poses a risk of recirculation. And secondly, that there will be less driving pressure at the secondary take off for the distal perfusion cannula (DPC) and thereby risking limb ischaemia. These risks can be mitigated by precise placement of the femoral venous drainage line to avoid recirculation and using a flow probe on the distal perfusion catheter in conjunction with a secondary limb monitoring tool (see Distal perfusion cannula). This configuration relies on SVC drainage alone and may not be sufficient for patients who need full ECMO flows.

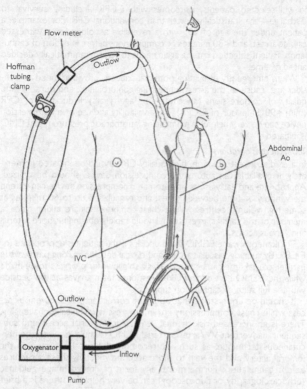

Fig. 8.4 Illustrating the VAV ECMO configuration with an upper body venous return cannula.

Of note, some patients with an underlying respiratory issue may also have profound sepsis and vasodilatory shock that may not be sufficiently management with VV ECMO and pharmacotherapy alone. If a patient is not responding to vasopressors, then VAV ECMO should be considered to better support end-organ perfusion. In these instances, the need for the haemodynamic support is usually transient and the patient can often be converted back to VV ECMO as the profound sepsis resolves.

Extracorporeal cardiopulmonary resuscitation (E-CPR)

Clinical decision-making

E-CPR falls under a special subsection of VA ECMO. In this scenario, patients who suffer cardiorespiratory arrest are emergently placed on peripheral VA ECMO during closed chest CPR or central VA ECMO while open internal massage is taking place (e.g. post-cardiotomy cardiac arrest).

In well-selected patients, outcomes with E-CPR—including survival to discharge—are statistically better than conventional CPR. For example, a patient under the age of 50, with a reversible aetiology for a witnessed cardiac arrest, and <30 minutes of compressions before initiation of cannulation. Patient selection criteria again needs to be programmatically decided ahead of time.

When emergently evaluating potential patients, providers need to consider age, cause of the arrest, underlying comorbidities, and duration and quality of compressions (anecdotal tip: 'age (years) + duration of CPR (min) <90' in favour of E-CPR). The availability and use of a compression device can be very helpful in maintaining intrathoracic pressure until ECMO is initiated.

Technical considerations

In a cardiac arrest situation, high-quality CPR should be initiated immediately. If available, an automated compression device, should be utilized. Appropriate and early use of an automated compression device can extend the window of time between arrest and cannulation up to 60 minutes at some high-volume centres. While chest compressions are taking place, a member of the cardiac arrest team should rapidly obtain fine-bore arterial and venous access.

Simultaneously, the ECMO team decides if the patient is appropriate for E-CPR. By running vascular access and clinical decision-making pathways in parallel, crucial time can be saved. This also allows for progress to be made while the ECMO cart or an ECMO response team arrives at the bedside with the full suite of cannulation supplies.

It should be understood that obtaining correct arterial and venous access while chest compressions are in progress is technically challenging. There is an increased risk of dual venous/dual arterial access and subsequent inadvertent VV/arterioarterial ECMO cannulation with the percutaneous technique; as such, we recommend surgical cutdown to the femoral artery and the vein to more accurately identify these structures before cannulation. Furthermore, any form of limited image guidance (echocardiography or fluoroscopy) can be very helpful. If there is a brief period of return of spontaneous circulation, then TTE can confirm wires in the IVC and aorta to guide further cannulation. Along those lines, if time and logistics allow, it may be helpful to place an X-ray board under the abdomen. Practically, it will mitigate against flexion at the waist or hips, which can make placing large femoral drainage cannulas more challenging. And then it offers the possibility of a quick X-ray should a technical difficulty arises. This becomes more important in large or morbidly obese patients who can sink into hospital beds designed to prevent pressure sores. If an X-ray plate is not available, a CPR board can prevent hip flexion.

In cardiac arrest situations, other practical cannulation tips to consider are using a stiff wire, using smaller cannulas, and less frequent stages of dilation. Due to anatomic considerations, the femoral venous drainage catheter during E-CPR should be preferentially placed into the right femoral vein if it is free. Also, having cannulators with refined endovascular wire skills and experience with standard ECMO cannulation is very helpful. They may be better suited to respond quickly to technical difficulties.

In E-CPR, the priority should be initiating femoral VA ECMO expeditiously. Once the patient has been stabilized on ECMO then an image-guided percutaneous DPC or an open surgically placed catheter can be considered. Some programmes may intentionally employ smaller arterial cannulas in E-CPR situations and elect to closely follow the leg for signs of ischaemia.

Clinical areas for ECMO cannulation

Intensive care unit (ICU)

The ICU, especially one that is already familiar with taking care of ECMO patients, is an excellent location for initial E-CPR deployment. For using E-CPR in an ICU, one needs to establish E-CPR protocols and then periodically rehearse them with the ICU teams. Practice and simulation are very important to having a well-functioning team. ICU providers should know which patients in code situations broadly meet ECMO inclusion criteria ahead of time.

Emergency department (ED)

In the ED, there should be a local ECMO chart and a primed ECMO circuit ready for imminent use. As in ICU settings, the ED teams should practice and drill simulated E-CPR codes periodically. There should be an available designated ECMO specialist who can help the ECMO team cannulate in the ED. A decision should be made ahead of time regarding which practitioner will undertake the cannulation, for example, designated providers in the ED teams or the surgical team. Also, programmes should have a policy regarding cannulating patients who have arrested prior to arriving at the ED. This is particularly important because quality of compressions in the field may vary and not every first response team has an automated compression device. However, the combined use of an automated compression device and an established ED ECMO cannulation may go a long way towards improving survival for patients who suffer out-of-hospital cardiac arrest. Some institutions have a protocol where such patients are identified en route to the hospital, akin to a 'code STEMI' patient, and they are directed to the cath lab or a hybrid operating room for emergent cannulation.

Operating room or cardiac cath lab

For patients who arrest in an operating room or in the cath lab suite before, during, or after a procedure, rapid deployment of ECMO can be lifesaving. This may be the optimal environment for a successful E-CPR deployment. The patient is already on the table; hence, the ergonomics are optimal. Image guidance is readily available or can be available should the need arise. In this scenario, open compressions (post cardiotomy) or closed compressions can be started immediately and vascular access may already be established and the ECMO supplies may be in close proximity. This logistical optimization can dramatically decrease time to cannulation.

Stepdown unit

Stepdown unit deployment of ECMO should be undertaken initially in a limited setting. Once the programme is comfortable deploying ECMO in the ICU and the ED, then expansion to the regular hospital wards and the stepdown unit is a reasonable next step. Again, ECMO carts should be located at set point throughout the hospital where a team can bring it to a bedside within 10–15 minutes of the code being called. In a stepdown unit situation where patients may not be as closely observed, it is important to know the period of 'downtime' prior to initiation of CPR. A witnessed arrest has a significantly better prognosis than a patient found down during periodic nursing rounds. Here patient selection can dramatically improve outcomes.

Once protocols have been established and this resource is available to hospital staff, the important thing will be careful patient selection. Strict criteria need to be established ahead of time and adhered to. Practical challenges include who fields the ECMO/E-CPR consults, who activates the ECMO team, and if there is an in-house ECMO specialist available who can come to the bedside during cannulation.

Technical considerations of ECMO cannulation

Once a determination has been made that a patient needs VV or VA ECMO cannulation, then the decision has to be made regarding cannula types.

An ECMO cannulation strategy needs to be planned ahead of time. The target vessels should be evaluated by ultrasound scanning in real time to determine the vessel calibre as well as the presence of a clot or stenosis. The size of the cannula should be based on the types of cannulas available, the patient's sex and body surface area (BSA), the projected needs of the cannula, and the patient's measured vessel size. The cannulator should be able to easily convert between French size and millimetres (3:1).

Tip: a quick way to calculate a ballpark estimated BSA = (weight(kg)/ 100) + 1.1.

Tip: a minimum cardiac output (L/min) needed to be delivered = BSA × 2.4 ('the ideal cardiac index'). This is a rough estimation of ECMO flow. In most cases there will also be some native heart output, albeit inadequate.

Cannulation strategy

Central ECMO

Central cannulation should be in the remit of cardiac surgeons only as it involves placing cannulas into the heart or sewing grafts onto the great vessels coming out of the heart. The cannulation strategy will be based on surgeon preference and likely related to the underlying cause of the need for ECMO.

Peripheral ECMO

Conversely, peripheral cannulation is now being performed by an expanding field of cannulators all with varying wire and endovascular skills.

ECMO cannula types

Broadly, cannulas can be split into arterial and venous, but select cannulas can have dual use. A cannula's performance is determined by its diameter (French size) and its length. As per Poiseuille's and Ohm's laws, a shorter, wider cannula flows better, and cannula diameter is a more important determinant of flow than its length. Before selecting a particular cannula, the operator should familiarize themselves with the cannula's published specifications. This should be done with the understanding that the published flows and fluid dynamics are in optimal settings, and often the data are based off of using water instead of the more viscous blood. Usually, a good rule of thumb is to subtract 0.25–0.5 L/min from the published flows to get the clinically anticipated flows. ECMO flows are most frequently limited by the venous drainage cannula. Certain clinical scenarios require high degrees of ECMO flows and so they may benefit from a second venous drainage line.

Arterial cannula

While they don't have as much of an impact on flow rates as venous drainage, an arterial cannula that is too small can lead to increased pressure drops that will limit flow. That being said, not all VA ECMO patients need full flow, and partial flow through a smaller cannula may be sufficient to address the problem. When placing an arterial cannula, operators should ask the question: what is the smallest cannula required to meet the patient's needs?

Tip: peripheral arterial cannula flow capacity (L/min) = cannula size (Fr) × 2/10 (for central cannulation add +1), for example, size 18 peripheral arterial cannula can deliver 3.6 L/min and when placed centrally, it can deliver as much as 4.6 L/min.

Aortic position

Aortic ECMO cannulas whether they are straight or angled are often CPB cannulas that have been repurposed for prolonged ECMO utilization. They have varying performance specifications based on their manufacturer, but usually run in 1–22 Fr sizes for adults. A common scenario is with post-cardiotomy cardiogenic shock (PCCS) where the patient is unable to come off of bypass (see Chapter 11). Some surgeons will elect to transition the patient to a VA ECMO circuit using the existing operative cannula configuration. Those patients will arrive in the ICU with an open chest and a temporary cannulation strategy that will need to be reconfigured to a more stable platform. Down the line when the patient has stabilized further and the chest can be closed, the patient may be transitioned to a peripheral configuration should ECMO still be required.

Axillary, subclavian, or innominate artery positions

These approaches allow for ambulation, physical therapy, and rehabilitation all of which are needed during the bridging period.

Axillary artery position

Usually a 6 or 8 mm chimney graft (note: French to millimetre conversion (3:1) to choose appropriately sized cannula for the chimney graft size) is sewn onto the axillary artery with a bevel. In turn, the graft is cannulated with a straight arterial cannula. The cannula can be tunnelled through the soft tissue surrounding the pectoralis muscles or brought through the primary subclavicular incision. When planning this tunnel, the graft should be examined with the retractors out and the arm in a natural position to ensure that there is no kinking. Extra care should be taken to limit the size of the arteriotomy and to precisely angle the bevel. The axillary artery approach is associated with a risk of brachial plexus injury, over-circulation to the ipsilateral arm, and bleeding requiring re-exploration.

Subclavian or innominate artery position

Technical approaches to the subclavian or innominate artery for central ECMO cannulation have been described. Typically, the grafts are sewn onto the artery and subsequently cannulated. Although a partial sternotomy may be required for the initial innominate artery cannulation, decannulation can be accomplished simply by ligating the graft.

Femoral position

The femoral artery can be cannulated directly percutaneously or through an open surgical approach. It can also be accessed indirectly through a surgical chimney graft as described previously. Depending on the manufacturer, the femoral cannulas often range from 14 to 20 Fr. They are often wire re-inforced along part of their length to minimize kinking.

Distal perfusion cannula

It is recommended that placement of an antegrade DPC guidewire is undertaken immediately after placement of the retrograde femoral wire and before placement of the arterial cannula (with the exception of E-CPR scenarios), see Fig. 8.3 (p. 83). This would ensure ultrasonic visualization and puncture of a filled superficial femoral artery with greater ease. Once the femoral and venous cannulas are in place and VA ECMO run is initiated, the DPC cannula is inserted over the previously placed guidewire. Backflow should be observed through the DPC. The ECMO run should be paused (maximum 15–30 seconds), the tubing lines clamped, and the DPC ad-equately de-aired and connected to the circuit using the special DPC high-pressure tubing and connectors. It is recommended that a wire-reinforced DPC cannula is utilized. Kinking is an issue with non-wire-reinforced DPC cannulas. We recommend that the non-wire-reinforced DPC is inserted at the time of cutdown for arterial cannulation. This would allow superficial femoral artery purse string placement facilitating removal of the DPC can-nula and would allow the DPC to be advanced into the superficial femoral artery run off all the way to the hilt of the sheath and buried in the wound closure leaving the outflow portion out of the wound and connected to the ECMO circuit. Burying the DPC cannula would eliminate any redundant length of the DPC cannula between the skin and the vessel entry site, which would be prone to kinking upon moving the patient's hip. Pulse oximetry, distal Dopplers, or near infrared spectroscopy (NIRS) can be used to con-firm distal flow. If there are concerns after placement of the DPC, an angio-gram can be performed through the catheter to confirm proper position.

Venous cannula

There are now a host of specially made, wire-reinforced femoral venous cannulas for ECMO. They are designed for the femoral position to prevent kinking and collapse at higher pressures. They come as multistage and single stage depending on the location of their fenestrations. The multistage can-nulas have fenestrations at the tip and along the distal portion of the cannula usually at 5 cm intervals. The single-stage cannulas have fenestration at the tip only; as such, they usually have a 2 cm tip that is not wire reinforced.

There are a variety of femoral venous cannulas on the market and each has differing performance specifications depending on their manufacturer. These cannulas usually come in two lengths: 38 and 55 cm. Both their length and diameter should be sized to a patient's BSA. Usually a 23 or 25 Fr multistage cannula fits most average sized adults. It is our experience that multistage cannulas provide better drainage than single-stage ones. To maxi-mize drainage, the cannula needs to terminate in the retro-hepatic IVC. The liver will help stent open the IVC and prevent it from collapsing around the drainage cannula if/when the patient is diuresed while on ECMO. An alter-native to a second venous drainage cannula is using a larger cannula such as a 29 Fr cannula in circumstances where flows >6 L/min are needed. It should be noted that these larger cannulas may be more technically difficult to place in the femoral position especially from the left side of a fem-fem VV ECMO configuration. In VV fem-fem cannulation, once wires have been placed up both femoral veins, it is recommended that the cannula be placed first on the left side. This is due to the acute angle that the left common iliac vein joins the right side for the IVC. The right iliac vein comes in at a new straight trajectory and if there is already a stiff cannula in place on the right it may be difficult to place a large multistage cannula up the left side.

Tip: venous cannula siphonage capacity (L/min) = cannula size (Fr)/5, that is, size 25 multistage venous cannula can drain up to 5 L/min.

Dual-lumen cannula

There are now several dual-lumen cannulas on the market. They all have a similar design, but slightly different flow dynamics. One lumen drains the IVC and SVC, and the other returns the oxygenated blood into the RA and across the tricuspid valve. They can be positioned in the right or left IJ vein, and for experienced operators in the left subclavian vein. Due to their large size and the importance of landing the drainage and return ports in the correct locations, image guidance is necessary. Care should be taken at time of placement that the cannula is oriented correctly to ensure that the RA opening is facing the tricuspid valve and not the side wall (see chapter 9 for further description and illustrations).

Cannulation sequence

ECMO cannulation, by nature, is an urgent or emergent procedure and is performed in patients in extremis. While the procedure has to be performed precisely and expeditiously, there is very little margin for error. Image guidance with ultrasound, TTE, TOE, or fluoroscopy is imperative.

There are six phases of ECMO cannulation according to the Extracorporeal Life Support Organization (ELSO): (1) preparation, (2) vascular access, (3) guidewire insertion and confirmation, (4) serial dilation, (5) cannula insertion, and (6) circuit connection and initiation.

Step 1: preparation

The operator must ensure that the patient has adequate IV access for administration of medications or blood products. The operator must ensure that unfractionated heparin, blood products, and resuscitative fluids are available, and that there is another clinical provider available to provide critical care management and heparin administration so that the operator can focus on the cannulation. All the supplies (the cannulas, wires, clamps, as well as back-up supplies must be available on the ECMO cart) must be prepared. The patient must be positioned appropriately depending on the intended vascular access site (e.g. shoulder roll placement to better expose the subclavian region) and access to imaging devices (ultrasound/fluoroscopy) and the ECMO circuit. The equipment and the patient's bed should be rearranged so as to optimize ergonomics during vascular access and cannulation. The operator should also plan ahead for potential back-up sites if he or she has unexpected difficulties with the primary cannulation sites.

Step 2: vascular access

Careful initial vascular access will facilitate later steps of dilation and cannulation. For example, if the vessel is accessed at too steep of an angle or off-centre then the wires are at higher risk of kinking or the side wall of the vessel is more likely to be injured during dilation or cannulation. It is recommended that the vessel should be accessed in two views using real-time ultrasound guidance at a 30° angle. Use of a soft-tipped micropuncture needle and a 0.14 microwire should be routine. The needle should enter the vessels at 12 o'clock.

Step 3: guidewire insertion and confirmation

Ultrasound should confirm that the wire is in the vessel in both the short and long axis. The guidewire should then be advanced to its target location under image guidance. If an ultrasound-only technique is being used, then it is critical that the wire be seen in real time on echocardiographic (TOE/TTE) evaluation of the heart or descending aorta. Fluoroscopy is an effective alternative for guiding advancement of the guidewire as well as further steps. Ideally, all the ECMO arterial, venous, and the DPC guidewires should be in place before progressing to the next stage.

Step 4: serial dilatation

Once the location of the proximal and distal tip of the guidewire is confirmed, systemic heparinization (usually 5000 IU of IV unfractionated heparin) is accomplished and then the operator can proceed with serial dilation. It is important to recognize that only the soft tissue between the skin and the vessel wall needs to be dilated and the dilator does not usually need to be inserted to its hub. Extra care must be taken to ensure that the rail system stays straight and that the wire does not kink or form S-shapes as it is being manipulated. A taut rail system is the only way to ensure that a vascular injury does not occur. In and out free movement of the wire as dilatation is being performed also reassures the operator that the wire is not kinked (especially in obese patients). For those less experienced with endovascular skills, real-time fluoroscopic guidance can allow for the wire to be visualized along its entire length during cannulation. It is also important to ensure that the wire length is maintained during various exchanges of the dilators. When working on the artery, it is important to avoid overdilation as this can lead to vascular injury or cannula site bleeding.

Tip: in the event of guidewire kinking during serial dilatation, the wire should be carefully withdrawn to expose the kinked portion. Then the smallest dilator is inserted past the kinked segment and into the vessel. The kinked wire is then removed while leaving the dilator in place. A new guidewire is then passed through the dilator and serial dilatation continued as above.

Step 5: cannula insertion

After serial dilation, the pre-selected cannula should be expeditiously placed over the wire, while maintaining the stiff rail system. When inserting the cannula, care should be taken to ensure that the inner cannula stylet is not inadvertently displaced. Specifically, the stylet can get held up on the skin edge or the soft tissue and lead to kinking of the wire or vascular injury.

Step 6: circuit connection and initiation

Once the cannula is placed, it should be flushed with sterile saline and clamped off. The cannula should then be connected to the correct side of the ECMO circuit using a wet-to-wet connection. Care should be taken to ensure that the circuit tubing is free of air bubbles. Once both limbs of the circuit are connected, ECMO should be initiated slowly. In parallel, the ECMO cannulas should secured to the patient at multiple points to mitigate against dislodgement. To minimize the risk of cannula site bleeding, a purse-string suture can be placed.

Arterial and venous decannulation

When cannulating the femoral artery, consideration should be given to plan for the final decannulation strategy. That is, whether a percutaneous closure device will be used or if the arteriotomy site will need open repair. If the femoral artery is surgically cannulated then pursue-string sutures may be placed to both help secure the cannula with Rummel tourniquets and later to close the puncture site. With a femoral artery cannula, care should be taken to not over-dilate the vessel and to ensure that the tapered portion of the cannula is not sliding back and forth. In this scenario, the patient can develop a large haematoma.

Venous cannula removal is generally more straightforward as this is a low-pressure system. Purse strings over the vein can be tied upon cannula removal if cannulation had been undertaken with an open technique. For decannulation of a venous cannula which was placed percutaneously (axillary, subclavian, or femoral), a deep figure-of-eight or mattress skin stitch usually suffices in achieving haemostasis.

Maintenance of ECMO and troubleshooting

Role of anticoagulation

Each programme should have a standardized anticoagulation protocol with set targets for VV and VA ECMO that includes a standardized monitoring regimen with activated clotting time (ACT), aPTT, or heparin level as well as a backup anticoagulation drug for patients who have heparin-induced thrombocytopenia (HIT), such as direct thrombin inhibitors (e.g. bivalirudin and chromogenic factor X assay measurements). HIT is a serious limb- and life-threatening complication of heparin and should be suspected in any patient on heparin with thrombocytopenia. A 'HIT screen' would stratify the likelihood of HIT in patients on heparin. Generally, aPTT could be maintained between 60 and 80 seconds. However, this can be down-titrated if there is bleeding. If ACT is used, it should be maintained around 150 seconds. It should be noted that if there is a concern for bleeding, holding anticoagulation in patients on VV and VA ECMO is possible for short periods of time. The tubing and connectors should be regularly examined for thrombus formation and tubing exchanged if thrombus is identified. Longer periods of heparin hold would risk thrombus formation in the circuit or the gas exchanger. Increased 'delta P' (pressure gradient across the membrane oxygenator) to >60 mmHg (normally <50 mmHg), would raise the possibility of gas exchanger thrombosis which leads to worse exchange manifested on the patient's arterial blood gases.

Blood product transfusion

Blood product transfusion should be minimized to avoid alloimmunization in BTT patients and to reduce the risk of transfusion-related lung injury. We recommend the threshold for red blood cell transfusion be haemoglobin concentration <7 g/dL. While on ECMO, platelets, fibrinogen, lactate dehydrogenase, and haemoglobin should be routinely checked and patterns monitored.

Haemodynamic monitoring on ECMO

On VA ECMO support, thermodilution cardiac output determination is erroneous. Frequent echocardiography is helpful to determine ventricular functional recovery.

Recirculation in VV ECMO

In recirculation, the cannulas are configured in such a way that the oxygenated return blood is immediately sucked back into the drainage cannula and pushed back through the ECMO circuit. Very little oxygenated blood actually makes it to the patient's left-sided circulation and, by extension, the patient's vital organs. This is diagnosed when the patient's oxygen saturation remains low or the systemic PaO_2 is unusually lower than what the flows would predict. On examination, the colour of both the oxygenated and deoxygenated ECMO tubes is either bright red or the inflow tubing blood flashes from dark to bright red. This indicates the proximity (<10 cm) of outflow and the inflow cannula and warrants repositioning.

Impaired gas exchange on ECMO

Impaired gas exchange (hypoxaemia or hypercarbia) on ECMO indicates one or a combination of the following factors: inadequate drainage or forward flow (inflow or outflow cannula too small for patient size), incorrect positioning of the inflow or the outflow cannula (e.g. recirculation, see previous paragraph), gas exchanger problem (raised delta P, see 'Role of anticoagulation' earlier in this topic), high cardiac output on VV ECMO (blood preferentially ejected by the heart rather than drained into the inflow cannula), or differential hypoxaemia on VA ECMO (see p. 82). In any case, efforts should be made to optimize oxygenation by correcting low haemoglobin levels. Increasing ECMO flows as much as possible may improve oxygenation and increasing sweep would reduce hypercarbia. If the ceiling is achieved with these measures, mechanical ventilation of the lungs can be optimized in order to oxygenate the blood that is ejected through the pulmonary circulation by the heart (more commonly an issue in VV ECMO). Finally, additional inflow or outflow cannulas (e.g. VAV ECMO in fem-fem VA ECMO, see pp. 82 and 84) can be inserted and connected to the circuit to improve gas exchange.

Left ventricular distention and venting strategies

LV distention may occur on VA ECMO support and is associated with increased pressurization of the pulmonary circulation and increased alveolar fluid. LV distention should be addressed quickly to avoid injury to the LV and to the lungs. LV distension leads to further irreversible myocardial damage due to LV wall stretching and could lead to pulmonary haemorrhage and/or LV thrombus formation. When the LV fails to eject and LV distention is detected, inotropes should be initiated and with the goal of achieving at least 20 mmHg of pulse pressure at all times. Should the patient fail to respond, LV venting can be undertaken surgically, that is, via the right superior pulmonary vein/LV apex and then connected to the inflow cannula or percutaneously using the Impella CP/2.5 (Abiomed, Danvers, MA, USA).

Low mixed venous oxygen saturation (SvO_2)

Low SvO_2 indicates increased oxygen extraction while on ECMO support. This is commonly due to low-flow states which can be mitigated by improving the perfusion pressures by means of inotropes/vasopressors and 'upsizing' (adding further) inflow and/or outflow cannulas. Other aetiologies could include low haemoglobin concentration which can be rectified with red blood cell transfusion and sepsis which prompt septic screen followed by targeted aggressive IV antibiotics. Increased delta P (see 'Role of anticoagulation' earlier in this topic) could indicate membrane gas exchanger malfunction.

ECMO pressure alarms

If flows drop off after initially being adequate then it can have one of several causes:

- Intravascular fluid depletion. If the circuit, including the patient's vascular system, is volume down as would be seen with diuresis then the lines will chatter or shake, and the pressures in the drainage cannula may drop below −100 mmHg (normal would be −50 to −80 mmHg). To fix this, pump speeds can be decreased and volume administered to the patient.
- Alarms could indicate transmembrane pressure elevations. Any pressures >60 mmHg should raise the possibility of thrombus formation in the gas exchanger.
- Alarms could indicate post-membrane pressure elevation. This pressure should ideally not exceed 300 mmHg; if so, this possibly indicates kinking, displacement, thrombosis of the outflow cannula, and/or that the cannula is too small a calibre for the patient and the need for upsizing.

Cannula site bleeding

The best way to avoid cannula site bleeding is to avoid over-dilation of the skin and vessel at the time of cannulation. For bleeding at a percutaneous venous cannula site, a correctly placed purse-string suture at the skin should be able to control the bleeding. For arterial site bleeding, the site needs to first be assessed for haematoma formation which could become a nidus of infection. Correct cannula positioning should be confirmed and partial dislodgment ruled out. Significant ongoing arterial site bleeding may warrant removal and repair of the site and relocation of the cannula to an alternative site.

ECMO weaning

A patient can be weaned from VV ECMO when their sweep gas requirements have decreased to the point that a formal sweep gas trial can be conducted. For this, the patient's ventilator is adjusted from 'rest' setting to lung protective ventilation strategy and the sweep gas is turned off. Most centres require at least 4 hours off of sweep before they proceed with VV ECMO decannulation. Once the 4 hours is achieved with acceptable gas exchange (at least PO$_2$ >60 mmHg and PCO$_2$ <40 mmHg and FiO$_2$ ≤50%) the patient can be decannulated.

VA ECMO weaning should always be undertaken using echocardiographic guidance. Weaning may also be facilitated by Swan–Ganz catheter readings during reduced support (1–2 L/min). Prior to weaning, low-dose inotropic pharmacological support or even IABP support may be initiated.

After removal of peripheral arterial cannulas, care should be taken to close the arteriotomy longitudinally to avoid narrowing. If the vessel is diseased or if the arteriotomy is >50% of the vessel diameter, then one may consider patch closure. With either surgical repair, attention must be paid to tact down any loose intima. After arterial repair, distal pulses should be checked with Dopplers in the operating room and postoperatively. If a graft has been applied to the artery for cannulation, a stump of the graft is left on the artery and oversewn.

Percutaneous mechanical circulatory support

Intra-aortic balloon pump

Description

An intra-aortic balloon pump (IABP) is the simplest form of MCS utilized commonly in both surgical and non-surgical HF. The IABP catheter is most commonly placed through the femoral artery. However, other insertion sites such as the right and left subclavian arteries, and surgical placement directly into the ascending aorta (with a chimney graft or direct) are possible.

Indications for IABP are as follows:
- Support in high-risk PCI or cardiac surgery.
- Acute management of cardiogenic shock (e.g. post myocardial infarction).
- Management of end-stage HF (e.g. dilated/ischaemic cardiomyopathy).
- PCCS (see Chapter 11).
- Bridge to OHT.
- Refractory LV failure.
- Mechanical complications of acute myocardial infarction (ventricular septal defect (VSD), papillary muscle dysfunction or rupture).
- Unstable angina refractory to medical management.
- Ischaemia-induced ventricular arrhythmias.

Contraindications
- Aortic dissection.
- Severe aortic insufficiency.
- Extensive peripheral vascular disease.

Methods of insertion

In an elective setting, an IABP should be placed in the cath lab using TOE or fluoroscopic guidance. However, it can also be inserted in more emergent settings in the coronary care unit or the cardiac surgical ICU without real-time imaging. In such cases, catheter position should be confirmed with a post hoc plain radiograph.

A femoral IABP is typically placed using the Seldinger technique with or without its accompanying 8 Fr sheath. The guidewire is fed into the descending aorta and the catheter tip is positioned distal to the take-off of the left subclavian artery.

An axillary IABP would allow for more liberal ambulation but is more technically challenging and requires the following considerations:
- Fluoroscopic positioning is generally required (C-arm, cath lab or hybrid operating room).
- Cutdown is performed onto the right or left axillary with a placement of a 6 mm side-arm graft onto this vessel.
- The guidewire is fed through the graft, into the aortic arch and into the descending aorta. Specialized angulated catheters may be required to manoeuvre the wire preferentially into the descending aorta. The IABP is then passed over the guidewire into the descending aorta. More recently percutaneous technique has become common practice.

Complications

IABP complications are relatively common and include:
- Limb ischaemia (ranges from 0.9% to 31%).
- Catheter migration (ranges from 40% to 60% in the axillary position).

- Catheter balloon rupture is a rare (<2%) but serious complication of IABP.
- Insertion site haematoma and infection (ranges from 8.6% to 40%).
- Formation of infective collection in type 1 diabetics (incidence as high as 37%).

Intravascular ventricular assist system (iVAS, NuPulseCV)

The iVAS (NuPulseCV, Inc., Raleigh, NC, USA) is a form of long-term counterpulsation VAD. It would allow the patient to ambulate and even be discharged from the hospital with the device. The components of the device include the blood pump, internal driveline tunnelled under the fascia and connected to a 'skin interface device', which in turn is connected to a 'drive unit'. The insertion technique is very similar to the insertion of the standard right axillary IABP (see p. 98) with the notable exception that the iVAS is inserted from the left axillary artery. Hence, a snare from the femoral artery would be required to guide the guidewire into the descending aorta due to the acute angle of the left subclavian artery take off from the aortic arch.

The iVAS is currently in the investigational stage and a feasibility clinical trial is underway.

Impella devices (Abiomed)

Description

The Impella (Abiomed, Danvers, MA, USA) VAD is a microaxial blood pump. Historically, the most common use of the Impella platform was for prophylaxis in high-risk PCI. However, more recently its utility has expanded to a multitude of uses including the management of cardiogenic shock. It is placed intravascularly in a retrograde fashion across the aortic valve with its inflow into the LV and outflow in the ascending aorta (LVAD). In addition, a right-sided device (Impella RP) is placed in an antegrade fashion across the pulmonary valve with its inflow at the RA/IVC junction and outflow in the main pulmonary artery (RVAD). The device can be used as a stand-alone support for cardiogenic shock or in combination with VA ECMO known as 'ECPELLA' where the Impella is utilized as an LV vent. However, it could be utilized to continue to support the patient's circulation once they have been completed weaned off ECMO. Other indications for its use include high-risk cardiac surgery and bridging decompensated patients to OHT or LVAD.

For the bridge indication, prior to insertion of the device each patient is assessed by a multidisciplinary team for candidacy for bridge to OHT or durable VAD.

The most commonly available percutaneous LVAD devices and their characteristics are as follows:
- The Impella 2.5 (9 Fr catheter and 12 Fr pump motor) can flow up to 2.5 L/min.

- The Impella CP (9 Fr catheter and 14 Fr pump motor) can flow up to 3.5 L/min. It can also be placed using a percutaneous approach. It can be placed for high-risk PCI or LV venting in the context of ECMO support.
- The Impella 5.0 (9 Fr catheter and 21 Fr pump motor) is a 'minimal invasive' VAD requiring surgical cutdown and sewing a 10 mm chimney graft onto the femoral or the axillary artery for insertion. It can flow up to 5 L/min.
- The Impella LD (9 Fr catheter and 21 Fr pump motor) is not a percutaneous device. It is centrally inserted through a typically 10 mm chimney graft into the LV through the ascending aorta.
- Impella 5.5 (9 Fr catheter and 19 Fr pump motor) is a more recently developed and popularized product with a goal of a longer-term temporary support. It is currently FDA licensed for 14 days of support for cardiogenic shock patients as compared to currently approved 10 days for Impellas 5.0 and LD. However, the FDA is currently considering a 30 day extension for patients supported on Impella 5.5. Like Impellas 5.0 and LD it is sited surgically and is capable of flowing as much as 6.2 L/min. It is projected that the Impella 5.5 will supersede Impellas 5.0 and LD as a higher support percutaneous device in the near future as it is able to be placed both peripherally and centrally. It has the advantage of significantly lower risk of haemolysis, thrombosis as compared to other Impella devices. The pump head portion in the 5.5 is more pliable with a shorter motor segment hence easily inserted than the Impella 5.0. Furthermore, as there is no pigtail at the tip of the device. Hence, there is less risk of thrombus dislodgement in cases of apical LV thrombus.

The Impella RP (11 Fr catheter and 22 Fr pump motor) is a percutaneous RVAD device. It is inserted under fluoroscopic guidance. The Impella RP is most commonly inserted through the femoral vein and across the pulmonary valve.

Contraindications

LV thrombus, intractable ventricular tachycardia, severe aortic regurgitation, severe aortic stenosis, mechanical aortic valve, and small artery access size.

Methods of insertion

- Standard right or left axillary artery approach through subclavicular exposure.
- Ideal size of the artery should be ≥6 mm and otherwise of good quality.
- Systemic heparinization (5000 IU of unfractionated heparin).
- A 10 mm Dacron graft is fashioned and anastomosed in an end-to-side fashion.
- Graft is de-aired and then tunnelled through a separate inferolateral stab incision.
- Impella sheath is placed into the Dacron graft and secured (Fig. 9.1).
- A 260 cm 0.035" guidewire is then passed through the sheath and into the ascending aorta through the aortic valve and in the LV apex under fluoroscopic and echocardiographic guidance (inlet should be 4–4.5cm from the aortic valve) with a 145° 6 Fr pigtail catheter (Fig. 9.2).

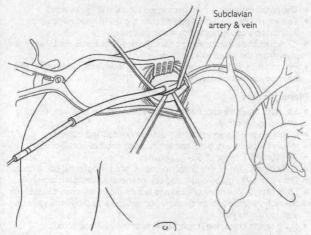

Fig. 9.1 Cutdown and placement of side-arm graft on the right axillary/subclavian artery.

Subclavian
artery & vein

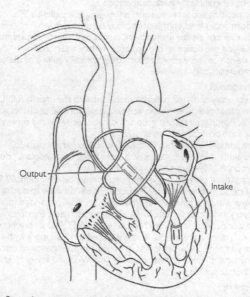

Output

Intake

Fig. 9.2 Optimal positioning across the aortic valve with the intake area placed approximately 3.5 cm below the aortic valve and away from the anterior mitral valve leaflet.

- The pigtail catheter is then exchanged for a 0.018" guidewire.
- The Impella device is then passed over the 0.018" guidewire under fluoroscopic and echocardiographic guidance.
- Care should be exercised to orient the device towards the LV apex and away from the mitral valve apparatus.
- Performance 'P' level is commenced at P9 level, echocardiogram, and haemodynamics are assessed.

Management

- Standard intensive care haemodynamic monitoring and lines including arterial line and PAC.
- Inotropes and vasopressors are used as needed and titrated.
- Wean sedation, extubate, and ambulate as soon as possible.
- Aim for aPTT range of 50–70 seconds.
- Daily monitoring of the axillary cutdown site for potential haematoma.
- Daily complete blood count and comprehensive metabolic panel.
- Daily plasma free haemoglobin and lactate dehydrogenase to assess for haemolysis (malpositioned inflow portion towards the mitral valve may lead to haemolysis).
- Daily serum creatinine (especially if haemolysis is suspected).
- SG catheter monitoring is helpful in determining total cardiac output and effectiveness of unloading of left heart.
- Echocardiographically guided repositioning.
- If the position appears adequate on imaging, the patient's 'P' (performance) level on the device may be turned down if tolerated.
- In the event of device malfunction, urgent replacement is performed by exchanging the device to the opposite axillary artery site.
- The device can be weaned echocardiographically guided as the patient haemodynamically improves.

Clinical outcomes

- A meta-analysis of 163 patients implanted with the Impella 5.0/LD use in cardiogenic shock reported an overall survival to discharge was 73.5%. Among the highest group of cardiac recovery and survival were those with post cardiotomy shock.
- In the authors' experience of their first 100 axillary Impella 5.0 placements, of those patients who were listed for transplant prior to insertion, 83.7% were successfully bridged to OHT.
- Among those patients in the bridge to durable device group, 60.9% went on to receive a durable VAD and 78.6% survived to discharge.
- Survival was 64% overall, and 50%, 48%, and 81% for bridge to recovery, bridge to durable VAD, and bridge to heart transplantation.
- Of those patients who were rescued with VA ECMO or biventricular support, many were able to be transitioned to LV support with an axillary Impella 5.0 with the added benefits including ease of removal during time of OHT compared to durable VAD and ability to ambulate/ rehabilitate patients.

Complications

Complications included stroke (10%), need for device exchange (13%), and clinically significant haemolysis (18.6%).

Dual-lumen VV ECMO cannula

Description

The dual-lumen VV ECMO cannula (e.g. the Avalon cannula (Avalon Laboratories, Rancho Dominguez, CA, USA)) is most commonly inserted through the right IJ vein. Alternative sites of insertion include the left IJ and the left subclavian veins. It has two inflow ports draining blood from the cavae to the oxygenator and one outflow port facing the tricuspid valve to the RA (Fig. 9.3).

Methods of insertion

The dual-lumen cannula is inserted with the Seldinger technique under C-arm fluoroscopic guidance.
- Commonly, the right IJ vein or the left subclavian vein is accessed with a 'micropuncture' needle.

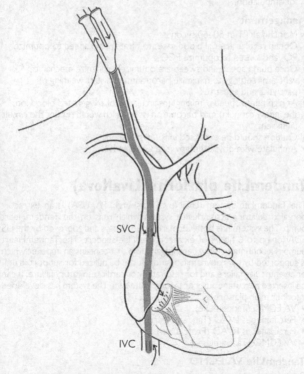

Fig. 9.3 Schematic presentation of the dual-lumen cannula (e.g. Avalon cannula) and its position (note the position of the outflow orifices facing the tricuspid valve).

- The guidewire is advanced well into the IVC.
- 5000 IU of unfractionated heparin is administered IV.
- Using the dilators (Avalon dilators for the Avalon cannula) the path into the IJ or the subclavian veins is serially dilated.
- Common Avalon cannula sizes are 31 Fr (suitable for most average sized males) can achieve up to 6 L/min and 27 Fr (suitable for most average sized females) can achieve up to 5 L/min.
- The cannula is advanced over the wire (Fig. 9.3).
- The cannula position is confirmed on fluoroscopy with the cannula tip in the IVC at the level of the diaphragm.
- The cannulas are primed and connected to the ECMO circuit and the pump started.
- Look for differential colour change within cannulas and look for immediate improvement in SpO_2 and PO_2 and reduction in PCO_2.
- Affix cannulas firmly to prevent dislodgement and in a manner to allow for ambulation.

Management
- Maintain aPTT at 50–60 seconds.
- Obtain regular arterial blood gases to titrate pump speed to optimize PO_2 and sweep to optimize PCO_2.
- Once pump speed and sweep are optimized, minimize mechanical ventilator settings to minimize barotrauma and start weaning off paralytics and sedatives.
- At high pump speeds, 'mixing' (recirculation of oxygenated blood into the inflow cannula) may become an issue which would render the circuit inefficient.
- Caution should be exercised in RV dysfunction.
- Ambulate with physiotherapy (see Chapter 19).

TandemLife platform (LivaNova)

The TandemLife system (LivaNova, Pittsburgh, PA, USA) is an extracorporeal circulatory assist device system which runs on the TandemHeart pump. The system has both CE marked for 30 days and approved by the US FDA for up to 6 hours of extracorporeal life support. The TandemHeart pump is a continuous-flow centrifugal pump that contains an impeller which is supported by hydrodynamic bearing. It can be utilized for support in uni- or biventricular failure and for respiratory or cardiorespiratory failure. It can be inserted percutaneously or through cutdown. The system has developed into four main platforms:
- VA ECMO (TandemLife).
- Percutaneous LVAD (TandemHeart).
- Percutaneous RVAD (ProtekDuo).
- VV ECMO (TandemLung).

TandemLife VA ECMO

Description
TandemLife is a percutaneous VA ECMO system that provides a kit with all the necessary components to allow a provider to initiate a patient on

VA-ECMO. The kit includes (1) TandemHeart pump, (2) membrane oxygenator, (3) sterile priming basin, (4) ProtekSolo arterial cannula (15 or 17 Fr), (5) ProtekSolo venous cannula (24 Fr), and (6) venous dilators (14, 18, and 22 Fr).

Methods of insertion

The TandemLife VA ECMO can be inserted percutaneously or through a surgical cutdown. The femoral artery and vein are identified either under ultrasound guidance or by direct visualization, and wire access is gained. Heparin bolus (50–100 units/kg) is administered. Using the Seldinger technique, arterial and femoral venous cannulas are inserted. The sterile priming basin is simultaneously used during this time to prime the TandemHeart pump and the membrane oxygenator. Once primed, the venous and arterial cannulas are connected to the pump via a wet-to-wet connection to remove all air from the circuit. The pump is then turned on and the patient is initiated on VA ECMO support with the speed adjusted to provide the desired level of support.

Management

The management of the TandemLife-supported patient can be broken up into two aspects: (1) the system and (2) the patient.

The system

The TandemLife system is managed very similarly to any centrifugal pump system with one notable difference which is the 'purge line'. The 'purge line' flows saline at 10 mL/hour through the motor chamber and completely surrounds the rotor towards the impeller to provide radial stability. Heparinized saline (90,000 U/L) flows around the impeller shaft–seal interface to flush the area, preventing thrombus formation. The pump rotates between 3000 and 7500 revolutions per minute (rpm) to provide up to 8 L/min of flow. When initiating the device, increase the rpm until the desired flow is achieved. The target ACT goal is 250 seconds which is achieved with systemic anticoagulation with heparin.

The patient

Management of a patient supported on the TandemLife system is identical to any patient support on VA ECMO. The patient needs to be adequately anticoagulated. Pump flows must be adequate for end-organ function recovery. This is achieved with close laboratory blood work and haemodynamic monitoring. Right arterial lines should be placed on all peripherally cannulated VA ECMO patients to avoid missing cerebral hypoxia as a result of differential blood perfusion to the right and left carotid. If cerebral hypoxia is noted, then the patient would require either a placement of an oxygenated venous return cannula to create a VAV ECMO circuit or conversion to central cannulation. Pulsatility (pulse pressure ≥20 mmHg) should be ensured (with inotropes) in peripheral cannulation for VA ECMO and frequent echocardiography is required to monitor for LV distension. If there is LV distension, LV venting can be accomplished by either open surgical LV vent placement or peripheral Impella device placement. When the LV recovery occurs, the next steps are to ensure adequate ventilatory function and haemodynamics on minimal inotropic support before weaning can begin. Weaning can be performed by decreasing the pump speeds until the flows are decreased by 0.5–1 L/min per day until the system flow is 2

L/min. Prior to pump removal a final echocardiogram is performed at 2 L/min. When adequate LV function is demonstrated, the patient can be weaned off fully and decannulated.

TandemHeart LVAD

Description

The TandemHeart system constitutes a temporary LA to aorta LVAD circuit. It utilizes a transseptal cannula (62 or 72 cm) that draws oxygenated blood from the LA and delivers blood to the body via the femoral artery or axillary providing a LA-to-femoral/axillary bypass. The TandemHeart system improves haemodynamic performance and increases end-organ perfusion for patients with LV failure.

Methods of insertion

The TandemHeart system can be inserted percutaneously using TOE and fluoroscopic guidance. The femoral vein is accessed by the Seldinger technique and the guidewire is passed into the SVC. Under imaging guidance, transseptal puncture is then achieved by using the Brockenbrough needle and a SL1 sheath. Once the transseptal puncture is made, heparin is administered to achieve a target ACT >250 seconds. Once the sheath is advanced

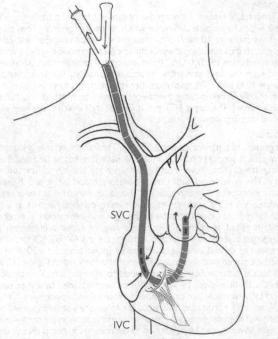

Fig. 9.4 The cannula position in the ProtekDuo.

in the LA, a stiff wire (0.035" Amplatz) is placed into the LA. The sheath is then removed, and the two-stage dilator is advanced into the LA. The dilator is then removed, and the tip of the 21 Fr cannula is left in the LA. The cannula tip contains three radiopaque marker discs to aid confirm the position of the cannula tip in the LA. TOE is also used to confirm placement.

The femoral artery is then accessed percutaneously using the Seldinger technique. A 15 or 17 Fr ProtekSolo arterial cannula is inserted. The pump and the cannulas are de-aired and are connected via a wet-to-wet connection to remove all air from the circuit. The pump is then turned on and the pump speed is adjusted according to the patient's needs.

The TandemHeart system can be placed in the axillary position to facilitate patient ambulation. The axillary artery and vein are exposed, and an 8 mm graft side-arm is sewn to the axillary artery. The arterial cannula is tunnelled through the skin and then placed within the graft and secured in place with a heavy tie. The pump inflow cannula is then tunnelled through the axillary vein and into the LA through direct visualization via a right atriotomy. The advantage of the axillo-axillary approach is that the patient can be ambulatory. This axillo-axillary approach describes an ambulatory LVAD strategy. However, if the inflow cannula is placed in the RA and a TandemLung oxygenator is added to the circuit, then the system consists of ambulatory VA ECMO.

Management

Adequate anticoagulation should be maintained on the TandemHeart (aPTT range: 60–80 seconds). Pump flows must be adequate for end-organ function recovery and optimum haemodynamics. Frequent echocardiography to monitor for LV recovery is required. Vigilant monitoring of SpO_2 is critical since severe life-threatening hypoxia can develop if the transseptal cannula is pulled back into the RA. Pump flow is determined by the patient's haemodynamic requirements. A PAC and an arterial line are essential tools of patient management and are extremely useful for weaning. Weaning can be initiated once the echocardiogram shows good LV function with the patient maintaining good haemodynamics on little inotropic or pressor support. The usual method of weaning is by 0.5–1 L/min every 12–24 hours.

TandemLung and ProtekDuo

Description

The TandemLung system comprises the Tandem pump, ProtekDuo cannula, and the TandemLung oxygenator. The ProtekDuo VV cannula set is intended for use as a dual-lumen single cannula for the RA venous drainage and PA reinfusion of blood. The combination of the ProtekDuo and the Tandem pump provides RV support making the ProtekDuo system a temporary RVAD (Fig. 9.4). The TandemLung oxygenator is intended for use in an extracorporeal circuit making the TandemLung a VV ECMO system.

The ProtekDuo is placed percutaneously via the right IJ vein under fluoroscopic guidance and comes in two different sizes: 29 Fr and 31 Fr. The 29 Fr ProtekDuo cannula is a wire-reinforced dual lumen with a 29 Fr proximal lumen draining deoxygenated blood from the RA to the pump while the 16 Fr distal lumen returns the deoxygenated blood to the PA to be oxygenated by the lungs. The 31 Fr ProtekDuo has a 31 Fr proximal drainage lumen and a 19 Fr distal lumen. Maximum flow across these cannulas are 4.5 L/min and 5 L/min respectively.

The ProtekDuo cannula provides percutaneous ambulatory RVAD support which makes it unique as compared to the CentriMag which requires an open approach, while the Impella RP despite being a percutaneous device is implanted femorally, impeding ambulation. In the VV ECMO arena the ProtekDuo is the superior platform. Compared to the standard two-cannula ('fem-IJ') approach, the ProtekDuo, being a dual-lumen cannula, requires only one neck access which allows the patient to potentially ambulate.

Methods of insertion

The right IJ vein is accessed using the Seldinger technique and 8 Fr sheath is placed. Then a 0.035" compatible balloon-tipped wedge catheter is advanced into the main PA and placed in either the left PA or the right PA. The 0.035" Amplatz super stiff wire is exchanged for the catheter and inserted into the PA and the sheath is removed. Systemic heparinization is then ensued for a target ACT >250 seconds. The path is serially dilated with the Tandem dilator kit and the ProtekDuo cannula is advanced under fluoroscopic guidance into the PA ensuring the distal tip is positioned in the main PA and the proximal drainage holes in the RA. Then the proximal (inflow-RA) and the distal (outflow-PA) tubes are connected to the Tandem pump. RVAD support is then initiated and progressively increased (as needed) to a maximum flow of 4.5 or 5 L/min depending on the calibre of the cannula used. If an oxygenator is required, this can be spliced into the circuit.

Management

The TandemLung system is unique as these patients are simultaneously on VV ECMO and RVAD support (i.e. oxygenated RVAD). The following considerations apply:
- LV function prior and during support must be frequently assessed to avoid acute LV failure and/or pulmonary oedema due to overflow (caution in poor LV function).
- All patients require judicious anticoagulation and ACT monitoring (range: 160–180 seconds).
- Arterial blood gas monitoring is crucial and will determine the level of CO_2 sweep, FiO_2, and flow needed from the system.
- Weaning can be initiated under echocardiographic guidance once adequate RV function and oxygenation is achieved.
- Low flows can result in pump thrombosis. If the pump flow is reduced to 2 L/min or less, consider higher anticoagulation targets.

The total artificial heart

Introduction

The SynCardia total artificial heart (TAH) (SynCardia Systems, Tucson, AZ, USA) is a biventricular, implantable, pneumatically driven, pulsatile device that orthotopically replaces both ventricles and all four valves (Fig. 10.1):
- The polyurethane-lined ventricles contain a four-layered diaphragm creating air and blood separation.
- Two tunnelled drivelines deliver compressed air.
- A maximal stroke volume of 70 mL results in a cardiac output of up to 9 L/min.

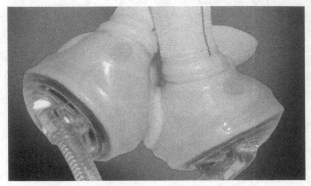

Fig. 10.1 SynCardia System's 70 cc TAH.

Indications for total artificial heart

The TAH is indicated as BTT for advanced biventricular HF that is worsening despite maximal medical and surgical therapies.[1] More than 75% of patients in the INTERMACS registry who have had TAHs implanted were profiles 1 or 2. The list of indications for TAH is lengthy:
- Irreversible biventricular failure (central venous pressure (CVP) >18 cmH₂O, RVEF <20%), that is unlikely to be sufficiently supported with a LVAD alone.
- Severe allograft failure, rejection, or heart transplant vasculopathy with cardiogenic shock.
- LVAD support with decompensated RV failure.
- Recurrent ventricular tachycardia/ventricular fibrillation.
- Hypertrophic, restrictive, infiltrative cardiomyopathy (i.e. small, non-dilated ventricles).
- Postinfarct VSD which cannot be repaired and ventricular failure.
- End-stage congenital heart disease.
- Cardiac tumour which requires resection of significant LV and RV.

1 The TAH is currently approved for BTT; clinical trials for use as destination therapy are ongoing.

- The most common indications in decreasing order of incidence are idiopathic dilated cardiomyopathy, ischaemic cardiomyopathy, congenital/genetic conditions, post-transplant graft failure, valvular cardiomyopathy, restrictive cardiomyopathy, and LVAD failure (including right HF).

Assessing for fit (70 cc vs 50 cc)

Obtain a CT scan of the chest and identify the anteroposterior distance from sternum to T10 vertebrae. If this is >10 cm, consider implanting the 70 cc TAH.

Preoperative and intraoperative management

- Continue preoperative management of cardiogenic shock and multisystem organ failure.
- Monitor routine arterial pressure and CVP; remove PAC.
  - These catheters can be exchanged if infection is a concern.
- Perform TOE preoperatively and perioperatively to assess venae cava compression, pulmonary vein compression, or both.
- Following chest closure, the device may shift and cause compression of the IVC, LA, or both. Findings of caval obstruction may include narrowing at the caval atrial junction; turbulent flow past the narrowing, into the RA, or both; decreased RA size; and flow acceleration across the stenotic portion.
- LA compression with resultant pulmonary venous obstruction can occur. Normal pulmonary vein velocities are in the range of 0.4 to 0.7 m/sec. The resulting pulmonary vein obstruction may manifest as high velocities of > 1.0 m/sec in systole or diastole.

Steps to implantation

- Monitor arterial blood pressure, CVP, pulse oximetry, temperature, and TOE.
- Prior to heparinization, prepare the atrial cuff and arterial grafts and tunnel drivelines:
  - Atrial cuffs:
    - Cut the quick connects to the atrial cuffs to 3–5 mm.
  - Arterial grafts:
    - Use a surgical sealant to cover the conduits; other techniques include exposing them to the patient's unheparinized blood and allowing to dry over 5 minutes in a stretched position.
    - Repeat the process 3 times to preclot.
    - Heparinized blood can be used with a combination of protamine and thrombin to preclot.
  - Driveline tunnelling:
    - Make an incision in the left midclavicular line 5–10 cm below the costal margin and create a tunnel from the subcutaneous layer into the anterior mediastinum.

- o Place the driveline at the end of a 40 Fr chest tube, and pass it through the tunnel.
- o Tunnel the right-sided driveline in a similar manner.
- o Wrap the LV and RV in antibiotic-soaked lap sponges and position laterally away from the wound.

Recipient cardiectomy

Heparinize, and proceed with ascending aortic and bicaval cannulation technique:

- Place umbilical tapes around the cavae.
- Limit dissection around the aorta and PA for future transplantation.
- Initiate total CPB and snare caval tapes.
- With a goal of preserving the tricuspid and mitral annuli but not the valves, make an incision on the RV side 1 cm below the atrioventricular (AV) groove and carry it towards the RV outflow tract proximal to the pulmonary valve; posteriorly, bring the incision to the intraventricular septum and across on the LV side of the AV groove, preserving the mitral annulus.
- Transect the great vessels just proximal to their respective valves.
- Trim excess muscle and chordae, and leave 2 mm of ventricular muscle around each annulus.
- Oversew the coronary sinus to prevent back bleeding through transected vessels; look for a PFO and oversew if encountered.

Atrial quick connect and graft attachment

- Invert the quick connect and place it into the LA cuff.
- Using 3-0 polypropylene (MH), sew the outer, atrial cuff to the quick-connect cuff in a running continuous fashion.
- Perform the right quick-connect anastomosis in a similar fashion.
- Evert both quick connects.

Testing the anastomosis for haemostasis

- Place the plastic testers that are fitted to the quick connects in place starting on the left side.
- Have the assistant surgeon compress the right and left pulmonary veins behind the LA as the surgeon injects a saline-blood admixture with a 60 mL syringe connected to a three-way stopcock.
- Assess the suture lines for leak and repaired as needed.

Great vessel anastomosis

- Measure the PA and aorta with the prosthetic ventricles brought into the field to mimic their natural placement.
- Cut the arterial grafts and then anastomose with a 4-0 polypropylene suture in a running continuous fashion.
- Take care to preserve as much length of native great vessels as possible just above the commissures.
- Pressure test the aortic and pulmonic anastomosis while cross-clamping the PA.

Postoperative management

- Monitor arterial blood pressure via arterial line (the waveform will be pulsatile).
- Precisely position the CVP monitor at the innominate–SVC junction to not impinge on the mechanical valve inflow via the RA.
- Monitor pulse oximetry.
- Have a low threshold for temporary chest closure given the propensity for postoperative mediastinal bleeding.
- At the time of chest closure, perform TOE to assess pulmonary vein compression, left bronchus IVC compression, or both.
- Provide standard postoperative mechanical ventilatory support and sedation with early extubation.

Management of preload

Patients may be hypertensive or vasoplegic when weaning from CPB:
- The use of vasodilators (rapid onset and short acting) including nitroprusside and nicardipine may be necessary.
- Nitroglycerine should be used with caution because of its greater degree of venodilation and decrease in preload.
- Treat vasoplegia with norepinephrine and vasopressin.

Management of volume status

Assess for signs of hypovolaemia, including decreased systemic blood pressure, decreased CVP, low fill volumes, metabolic acidosis, and elevated serum lactate levels:
- Caution should be exercised when assessing the patient's volume status because changes can be made to the device settings that may alter cardiac output to normal values.
- Sudden changes to device fills, flows, and output may indicate an acute driveline or inflow obstruction.
- Atrial tamponade may manifest as decreased flow, fill volumes, or cardiac output and elevated CVP.
- Pulmonary vein obstruction is also a possible cause manifesting as pulmonary venous congestion, pulmonary oedema, and hypoxia:
  - Promptly evaluate all such cases with TOE.
  - Perform expeditious surgical re-exploration and relief of obstruction if necessary.

Anticoagulation

Anticoagulation practices are typically institutional specific but, in general, utilize an antithrombotic approach including antiplatelet and anticoagulant agents:
- Most commonly initiate with unfractionated heparin at 2–5 units/kg per hour following chest closure when there is minimal chest tube drainage:
  - Target an aPTT value of 40–60 seconds or heparin levels from 0.11 to 0.27 units/Ml.
- TEG is useful in the early postoperative period:
  - The coagulation index should be maintained at <1.2.
  - TEG with platelet mapping should also be used to keep the maximum amplitude (arachidonic acid, adenosine diphosphate) at <50 mm.

- Begin antiplatelet agents early if the platelet count is >100,000 × 10⁶/L.
- Prescribe aspirin at 81 mg/day up to 325 mg/day with TEG guidance.
- Institute dipyridamole 50 mg every 8 hours up to 400 mg every 6 hours if necessary, as directed by TEG platelet mapping.
- Begin warfarin once the patient's condition is haemostatic and end-organ recovery is achieved:
  - Target a goal INR of 2.0–3.0.
- If a high degree of haemolysis is evident, pentoxifylline may be used at 200–500 mg every 8–12 hours:
  - This may be initiated early in the postoperative period.
- HIT is a potential risk in these critically ill patients:
  - Use direct thrombin inhibitors such as argatroban or bivalirudin.

Postoperative complications

Renal dysfunction

Renal dysfunction after TAH implantation occurs in up to one-third of patients. Proposed mechanisms include the lack of BNP and its compensatory mechanism due to removal of the ventricles.

- IV infusion of nesiritide was previously utilized to maintain urine output and renal function but is no longer available.
- Intermittent ultrafiltration is the current standard of practice.

Postoperative anaemia

The aetiology of immediate postoperative anaemia is multifactorial. Bleeding in the first few days postoperatively requires mediastinal exploration in nearly a quarter of patients. A small proportion of patients have GI bleeding. Inflammation has been proposed as another cause of anaemia after TAH, as is evidenced by elevated levels of inflammatory biomarkers. Another haematological finding is haemolysis, demonstrated in laboratory findings as decreased haptoglobin, increased lactate dehydrogenase, and increased plasma-free haemoglobin.

- Target a haemoglobin level as low as 6 g/dL (a common threshold for transfusion and tolerated by many patients).
- Avoid transfusion as much as possible given the risk of anti-HLA antibody formation in patients being bridged to transplantation.

Outcomes

A recent review of INTERMACS data provides an overview of the TAH population, factors associated with survival, and rates of adverse events.

Overview

Patients with TAHs were found to be much sicker when compared to patients receiving an LVAD, with the majority being INTERMACS 1 and 2. RV failure was present in 82% of patients implanted. Before implantation, 11% of patients required haemodialysis; an additional 29% required haemodialysis after TAH implantation.

Survival

The SynCardia TAH paired with the Freedom Driver (Fig. 10.2) allows patients to be discharged from the hospital (new drivers are also being designed); 24% of patients in the INTERMACS registry who were implanted with the TAH were discharged (91% to home, 4% to a rehabilitation setting, 5% to other). The median length of stay from implant to discharge was 1.6 months.

The most commonly identified causes of death were multisystem organ failure (36%), neurological injury (18%), and elective withdrawal (12%). Significant risk factors for early mortality included older age and the need for dialysis before implantation. Mortality was associated with the patient's medical condition (poor nutrition, renal dysfunction), as well as management. Risk factors associated with late mortality were high creatinine and low serum albumin levels.

Centre volume was also associated with mortality rates as well as heart transplant rates. Centres implanting ten or more TAHs had a 12-month survival of 64.8%, compared with 36.7% in those centres implanting fewer than ten TAHs. Similarly, transplant rates within the 12 months after TAH implantation were higher in the higher-volume centres: 58.4% in the centres implanting ten or more TAHs, versus 43% for low-volume centres. Overall survival at experienced centres at 12 months was approximately 73%, transplanted plus still on device.

Adverse events

The most common adverse events in the early phase after TAH implantation (<3 months) were bleeding and infection; in the later phase (within 6 months), infection and minor device malfunction were most prevalent (Table 10.1).

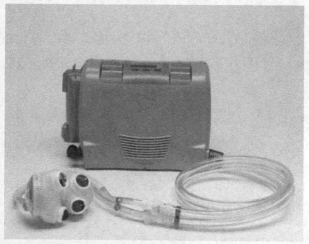

Fig. 10.2 SynCardia System's TAH Freedom Driver, portable driver.

Table 10.1 Adverse events occurring in TAH patients

Event	Early[a]		Late		
	Events	Rate[b]	Events	Rate[b]	p-value[c]
Thromboembolism:					
Venous	17	1.7	3	0.2	0.0001
Arterial non-CNS	20	2.0	2	0.1	<0.0001
Bleeding	414	41.3	96	7.1	<0.0001
Device malfunction:					
Major	13	1.3	34	2.5	0.04
Minor	50	5.0	203	14.9	<0.0001
Pump thrombus	4	0.4	3	0.2	0.4
Hepatic dysfunction	52	5.2	11	0.8	<0.0001
Infection	389	38.8	167	12.3	<0.0001
Neurological dysfunction	148	14.7	40	2.9	<0.0001
Pericardial drainage	63	6.3	1	0.1	<0.0001
Renal dysfunction	162	16.1	21	1.5	<0.0001
Respiratory failure	219	21.8	38	2.8	<0.0001

[a] Early indicates ≤3 months of device implantation. Late indicates >3 months after device implantation.

[b] Rates are reported per 100 patient-months.

[c] The p-values compare early and late rates.

Post-cardiac surgery cardiogenic shock

Introduction

Post-cardiotomy cardiogenic shock (PCCS) occurs after about 2–6% of all adult cardiac operations. While most patients are salvaged and maintained on maximal inotropic support and IABP leading to recovery of the myocardium, around 1% do not respond to such initial therapies and decline rapidly with worsening cardiogenic shock ('refractory PCCS'). In a select cohort of patients, advanced MCS such as VA ECMO and short-term VADs have been utilized with variable success over the years.

In this chapter, our focus will be placed on discussions surrounding management of 'refractory PCCS' in the adult age group with short-term MCS. Management of cardiogenic shock following OHT is covered in Chapter 17.

Definitions

The normal range of CI in healthy adults is 2.5–4.5 L/ m²/min. PCCS is defined as systolic blood pressure persistently <90 mmHg and MAP 30 mmHg below baseline in tandem with CI <1.8 L/m²/min without haemodynamic support and <2.0 L/m²/min with support while filling pressure should be adequate or elevated (LVEDP >18 mmHg and RVEDP >10 mmHg).

While all aforementioned values could be measured by means of a PA catheter, the clinical features of PCCS are manifested by end-organ dysfunction in the form of oliguria, cool extremities, increasing serum lactate, and worsening metabolic acidosis. PCCS becomes 'refractory' when the worsening haemodynamic and metabolic parameters do not improve with high doses of inotropic support and IABP and the patient demonstrates progressive decline leading to multiorgan failure and demise.

Management of post-cardiotomy cardiogenic shock

Early shock

The most common scenario is acute PCCS (within minutes) upon separation from CPB ('early PCCS') with progressive decline in haemodynamic parameters as mentioned previously and worsening metabolic acidosis. Prolonged CPB and aortic cross-clamp times, recent myocardial infarction, diffuse CAD, poor baseline LV or RV function, and suboptimal myocardial protection are predictive factors for early PCCS. TOE may demonstrate regional wall motion abnormality or generalized hypokinesis of the LV, the RV, or both.

Latent shock

'Latent PCCS' represents a more insidious onset of myocardial failure in the hours or days following cardiac surgery which is usually manifested by borderline or slowly declining haemodynamic or metabolic parameters with accompanying end-organ dysfunction/failure. Echocardiography and invasive haemodynamic measurements are indispensable tools to rule out mechanical causes of HF (i.e. progressive cardiac tamponade).

Step-wise approach to the high-risk patient

There is no universally agreed protocol in the management of PCCS. The step-wise approach detailed below provides a safe and systematic strategy in the perioperative period for the patients who are high risk for PCCS and the necessary measures that should be taken in PCCS/impending PCCS in order to optimize end-organ (including myocardial) perfusion.

During all stages of management, TOE by a skilled anaesthesiologist and appropriately positioned PAC are indispensable tools in real-time assessment of haemodynamic parameters and myocardial response to treatment.

Step 1: preoperative optimization

- Anticipation of PCCS and appropriate discussion with patient and family regarding wishes and 'ceiling of care' can aid decision-making intraoperatively.
- Depending on the PA pressure, mixed venous saturation (SvO_2), and biventricular function, preoperative management of the high-risk patient in the ICU with an appropriate inotrope/inodilator support, diuretic therapy, and IABP is an important aspect of preoperative optimization, thereby reducing the risk of PCCS.

Step 2: measures prior to separation from CPB

- Consider and correct any potential reversible aetiology/ies as a result of technical errors (e.g. significant para-prosthetic valvular regurgitation or occluded coronary graft/s).
- Adequate intracardiac de-airing with LV and aortic root vents.
- Rewarm and correction of any metabolic and electrolyte derangements (artificially correct residual metabolic acidosis to achieve base excess below −2 and haemoglobin >100 g/dL).
- Consider half-tidal volume ventilation of lungs while on CPB to reduce the risk of pulmonary atelectasis and high PVR.
- Achieve sinus rhythm, if possible, medically or with DC cardioversion.
- Epicardial pacing to heart rate of 90 bpm with ideally AAI or DDD.
- Adequate filling to maintain euvolemia.
- Initiation of positive inotropes with β_1-adrenergic agonist (epinephrine/dobutamine/dopamine) activity while on CPB support.
- Once the aortic cross-clamp is released, consider priming the myocardium with an inodilator/phosphodiesterase-3 inhibitor such as milrinone/enoximone particularly in patients with preoperative evidence of RV dysfunction with or without PH.
- Allow adequate reperfusion of the myocardium after release of cross-clamp before attempting weaning off CPB.
- Placement of IABP. Timing of inflation should be optimized to the dicrotic notch.

Step 3: measures during separation from CPB

- Ensure lungs are fully expanded (if suboptimal expansion, check endotracheal tube, perform bronchoscopy prior to weaning attempt).
- Pace atrially or dual chamber at a rate of 80–90 bpm ensuring enough diastolic coronary perfusion time. In certain circumstances, a rate of

100–110 bpm might be necessary—in particular, higher pacing rates are beneficial for RV dysfunction.
* Gentle weaning from CPB, that is, reduction of CPB support by 500 mL/min increments while monitoring the filling pressures and avoiding ventricular distention.

Step 4: measures following separation from CPB

* Avoid hypoxaemia or hypercarbia.
* Correct any metabolic/respiratory acidosis.
* If low, the CVP should carefully be optimized to between 10 and 15 mmHg.
* Titration of vasoactive catecholamine and inodilator infusions to achieve a CI of 2.5 L/m²/min with a SVR of 800–1200 dynes/sec/cm⁵ or indexed SVR (SVRI) of 1500–2000 dynes/sec/cm⁵ per m².
* Protamine should be administered very cautiously and slowly.
* Reduction of PA pressures utilizing the following:
  * Inhaled pulmonary vasodilators (nitric oxide or epoprostenol/ iloprost) can be used to reduce pulmonary vasoconstriction and reduce RV afterload especially when there is RV dysfunction.
  * Infusion of phosphodiesterase-3 inhibitors (e.g. milrinone) can aid improve biventricular contractility and their energy reserves while reducing the RV and systemic afterload (although these may induce deleterious systemic hypotension).

Step 5: mechanical support strategies

Short-term strategy: CPB

If the strategies in previous steps fail, recommencing CPB is the safest and most expedient, short-term 'fall-back' strategy while the team conducts further evaluation and planning. CPB would also allow for further myocardial recovery with further reperfusion and resting of the heart in cases of myocardial stunning as a result of suboptimal myocardial protection during the initial surgery. This also allows correction of any electrolyte abnormality before attempting further weaning of CPB. If coronary air embolism is suspected, mild permissive hypertension while on CPB could improve coronary perfusion for the next attempt at weaning. Furthermore, CPB would allow time for 'bridging to decision' in such acute settings. If there is persistent regional LV dysfunction or ST-segment changes consistent with ischaemia, coronary grafting should be considered. If there is significant valvular dysfunction, operative correction should be considered at this time.

Longer-term strategies: MCS

Depending on which ventricle is failing, the following strategies can be employed as salvage strategies. More details regarding insertion techniques have been covered in Chapters 5, 8, and 9. The pros and cons for each strategy are as follows:

ECMO

VA ECMO (see Chapter 8): can be achieved centrally (transition from central CPB → central VA ECMO) or peripherally (typically femoro-femoral/ axillo-femoral).
   Pros: expedient, familiar and safe, allows for complete (heart–lung) support, femoral or axillary cannulation would allow for chest closure.

Cons: need for heparin (bleeding risk), limb ischaemia (peripheral ECMO), North–South syndrome (in peripheral VA ECMO → need for VAV ECMO), need for pulsatility (LV vent may be required to prevent LV stasis). Concomitant use of mild dose of inotrope and/or IABP is important to facilitate LV contractility and aortic valve opening in order to avoid LV stasis and thrombosis. Finally, risk of prosthetic mitral valve (mechanical or bioprosthetic) thrombosis due to blood stagnation.

Short-term VADs
(See Chapter 5.)

Surgical short-term VAD
Can be utilized to selectively support right, left, or both sides of the heart (RVAD/LVAD/BiVAD, respectively) depending on the failing chambers and with or without an oxygenator depending on the functioning state of the lungs. LVAD is usually established with inflow through the LV apex and outflow into the ascending aorta. Alternatively, a cannula inserted through the right superior pulmonary vein or roof of LA passed into the LV cavity past the mitral valve can be used as the inflow port. Alternative outflow ports to the ascending aorta include the axillary artery or femoral artery. RVAD is established with inflow through the RA and outflow into the main PA. Alternatively, inflow can be established using a long two-stage venous cannula inserted through the common femoral vein into the RA past the IVC. The outflow in the PA could be either by direct cannulation or through a side-arm PTFE/Haemashield graft anastomosed to the main PA and exteriorized through the left second/third intercostal space in the parasternal region.

Pros: expedient with open chest following termination of CPB, lines can be tunnelled through the skin allowing for chest closure, direct cardiac chamber cannulation (no need for venting), allows better ambulation and physical therapy, and less risk of mitral prosthetic valve thrombosis from blood stagnation as the LV is well vented.

Cons: can only be placed centrally (typically sternotomy), LV apex incision (in LVAD), need for heparin (bleeding risk), pulmonary haemorrhage (RVAD), no oxygenator by default, and thrombosis.

Percutaneous VAD
Percutaneous VADs (see Chapter 9) are available for left and right heart support (Impella 2.5 and 5.0 (Abiomed, Danvers, MA, USA)). They work with an 'impeller/micro-axial pump'. In the left heart position, they work by propelling blood from the LV into the ascending aorta. Placement requires general anaesthesia and fluoroscopy to ensure that the propeller has appropriately crossed the aortic valve and is positioned in the LV outflow tract.

The percutaneous right heart support can be in a form of an impeller (as for the left heart Impella described above, e.g. the Impella RP) which can be placed through a 23 Fr peel away sheath into the femoral vein and fluoroscopically guided across the PA. Alternatively, it can also be in form of a centrifugal pump e.g. the ProtekDuo (TandemLife, LivaNova, Pittsburgh, PA, USA) which is typically placed through the right IJ vein and floated to the PA fluoroscopically such that the inflow orifice sits in the RA and the outflow in the main PA thereby bypassing the RV.

Pros: less invasive since removal does not require sternal entry/re-entry.

Cons: haemolysis, limb ischaemia (left heart support), vessel perforation, bleeding, cutdown needed for left heart Impella arterial removal, malposition is common, and post-insertion ambulation is difficult.

Clinical considerations for mechanical circulatory support

Given the complexity of the clinical situations when faced with 'refractory PCCS' requiring consideration for MCS, there is lack of set protocol in patient selection and the subsequent management. There are pre- and post-MCS clinical considerations that can be taken into account as follows:

Pre-MCS clinical considerations

There is no agreed protocol to aid decision-making and all cases should be looked at individually. Given the complexity of such clinical settings and major implications on the patient and the service at large, we advocate multidisciplinary (surgical, anaesthesia, perfusion, and critical care) decision-making. Consideration of the wishes of the patient and family, at this time, should be factored into decision-making.

Some of the considerations to be taken into account are as follows:
- MCS can be resource intensive.
- 'MCS to where?', that is, the aim of the MCS should be determined:
  - Does the patient qualify for 'bridge to decision,' 'bridge to transplant' or 'bridge to durable LVAD'? Also, what are the chances of 'bridging to recovery'?
- The 5-year survival rate after advanced MCS in the PCCS setting can be as low as 17% (see Table 11.1, p. 124).
- In contrast, delayed institution of MCS (often end-organ injury has begun) is unlikely to rectify the patient's course. Therefore, early support is critical to success.
- Complications which are life-threatening include:
  - Major haemorrhage requiring re-exploration.
  - Renal failure requiring renal replacement therapy.
  - Thromboembolism.
  - Stroke.
  - Severe sepsis.
  - Limb ischaemia.
  - Infection (bacterial and fungal).
- Some of the reported adverse prognostic indicators (see Table 11.1, p. 124) are as follows:
  - Advanced age >70 years.
  - Female sex.
  - Chronic kidney disease.
  - Advanced pulmonary disease.
  - Diabetes mellitus.
  - Obesity.
  - High EuroSCORE >20.
  - Prolonged ECMO support >48 hours.
  - Rising serum lactate levels while on MCS.

Post-MCS clinical considerations

Following institution of MCS, the following should be considered:

- Unfractionated heparin can be held to control bleeding and until correction of coagulopathy. It can be safely started after 24 hours with aPTT range of 60–80 seconds. Convert to direct thrombin inhibitors (e.g. bivalirudin or argatroban) if HIT is suspected.
- Distal limb protection with a DPC should be used with peripheral VA ECMO and femoral arterial cannulation.
- Attempt to achieve contractility and ejection with positive inotropic infusions while on VA ECMO of at least 20 mmHg pulse pressure in order to prevent LV blood stagnation and thrombosis, pulmonary haemorrhage, and/or ventricular distention and myocardial damage.
- While on VA ECMO in the absence of LV ejection, LV venting should be strongly considered. Venting in peripheral VA ECMO can be achieved through the following routes:
  - Right superior pulmonary vein.
  - LV apex.
  - Percutaneously (e.g. Impella 2.5/CP)—short-term venting due to haemolysis and limb ischaemia complications.
  - Use of IABP and mild inotrope infusion.
- Prevention of differential hypoxaemia (i.e. North–South syndrome)— right radial arterial line is essential for objective PO_2 measurement. If this PO_2 is abnormally low, optimize mechanical ventilator support. VAV ECMO (see Chapter 8) may be required to overcome this complication.
- Any cardiac rhythm disturbance should be treated aggressively with the goal of the rate of 80–100 bpm and AV synchronous rhythm.
- Patients supported on VA ECMO or short-term VADs should be considered for diagnostic coronary angiography. Furthermore, if there is a major issue with the coronary circulation, PCI should be considered.
- For VA ECMO weaning, see Fig. 11.1.
- Wean potent vasopressors (e.g. norepinephrine) as much as possible to maintain systemic vascular resistance at 800–1200 dyne/sec/cm⁵. Adding volume expansion may lead to better flow rates, enabling the weaning of vasopressors.
- Daily TOE to monitor ventricular recovery.
- Weaning of sedation for neurological evaluation. If unarousable following sedation hold consider head CT scan to assess prognosis for neurological recovery.
- Patients who show ventricular recovery on echocardiography, should have VA ECMO/short-term VAD flows weaned down to 1–2 L/ min. Consider anticoagulation during the weaning process. Continue echocardiographic assessment. If stable at low flows for 1–2 hours, VA ECMO/short-term VAD should be removed. After weaning of VA ECMO/short-term VAD, support circulation with IAPB and/or moderate inotropic agent (dopamine, dobutamine, or epinephrine).
- If weaning of MCS failed and the patient meets criteria for durable VAD or transplantation, optimize and proceed accordingly.
- If weaning of MCS fails and the patient does not qualify for destination MCS or transplantation → discussion with family regarding end of life care.

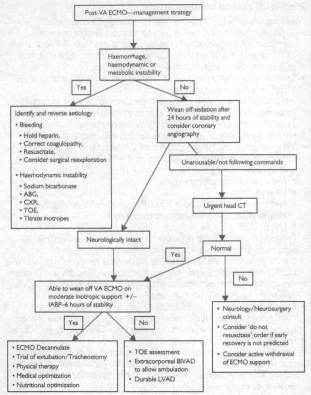

Fig. 11.1 Illustrating 'post-VA ECMO' management strategies.

Outcomes and adverse prognostic indicators

The literature on refractory PCCS is very heterogeneous. The outcomes data have been derived mainly from retrospective observational studies and small case series. The reported patient groups range from complex heart transplant, redo cardiac surgery, to routine first-time open-heart surgery making the data difficult to interpret. Rastan and colleagues reported one of the largest case series with one of the longest follow-up periods of 5 years for refractory PCCS salvaged with MCS. They reported survival to hospital discharge and 5-year survival to be 39% and 17% respectively. However, a meta-analysis performed by the authors of this chapter (Khorsandi and colleagues) found the pooled survival to hospital discharge was lower (~30%).

A large body of evidence suggests survival benefit from MCS for refractory PCCS. Some reports claim post-transplant MCS results in better survival rates than when used for PCCS after other forms of adult cardiac surgery. As PCCS has a universally high mortality without MCS, one should consider early institution of MCS in these patients, particularly in the absence of negative predictive factors. Timing is critical; MCS to rectify the circulation must be initiated before end-organ injury. Recent studies (Table 11.1) found that survival following ECMO was significantly better in OHT patients compared to post-cardiotomy patients. Adverse prognostic indicators common to a few of the studies have been reported as advanced age (>70 years), elevated serum lactate levels, and multiorgan dysfunction.

Table 11.1 Pertinent studies looking at outcomes of MCS utilization for refractory PCCS

Author, year, and country	Study period	Patient cohort	Results	Adverse prognostic indicators
Rubino et al., 2018, UK	2008–2016	101 patients: • PTE (28.7%) • OHT (21%) • CABG and valve (15%) • CABG and other (12%) • Valve (11%) • Other	Weaned from ECMO: 57% In-hospital survival: 33% (OHT: 63%) 1-year survival: 27.7% (OHT: 54%) Survival considerably higher in OHT	Age >70 years, persistently elevated lactate, multiorgan dysfunction
Hernandez et al., 2007, UK	1995–2004	Multicentric retrospective cohort from STS database of 5735 patients who had post-cardiotomy VADs	Operative mortality: 45.9% Reduction in mortality and major morbidity over time with newer cardiac surgical techniques, perioperative management, and advances with devices	Urgency of operation, renal failure, myocardial infarction, aortic stenosis, female sex, race, peripheral vascular disease, NYHA class IV, left main coronary disease, and valve procedure
Rastan et al., 2010, Germany	1996–2008	• 516 patients: • CABG (37.4%) • CABG and AVR (16.6%) • AVR (14.3%) • Heart/lungtransplant (6.5%) • Other (25%)	Weaned from ECMO: 63.3% Discharged home: 24.8%	

continued

Table 11.1 *Continued*

Author, year, and country	Study period	Patient cohort	Results	Adverse prognostic indicators
Doll et al., 2004, Germany	1997–2002	219 patients: • CABG (n = 119) • CABG and AVR (n = 240) • MVR (n = 110) • Other (n = 44)	30-day mortality: 76% (n = 167) Discharged from hospital after 29 ± 24 days: 39% (n = 52) 5-year follow-up: 74% (n = 37) were alive	
Slottosch et al., 2013, Germany	2006–2010	77 patients: • CABG (n = 43) • Valve (n = 10) • CABG and valve (n = 11) • Aortic surgery (n = 5) • Heart transplant (n = 2) • Other (n = 6)	Weaned from ECMO: 62% 30-day mortality: 70%	Advanced age (p = 0.003); rising serum lactate, prolonged ECMO course, and ECMO-GI complications were independent predictors of 30-day mortality (p <0.05)
Wu et al., 2010, Taiwan	2003–2009	110 patients: • CABG (n = 31) • Valve (n = 16) • Multiple valves (n = 26) • Combined valve and other (n = 19) • Aortic surgery (n = 8) • Post-infarction VSD (n = 3) • Pulmonary endarterectomy (n = 4) OHT (n = 3)	Weaned from ECMO: 61% (n = 67) Survival to hospital discharge: 42% (n = 46)	Age >60 years, renal failure, serum bilirubin >6 mg/dL, and duration of ECMO >110 hours; persistent HF (EF <60%) was a predictor of mortality after hospital discharge
Elshar kawy et al., 2010, USA	1995–2005	233 patients: • CABG (n = 86) • Any valve (n = 69) • AVR/repair (n = 42) • MV repair/MVR (n = 44) • TV repair/TVR (n = 16)	Survival to hospital discharge: 36%	Advanced age, known diabetes, CABG, longer CPB time

Author, year, and country	Study period	Patient cohort	Results	Adverse prognostic indicators
Li et al., 2015, China	2011– 2012	123 patients: • CABG (n = 44) • CABG and other (n = 15) • Valve (n = 40) • OHT (n = 11) • Other (n = 13)	Survival to hospital discharge: 34.1%	

AV, aortic valve; AVR, aortic valve replacement; MV, mitral valve; MVR, mitral valve replacement; TV, tricuspid valve; TVR, tricuspid valve replacement.

Heart transplantation

Patient selection criteria and bridging support for cardiac transplantation

Medical assessment
of transplant candidates

Cardiac transplantation remains the gold standard treatment for patients with end-stage HF refractory to medical therapy. The decision to list for transplantation is most commonly achieved through multidisciplinary evaluation to ensure the patient meets an indication for transplant and to vet any alternative therapies that may be less invasive. This assessment also includes a review of potential contraindications, the collection of clinical data, the weighing of the risks of the transplant itself against the benefits provided, and timeframe for ongoing reassessment. The ISHLT first issued formal guidelines for selecting transplant candidates in 2006 and updated these recommendations in 2016.

Common causes of HF that may ultimately warrant cardiac transplantation include NICM including RCMs, CAD leading to ischaemic cardiomyopathy, congenital heart disease, and transplant recipients requiring re-transplantation. In an era where long-term MCS devices are commonly used to support end-stage HF, device complications can become a strong indication even in the absence of refractory symptoms.

Common indications for referral for cardiac transplantation evaluation are illustrated by the following clinical scenarios or syndromes (Box 12.1):

- Cardiogenic shock requiring continuous IV inotrope support or MCS to prevent end-organ malperfusion.
- NYHA class IV HF symptoms refractory to optimal medical management and limited 1-year survival. Typical criteria to define this degree of HF in the ambulatory population include CPX testing with peak VO$_2$ <14 mL/kg/min or <12 mL/kg/min on BB therapy, SHFM suggesting 1-year survival <80%, or HFSS with medium to high risk:
  - The SHFM is a prospectively validated score that predicts survival and includes the following predictors: age, sex, NYHA class, weight, EF, systolic blood pressure, medication usage including diuretic usage, laboratory parameters, and presence of devices.
  - The HFSS is a prospectively validated score that predicts survival without transplant and includes the following predictors: presence of CAD, resting heart rate, LVEF, mean arterial blood pressure, presence of conduction delay on ECG, serum sodium, and peak VO$_2$. The three strata are low (1-year survival 88%), medium (60%), and high risk (35%).
- RCMs with NYHA class III–IV symptoms particularly when caused by infiltrative processes that have limited extracardiac involvement at the time of evaluation.
- Unstable arrhythmias (typically ventricular in origin) that have become refractory to antiarrhythmic drug therapy, transcatheter ablations, defibrillator implantation, or surgical correction.
- Complex congenital heart disease causing NYHA class IV symptoms refractory to medical management or further surgical palliation including cyanotic heart disease and failing Fontan physiology after correction of a single ventricle circuit. This indication is particularly important to identify before the development of irreversible pulmonary hypertension.
- Cardiac transplant recipients with severe cardiac allograft vasculopathy, severe and persistent primary graft dysfunction, or severe restrictive physiology.

Other indications for cardiac transplantation include intractable severe angina not amenable to revascularization, HF with major limitation of daily activities and VO_2 <55% of predicted, and patients with AL or TTR amyloidosis.

Box 12.1 Common indications for cardiac transplantation

- Cardiogenic shock requiring IV inotropes or MCS.
- NYHA class IV symptoms refractory to optimal medical management.
- RCM with NYHA class III–IV symptoms.
- Unstable arrhythmias refractory to other management.
- Complex congenital heart disease with NYHA class IV symptoms refractory to other management.
- Cardiac transplant recipients with severe graft dysfunction.
- Intractable severe angina not amenable to revascularization.
- Cardiac amyloidosis.
- Candidacy for multiorgan transplantation:
  - Heart–lung: irreversible pulmonary vascular disease, hypoplasia of vasculature.
  - Heart–kidney: combined HF and end-stage renal disease.
- Heart–liver: congenital heart disease with chronic venous congestion leading to irreversible liver disease.

Patients possibly eligible for multiorgan transplantation should be referred to experienced transplant centres. Indications for combined heart–lung transplantation include irreversible pulmonary vascular obstructive disease and hypoplasia of pulmonary vasculature. Combined heart–kidney transplantation may be considered for patients with end-stage renal failure and appropriate indication for kidney transplantation, as well as heart–liver transplantation in congenital heart disease patients with chronic venous congestion leading to cirrhosis. TTR amyloidosis has previously been considered an indication for heart–liver transplantation due to the fact that the TTR protein is produced by the liver, but novel pharmaceutical therapies may absolve the need for concurrent liver transplantation.

Congenital heart disease represents another separate consideration in evaluating recipients for heart transplantation. While this indication is discussed in other chapters, the following considerations are essential:

- Assessing PVR that, if elevated, may lead to rapid RV failure after transplantation. Calculating PVR is difficult in patients with persistent shunts and collateral circulation.
- Multiple prior cardiac operations may lead to prohibitively long and risky explants, specifically in relation to right-sided structures that may lie directly behind the sternum.
- Other end-organ failure (hepatic failure being the most common).

Contraindications to transplantation (Table 12.1) are divided into absolute and relative; those with reversible contraindications may be appropriate candidates for bridging MCS to allow the patient to be re-evaluated in the future.

Table 12.1 Contraindications for cardiac transplantation

Absolute contraindications	Relative contraindications
Irreversible severe PH	Advanced age
Life expectancy <2 years secondary to unrelated illness	Obesity
Chronic uncontrollable infection	Active smoking
Severe cerebrovascular disease	Diabetes mellitus with poor control or significant end-organ damage
Prohibitive risk factors identified in psychosocial assessment	Renal dysfunction
	Active infection
	Anatomic features prohibiting surgery
	Prohibitive risk factors identified in psychosocial assessment

Absolute contraindications to cardiac transplantation are those that have been adopted at most transplant centres and include the following:
- Irreversible severe PH with PVR >5 Wood units. These patients may be considered for heart–lung transplantation but will not tolerate isolated heart transplantation. Chronic LVAD unloading may result in improvement of PVR over months. Some centres have reported successful outcomes when PH can be reduced pharmacologically, but a useful threshold for PH remains to be clearly defined.
- Life expectancy <2 years secondary to an unrelated severe systemic illness including malignancy, refractory infection, and other systemic illness not corrected or modifiable by cardiac transplantation.
- Chronic extracardiac infection that cannot be definitively controlled.
- Cerebrovascular disease that impairs cognitive function and may limit survival.
- Active substance abuse or medical non-compliance, identified through the psychosocial assessment described on p. 135.

Relative contraindications to cardiac transplantation are often more centre specific or modified slightly based on centre expertise and resources, and variability among centres has been shown to be significant in programme surveys. While individually not absolute, the cumulative risk of multiple relative contraindications can be high and should be considered. They include the following:
- Advanced age: careful selection of patients over the age of 60–65 and extremely careful selection of patients aged >70 may yield candidates who are suitable for transplantation.
  - In general, transplantation in this age group results in reduced but acceptable post-transplant survival compared to younger recipients. Since the cause of death in many of these patients is recipient driven, many centres focus on the absence of comorbid conditions and frailty as potential indicators of success rather than chronological age.
- Obesity: while each centre may have a different cut-off, a BMI of ≥35 kg/m² is typically prohibitive as the recipient is at higher risk.

- Active smoking.
- Diabetes mellitus with inadequate control or significant end-organ damage.
- Renal dysfunction not attributed to cardiac failure such as estimated glomerular filtration rate (eGFR) <30 mL/min/1.73 m². This comorbidity may prompt evaluation for combined heart–kidney transplantation.
- Active infection or colonization with multidrug-resistant organisms that would jeopardize successful transplantation particularly in the face of immunosuppression. Patients with chronic, controlled infection such as hepatitis B, hepatitis C, and HIV may be suitable candidates for transplantation if they have mild forms of disease and no evidence of end-organ dysfunction.
- Prior substance abuse and high risk for relapse as identified through the psychosocial assessment described in the following section (see p. 136).
- Advanced peripheral vascular or cerebrovascular disease.
- Advanced primary lung disease, regardless of pulmonary vascular resistance can complicate recovery from cardiac transplantation.
- Anatomic features that would make the transplant operation prohibitive. This may stem from prior operations for acquired heart disease, but is especially important in congenital heart disease. Chronic cyanosis can cause significant systemic–PA collaterals, which can complicate surgery or persist after surgery and compromise the outcome.
- Other systemic illness which may interfere with postoperative rehabilitation.
- The presence of extensive anti-HLA antibodies.

Psychosocial assessment of transplant candidates

Due to the scarcity of organ donors as well as the complexity and costs of post-transplant care, selection of heart transplant recipients must include a thorough psychosocial evaluation. Recipients must be able to adhere to treatment recommendations for life; these include frequent clinic visits, laboratory assessments, routine catheterizations and biopsies, and potential hospitalizations for complications. The psychosocial assessment includes identification of risk factors for poor post-transplantation outcomes; assessment of factors related to knowledge, understanding, and ability to engage in decision-making; and an assessment of patients' personal, social, and environmental resources and circumstances. These components when assessed in totality have been demonstrated to play an important role in clinical outcomes. The ISHLT has made specific recommendations for the psychosocial evaluation of potential recipients of heart transplantation (or lung transplantation or MCS).

Key domains for assessment include treatment adherence, mental health history, substance use history, cognitive status and capacity to give informed consent, knowledge and understanding of current illness, knowledge and understanding of current treatment options, coping with illness, social support, and social history (Box 12.2).

> **Box 12.2 Psychosocial assessment domains for cardiac transplant evaluation**
>
> *Domain*
> - Treatment adherence and health behaviours.
> - Mental health history.
> - Substance use history.
> - Cognitive status.
> - Knowledge and understanding of current illness.
> - Knowledge and understanding of treatment options.
> - Ability to cope with illness.
> - Social support.
> - Social history.
>
> Reproduced from Dew MA, DiMartini AF, Dobbels F, et al. The 2018 ISHLT/APM/AST/ICCAC/STSW recommendations for the psychosocial evaluation of adult cardiothoracic transplant candidates and candidates for long-term mechanical circulatory support. J Heart Lung Transplant. 2018 Jul;37(7):803–823. doi: 10.1016/j.healun.2018.03.005.with permission from Elsevier.

The recommended procedure for psychosocial evaluation of transplant candidates includes (1) selection of a qualified evaluator, (2) performance of the psychosocial evaluation and identifying when further evaluation is needed, (3) communication of findings back to the transplantation team, and (4) monitoring/mitigating identified risk factors to optimize transplant outcomes. The evaluator should be formally trained and licensed in their healthcare discipline and familiar with local transplant policies and procedures. The psychosocial evaluation should be presented to the patient as one of many elements in his/her overall evaluation, ideally with the patient directly interviewed in a language in which the potential recipient as well as support system members can converse interactively.

Risk factors for poor post-transplantation outcomes

Treatment non-adherence, mental health history, and substance use history have been identified as risk factors for poor post-transplantation outcomes. Assessment of the candidate should include assessment of past medical adherence, knowledge of the regimen that is required, and willingness to participate. Poor treatment adherence has been shown to increase the risk of post-transplant morbidity and mortality. Psychiatric conditions range from prohibitive to transplant to relatively common within the transplant population. Assessment of the psychiatric condition's interference with the patient's ability to adhere to the medical regimen and the degree to which the condition is controlled is important. Depression and anxiety are common in the pre-transplant population. Depression predicts post-transplant mortality. Anxiety, bipolar disorder, and personality disorders have not been shown to directly correlate with increased mortality but likely have effects on medication compliance, substance abuse, poor social support, and/or poor coping skills.

Illegal substances, tobacco, and alcohol abuse have been shown to increase risk for post-transplant mortality, and active abuse is an absolute contraindication to transplantation. Assessment should include review of all substances used in the past, current status of use, treatments received, and insight/willingness to abstain. With the legalization of marijuana use in some parts of the world without clear evidence for whether it is a risk factor for postoperative outcomes, assessment should focus on manifestations of substance abuse.

Assessment of factors related to understanding, and ability to engage in decision-making

The patient's cognitive ability to comprehend their condition, the medical and surgical treatment, and postoperative regimen should be assessed. Intellectual disability does not necessarily portend worse outcomes, and can be mitigated by increased social support, although dementia is a contraindication to transplantation. However, the complex interaction between HF and cognitive function is not clear, and defects in cognition need to be formally assessed prior to transplantation. This is true not only to avoid inappropriate transplantation in a patient not able to reap the benefit, but to provide a baseline since immune suppression may cause long-term changes in cognition. One must determine the patient's level of understanding of their medical condition and the current treatment options, which is not only critical to informed consent and shared medical decision-making but also can identify gaps in knowledge or support which could help optimize the patient's condition. Knowledge deficiencies in one's medical condition have been associated with worse self-care and medical adherence.

Assessment of patients' personal, social, and environmental resources and circumstances

A thorough social history elucidating the patient's education level, financial resources, living situation, and legal history is important to understanding the context which will affect the patient's overall health. Lack of sufficient social support is a contraindication to transplantation. Lastly, the patient's ability to cope with their illness may help predict their post-transplant success, as optimism, a greater sense of self-efficacy, and active problem-solving skills have been tied to improved clinical outcomes.

Bridging support for transplant candidates

Bridging support devices, ranging from femoral catheter IABPs to durable LVADs to TAHs, can provide a bridge to decision regarding transplant candidacy or a support strategy for patients already listed, who are threatening to die as a result of cardiogenic shock. Longer-term bridging devices such as LVADs can allow time for relative contraindications such as obesity, PH, substance use, or insufficient social support to be reversed or resolved. Renal, pulmonary, and hepatic function frequently improves during LVAD support. LVADs can also become destination therapy for those ultimately deemed ineligible for transplantation either due to irreversible contraindications or loss of candidacy for new medical/psychosocial reasons.

Temporary bridging devices such as an IABP, percutaneous VADs (e.g. Impella (Abiomed, Danvers, MA, USA), TandemHeart LivaNova, Pittsburgh, PA, USA)), and ECMO are typically used for patients presenting with haemodynamic collapse. These devices provide short-term haemo-dynamic support and can help with preoperative optimization. IABPs are inserted and removed easily, require less technical support, and are rela-tively inexpensive. While this strategy is best utilized for patients waiting days before a suitable organ is identified, modifications in the placement technique (axillary artery rather than femoral artery) may allow ambulation and rehabilitation while on support. Furthermore, newer counterpulsation devices in development, may not only enable ambulation but are also de-signed for the option of discharge from the hospital setting.

Other percutaneous circulatory assist devices (e.g. Impella, TandemHeart) are generally considered to provide greater haemodynamic support than IABPs and are usually placed in the cardiac catheterization laboratory or in the operating room. The Impella platform is an axial pump that res-ides in the LV outflow tract and pumps blood from the LV into the aorta. A number of devices with increasing support (2.5 L/min, 3.5 L/min, or 5 L/min) are available on this platform which resembles a catheter sitting across the aortic valve. The TandemHeart relies on a drainage cannula situated in the LA across the intra-atrial septum; it provides antegrade flow utilizing an extracorporeal centrifugal flow pump which delivers blood back via a femoral arterial cannula. These devices typically provide bridging therapy from days to 1 week.

VA ECMO, used in cases of cardiogenic shock, is an extracorporeal car-diopulmonary support system that drains deoxygenated blood from the venous system, oxygenates it via an artificial membrane lung, and returns it to the systemic circulation. Cannulas may be placed centrally via sternotomy or thoracotomy, or peripherally, typically via the femoral vessels. Patients are typically supported for no longer than 1 week. Extracorporeal VADs and VA ECMO have a high rate of infection, bleeding complications, and thromboembolic complications including stroke. Short- and mid-term sur-vival outcomes of patients bridged to transplantation with VA ECMO are inferior compared to propensity-matched controls bridged to transplant-ation via continuous-flow LVAD.

Durable LVAD implantation has continued to increase since its inception in the early 1990s and offers patients the ability to be bridged for months to years. The 2015 ISHLT registry indicated that at least 50% of patients are bridged to transplantation with MCS, the vast majority utilizing LVAD. This affords transplant candidates with longer expected waiting list times the ability to stabilize with reduced risk of clinical deterioration. It also pro-vides for reversal of some relative contraindications. Single-centre studies exist that show improved post-transplant survival when patients are bridged with MCS. However, some patients become sensitized related to required transfusions with LVAD implantation; infection and thromboembolic ad-verse events may also occur during LVAD support.

Cardiac donor selection and management

Pathophysiology of brainstem death

Knowledge of the underlying physiological changes of brainstem death (BSD) is crucial to understanding the different aspects of donor management and optimization. Several physiological changes occur in association with the rising intracranial pressure that usually precedes BSD and these consist of cardiovascular, respiratory, endocrine, and metabolic responses detailed below.

Cardiovascular

- In response to raised intracranial pressure and reduced cerebral perfusion pressure, a hypothalamic-induced catecholamine storm occurs resulting in intense vasoconstriction, raised systemic vascular resistance, tachycardia, and systemic hypertension. This aims to restore cerebral blood flow by improving cerebral perfusion pressure.
- Myocardial oxygen demand increases as a result without a simultaneous increase in oxygen supply due to coronary vasoconstriction. This is implicated in the impairment of cardiac function seen early after BSD:
  - Acute myocardial injury occurs in a quarter of donation after brain death (DBD) donors and myocardial dysfunction in 40%. Severity of injury relates to the speed of onset of BSD with rapid rises in intracranial pressure resulting in exponential increases in catecholamine release and therefore a higher incidence of myocardial damage.
- Systemic hypertension stimulates carotid baroreceptors resulting in slowing of the heart rate often to bradycardic levels.
- Along with respiratory irregularities, which occur secondary to reduced brainstem perfusion or possible brainstem herniation, hypertension and bradycardia represent the classic Cushing's triad.
- As BSD proceeds, sympathetic tone diminishes, leading to a period of hypotension and global hypoperfusion due to loss of vasomotor tone and an impaired cardiac output.

Respiratory

- Pulmonary oedema occurs secondary to raised pulmonary hydrostatic pressure and catecholamine-induced endothelial injury.

Endocrine and metabolic

- Posterior pituitary function is commonly lost resulting in diabetes insipidus. Anterior pituitary function may be preserved or partially affected.
- Hyperglycaemia develops secondary to reduced insulin levels and increased insulin resistance.
- Temperature control is lost due to hypothalamic failure with initial hyperpyrexia and subsequent hypothermia.
- A generalized inflammatory response, ischaemia-reperfusion injury, and coagulopathy occur secondary to release of tissue thromboplastin from necrotic neural tissue in the brain-dead donors.

Cardiac donor assessment and selection

Principles of donor selection

Selection of donor hearts is based on two core principles:
- Assessment of donor heart quality including both structure and function.
- Recipient individual requirements and donor–recipient compatibility.

Donor selection is rarely a black-and-white process and a degree of 'balancing' between the two principles is required.

Assessment of donor quality

Assessment should include a review of the donor's history, clinical examination findings, haemodynamic status, and laboratory values and imaging (echocardiogram, possible cardiac angiography). The desirable and undesirable donor characteristics are summarized in Table 13.1.

Table 13.1 Summary of desirable (classical cardiac donor selection criteria) and undesirable donor characteristics.

Characteristic	Desirable (classic selection criteria)	Undesirable[a]
Age (years)	<55	>55
History of chest trauma or cardiac disease	Nil	Congenital or valvular heart disease
History of malignancy or current sepsis	Nil	Metastatic cancer; uncontrolled sepsis or aspergillosis
History of prolonged hypotension or hypoxaemia	Nil	History of hypoxaemia (e.g. drowning), hypotension, ventricular fibrillation, and CPR
Meets haemodynamic criteria: MAP >60 mmHg; CVP 8–12 mmHg; inotropic support <10 mcg/kg/min (dopamine or dobutamine)	Yes	High dose of catecholamines (dopamine >10 mcg/kg/min, need for epinephrine or norepinephrine)
ECG	Normal	Signs of infarction (Q waves), LVH, and atrial fibrillation
Echocardiogram	Normal	Regional wall motion abnormalities, valvular abnormalities, LVH (>13 mm), and cavity enlargement
Coronary angiography (if indicated by donor age and history)	Normal	Presence of CAD (or risk factors for CAD if angiogram unavailable)
Serology: hepatitis B surface antigen (HBs-Ag), hepatitis C virus (HCV), and HIV virus	Negative	HBs-Ag positive, HIV positive, or anti-HCV positive. History of high-risk social behaviour (e.g. incarceration, substance misuse)

[a] Majority of quoted undesirable characteristics are considered relative rather than absolute contraindications to donor utilization.

Adapted from Sabiston & Spencer Surgery of the Chest, 8th ed. Sellke FW, del Nido PJ, Swanson SJ, et al. eds. Philadelphia: Saunders Elsevier, 2016.

History and examination

Donor age

- Independent predictor of postoperative mortality and the likelihood of donor heart use.
- Upper age cut-off has gradually shifted upwards with most centres accepting donor age <55 years as a cut-off. Some centres procure hearts from those aged ≥65 years (see Chapter 14).
- Utilization of hearts form older donors mandates meticulous donor assessment and assessment of the risk–benefit ratio for each recipient balancing the anticipated waiting list mortality against the expected reduced post-transplant survival with older donors.

Assess donor comorbidity

- Diabetes mellitus, CAD, or associated risk factors (hypertension, hyperlipidaemia, peripheral vascular disease, smoking, obesity, family history, substance misuse), valvular heart disease, and LVH.

Cause of death and associated circumstances

- Deaths secondary to cerebrovascular events have been associated with reduced transplant survival.
- Causes of death deemed unfavourable for cardiac procurement include drowning, electrocution, hanging, strangulation, and carbon monoxide poisoning.
- Preceding cardiac arrest and CPR is associated with reduced post-transplant survival but is not an absolute contraindication to donor use.

Blood investigations

Serology

- Test for hepatitis B surface antigen, HCV, and HIV virus.
- Hepatitis B- or C-positive donors may be appropriate in selected higher-risk recipients.
- For hepatitis C, serology does not specifically differentiate the presence or absence of viraemia. Positive serology indicates current or past infection.

Nucleic acid amplification testing (NAAT)

- Directly measures viral RNA using polymerase chain reaction (PCR) or transcription-mediated amplification.
- More accurate assessment of transmission risk.
- PCR testing of donor blood for HCV and HIV viral DNA is now performed routinely in addition to serological testing.
- Differentiates past from current HCV infection:
  - HCV-seropositive donor who is NAAT negative (non-viraemic) indicates a spontaneously cleared or successfully treated infection or a false-positive antibody result.
  - HCV-seropositive donor who is NAAT positive (viraemic) indicates active infection with high infection risk.

Cardiac enzymes

- Elevated cardiac enzymes in isolation should not be used to justify donor non-use.
- Conflicting evidence regarding their association with post-transplant survival and outcomes.
- Raised cardiac enzymes have been associated with increased rates of rejection.
- Higher troponin levels are seen closer to the time of coning and levels fall subsequently.
- Although troponin levels are inversely correlated with CI and ventricular function, elevated cardiac enzymes in the presence of normal cardiac function is commonly encountered.
- Normal troponin levels in the presence of echocardiographic evidence of dysfunction is helpful and reassuring against recent myocardial injury.

Electrocardiogram

- Need to correlate ECG findings with cardiac enzyme levels and echocardiographic assessment.
- Look for evidence of ischaemia (ST-segment changes, Q waves), conduction abnormalities (e.g. left bundle branch block), rhythm abnormalities (e.g. atrial fibrillation), LVH, and acute strain patterns.
- ST-segment, T-wave changes and prolongation of the corrected QT interval are described in BSD and are not considered sensitive indicators of suboptimal donor heart quality. Non-specific ST changes are also commonly seen in patients who have undergone CPR, experienced chest trauma or neurological insult, or are currently being treated with vasoactive medication.
- Q-wave formation and left bundle branch block are more suggestive of underlying disease.

Echocardiogram

- Echocardiography (transthoracic or transoesophageal) is the most important tool in assessing donor heart function and structure.
- Should be performed in all donors particularly older donors (>40 years) and those with a history of hypertension, and substance abuse or CAD risk factors.
- Allows for real-time assessment of heart function and structure.
- Initial echocardiography should only be performed *after* initial haemodynamic resuscitation. Serial echocardiograms may be required to assess response to treatment (see later in topic).

Functional assessment

- RV function.
- LV function.
- Wall motion abnormalities:
  - Global myocardial depression can be seen initially and this in isolation should not preclude subsequent procurement.

- Transient regional wall motion abnormalities occur commonly and segmental systolic inward motion and thickening abnormalities may resolve with resuscitation.

Pharmacological stress assessment (PSE)

- Use of PSE in marginal heart donors and those with a high cardiovascular risk shows potential for extending donor criteria in heart transplantation:
  - Dobutamine or dipyridamole PSE in 'marginal' donors defined as age >50 years or <50 years with concomitant risk factors such as cocaine use, hypertension, and diabetes.
  - Majority of patients with normal resting and PSE echocardiograms had good outcomes following transplantation.
  - Patients with normal resting echocardiograms and abnormal PSE may have CAD or other cardiac pathology.

Structural assessment

- Chamber size: significant dilation of the RV or LV is a contraindication to donor organ utilization.
- LVH:
  - The observer must ensure adequate filling of the LV when assessing for hypertrophy as pseudohypertrophy can be encountered in underfilled subjects and does not represent a contraindication to transplantation.
  - Mild LVH (wall thickness ≤13 mm) is not a contraindication to transplantation.
  - Transplantation is not advisable in presence of both echocardiographic (>13 mm) and ECG criteria for significant LVH.
  - Studies have suggested decreased survival in heart transplant recipients whose donor heart LV wall thickness exceeded 1.4 mm.
  - Combination of LVH and prolonged total ischaemic time may be associated with higher rates of primary graft dysfunction.
- Congenital or valvular abnormalities:
  - Classically. most valvular and congenital cardiac abnormalities represent a contraindication to procurement.
  - 'Bench' repairs for mild abnormalities such as secundum ASD and mild–moderate MR or TR can be performed on the donor heart to enable its utilization.
  - Normally functioning bicuspid aortic valves are commonly seen and do not represent a contraindication to procurement.

Limitations of echocardiography and importance of serial imaging

- Accuracy of TTE interpretation at the donor hospital may be suboptimal.
- A single echocardiogram may provide initial information that is not representative of the true function of the donor heart and should be repeated to assess response to intervention. An important fraction of hearts with reduced ventricular function will show normalization on serial echocardiography studies, commonly performed at 4–8-hour intervals.

Pulmonary artery catheterization

- Aggressive haemodynamic management with the use of PAC, among other metabolic and hormonal interventions, yields a 30% increase in the donor pool and is linked to better transplant outcomes.
- With 42% of donor hearts exhibiting some form of cardiac dysfunction on echocardiography, the correlation between these abnormalities and actual underlying pathology is often lacking. PAC should be therefore considered particularly if the initial evaluation of cardiac function confirms an EF ≤45%.
- Tailored therapy should be instituted to achieve the following targets:
  - PCWP 8–12 mmHg.
  - CI >2.4 L/min/m².
  - SVR 800–1200 dyne/sec/cm⁵.

Coronary angiography

Coronary angiography can be considered if this is available at the donor hospital to assess for CAD in donors with the following characteristics:
- Male donors aged 35–45 years and female donors aged 35–50 years if there is a history of cocaine use or in the presence of three or more risk factors (Box 13.1).
- Male >45 years and female >50 years. Angiogram is strongly recommended particularly in donors >55 years old.
- In the presence of CAD, there are no specific absolute contraindications to donor use and decisions should be made taking into consideration the recipient's status (e.g. urgent or elective, uncontrollable arrhythmias, haemodynamic deterioration without mechanical support options), donor cardiac function, and the feasibility of 'bench' CABG.
  - The combination of increased donor age and CAD correlates significantly with subsequent coronary allograft vasculopathy.
  - Mild CAD should be restricted to high-risk recipients.
  - Bench CABG is associated with a 65% graft patency at 2 years.
- The inability to perform a coronary angiogram at the referring hospital should not be considered a contraindication to donor use and suitability should continue to be based on echocardiographic assessment of

---

Box 13.1 Risk factors for ischaemic heart disease

- Smoking.
- Hypertension.
- Diabetes mellitus.
- Dyslipidaemia.
- BMI >32 kg/m².
- Positive family history of premature CAD.
- Previous history of ischaemic heart disease.
- Evidence of ischaemia on ECG.
- Anterolateral regional wall motion abnormalities.
- EF ≤45%.

cardiac function, haemodynamic stability, and surgical findings during
procurement (see p. 171 for surgical aspects of organ procurement).
Risk factors for CAD should be factored into the decision to use a
donor heart for a specific recipient.
• To reduce the risk of significant nephrotoxicity in the donor, contrast
left ventriculography should be avoided if echocardiographic images are
deemed adequate.

Intraoperative assessment

Remains an integral part of donor assessment and allows:
• Visual assessment of dynamic cardiac function.
• Palpation for the presence CAD.

Post-procurement assessment

The donor heart can also be assessed following procurement prior
to implantation, using an extracorporeal circulation, known as ex vivo
heart perfusion (see Chapter 14). Observation of cardiac function and
measurement of serum lactate can be performed during ex vivo heart
perfusion.

Recipient individual requirements and donor–recipient compatibility

When matching donors to recipients, it is important to select a donor heart
that meets the needs and characteristics of the recipient. Factors that need
to be considered include the following:

Donor-recipient organ matching Histocompatibility
• ABO compatibility:
  • Donor and recipient must be ABO compatible to prevent hyperacute
    rejection. Some ABO incompatible transplants have been performed
    in neonates with immature immune response.
• HLA compatibility:
  • HLA mismatch is not a contraindication.
  • HLA-A1, -A2, and -A3 mismatch is associated with an increased risk
    of chronic rejection.
  • If >10% reactivity on lymphocyte toxicity screen, a prospective
    lymphocyte cross-match between donor lymphocytes and recipient
    serum is required by many centres. A positive lymphocyte cross-
    match indicates a high risk of hyperacute rejection and the heart is
    rejected for that recipient.
  • Other centres rely more heavily on predetermination of specificity
    of recipient antibodies and antibody concentrations, enabling a virtual
    cross-match with prospective donors.

Urgency

- How urgent is the transplantation? For example, 'super' urgent, urgent, or elective.
- What is the waiting list mortality? What is the SHFM or HFSS? Recipients with a higher waiting list mortality include patients of older age, or those with congenital heart disease, RCM, or a previous failing allograft, obesity (BMI >35 kg/m²), or HIV.
- Extended criteria donor (ECDs) or 'marginal' donors should be considered for sicker recipients without alternatives and poor physiological reserve in urgent need of transplantation (see Chapter 14).
- Multiple studies have demonstrated the success of utilization ECD hearts for heart transplantation (also referred to as extended criteria cardiac transplantation (ECCT)) in the high-risk recipient group. This strategy improved patient survival in this cohort when compared to optimal medical therapy alone.
- Benefits of ECCT should be weighed against the downside of increased donor-related complications such as graft dysfunction, future CAD, and infection risk with ECD organs.

Expected recipient size and power requirements (consider current power use)?

- Is the donor heart suitably powerful to support the recipient circulation?
- Greater requirements in males, higher BMI, and greater muscle mass.
- Lesser requirements in female patients, and/or lower BMI.
- Size and sex mismatch:
  - A normal sized adult male (>70 kg) donor is suitable for most recipients.
  - With small donors, size matching with BMI or height is more accurate than weight.
  - Donor heart undersizing must not exceed a 30% mismatch in predicted heart mass. See Box 13.2.
  - Any donor undersizing is undesirable for recipients with known PH.
  - Donor heart oversizing must also not exceed a 30% mismatch in recipients where the pericardial space is likely to be restrictive (e.g. multiple previous sternotomies, recent large myocardial infarction, current LVAD in place).
  - Sex mismatch downsides are observed mainly in male recipients who are matched with female donors.

Box 13.2 Predicted heart mass

Predicted LV mass (g)	$a \times \text{height}^{0.54}(m) \times \text{weight}^{0.61}(kg)$ where $a = 6.82$ for women and 8.25 for men
Predicted RV mass (g)	$a \times \text{age}^{-0.32}(\text{years}) \times \text{height}^{1.135}(m) \times \text{weight}^{0.315}(kg)$ where $a = 10.59$ for women and 11.25 for men

Anticipated ischaemia times

- Distance from donor to transplant centre must be considered as longer distances will lead to increased cold and total ischaemia times which are important predictors for primary graft dysfunction.
- Ischaemia time is an independent risk factor for survival. Total ischaemia times <4 hours are considered optimal.
- Longer ischaemia times are associated with higher recipient mortality particularly in combination with other undesirable donor characteristics (e.g. significant LVH).

Other considerations

Viral-infected donors can be used in infected recipients and in selected non-infected recipients. In a recent trial (DONATE HCV), hearts procured from HCV-infected donors showed excellent graft function with undetectable hepatitis C viral load at 6 months after transplantation (direct acting antiviral agents were initiated within a few hours of transplantation).

Cardiac donor optimization

What is donor optimization?

Prior to BSD testing, the goal of donor management is directing at maximizing survival rather than specific optimization for individual organs. Following BSD confirmation, the emphasis shifts from maintaining patient survival to specific organ optimization for procurement and subsequent transplantation. This is termed donor optimization.

Key facts

- Optimization of donor physiology increases the number of transplantable organs by creating the optimal milieu for organ preservation and recovery of function.
- Aggressive donor management protocols (PAC-assisted haemodynamic management, and hormonal/metabolic therapy) can increase donor use by 30%.

Donor optimization set-up and goals

- Most patients will be in an ICU environment during confirmation of BSD and, if not, they should be transferred after BSD is confirmed.
- Following initial stabilization, BSD confirmation and death certification, and confirmation of consent, focus should be directed at specific organ optimization.
- In the UK and elsewhere, Specialist Nurses for Organ Donation (SN-ODs), or similar practitioners, should be present at the donor centre to assist in the delivery of donor care.
- In the UK specifically, specific cardiothoracic 'scouting' teams of trained personnel are sent from the transplant centre to locoregional (within 2 hours' travel distance) donor ICUs as soon as a potential heart donor is identified. The scout team becomes in charge of subsequent donor care and will perform serial diagnostic and therapeutic procedures, including TTE/TOE, PA catheterization, along with careful titration of vasoactive drugs and fluid resuscitation.

- In the USA, specialists from organ procurement agencies assume care and manage the donor with input from transplant surgeons.
- Regional organ procurement centres are available in some regions and assume management after donors are transported from outlying hospitals; these centres relative to other hospitals are able to focus entirely on donor management.
- The *three primary facets* of donor optimization include:
  - Circulatory and endocrine management (including hormonal resuscitation and management of diabetes insipidus).
  - Respiratory management and lung recruitment procedures.
  - General critical care management including temperature management and thromboembolic prevention.
- Donor management aims (Box 13.3) to optimize preload (by achieve an adequate effective circulating volume while avoiding fluid overload), afterload (by adjusting vasoconstrictors and vasodilators) and cardiac output (by normalizing cardiac function without relying on high doses of beta-adrenergic agonists or other inotropes that increase myocardial oxygen demand), and to correct acidaemia, anaemia, hyponatremias and respiratory gas exchange.

Box 13.3 Rule of thumb—goals of donor optimization

'Rule of 100': systolic arterial pressure >100 mmHg, urine output >100 mL/hour, PaO_2 >100 mmHg, haemoglobin concentration >100 g/L, and a 'blood sugar 100% normal'.

Circulatory and endocrine management

Regular clinical monitoring of response to treatment is essential. Fluids, inotropes, and vasopressors should be adjusted every 15 minutes to achieve target haemodynamic values listed here with alpha-adrenergic agonist use kept to a minimum:

- Sinus rhythm 60–100 bpm.
- MAP 60–80 mmHg.
- CVP 4–12 mmHg.
- PCWP 8–12 mmHg.
- CI >2.4 L/min/m².
- SVR 800–1200 dyne/s¹/cm⁵.
- SvO_2 >60%.
- Urine output 0.5–2.0 mL/kg/hour.

Monitoring and investigations

Adequate monitoring equipment should be installed, and these include:

- Invasive arterial and central venous pressure lines.
- PA catheterization and cardiac output monitoring particularly if LVEF <45%.
- Continuous ECG monitoring.
- Urinary output measurement.

Investigations

- Blood investigations—renal function and troponin measurements particularly if there is a history of a preceding cardiac arrest.

- Twelve-lead ECG (see Cardiac donor assessment and selection, p. 141).
- CXR *following* recruitment procedures.
- Serial TTE/TOE is essential in assessing cardiac function and responses to treatment, and in excluding any significant structural abnormalities (see Cardiac donor assessment and selection, p. 141).

Management strategy

See Fig. 13.1.

- *Restoring adequate circulating volume* should be the primary priority initially:
  - Correct hypovolaemia with fluid boluses (3–5 mL/kg of a balanced crystalloid or colloid as a rapid bolus; repeat as necessary) while avoiding fluid overload.
  - No specific class of fluid resuscitation has been proven to be superior to the rest but some have expressed concerns about the use of starch-based products due to their potential association with graft dysfunction.
- *Restoring vascular tone*:
  - If hypotensive despite restoration of circulating volume, commence vasopressin where vasopressin is required and wean catecholamine vasopressors as able.
- *Restoring cardiac contraction*:
  - If hypotensive despite restoration of circulating volume and vascular tone, introduce inotropic therapy.
  - Myocardial stunning is not uncommonly encountered and reversal can be achieved with supportive therapy.
  - If LVEF <45% then PAC placement and hormonal resuscitation is strongly recommended (see later in list).
  - Dopamine is considered first line when inotropic therapy is required followed by dobutamine.
  - Use of high-dose catecholamine therapy, especially norepinephrine, is associated with impaired graft function and a reduced rate of cardiac retrieval. Catecholamines should therefore be weaned as soon as possible in favour of dopamine or dobutamine.
- *Hormonal resuscitation*:
  - Inotropic requirements may be reduced with hormonal therapy, and hormonal resuscitation should be considered in all donors.
    - If response to catecholamine therapy is suboptimal, consider a trial of IV hydrocortisone (50–100 mg).
    Triiodothyronine (T3; 4 mcg bolus at the onset of the infusion followed by an infusion of 3 mcg/hour) use has been associated with increased organs retrieval rates and improved organ function post-transplantation. Some advocate its use only in patients with persistently impaired cardiac performance despite initial measures of volume resuscitation and vascular tone restoration, while others advocate its use as first-line treatment.
  - Administer IV methylprednisolone (15 mg/kg, max 1 g) to reduce the general proinflammatory response and reduce the accumulation of extravascular lung water.

- Start insulin infusion to ensure good glycaemic control with the added anti-inflammatory benefits including reduced cytokine release:
  - Keep blood sugar at 4–10 mmol/L (70–180 mg/dL) (minimum 1 unit/hour).
  - To avoid hypoglycaemia, add a continuous infusion of 20% or 50% dextrose at 25 or 10mL/hour, respectively.

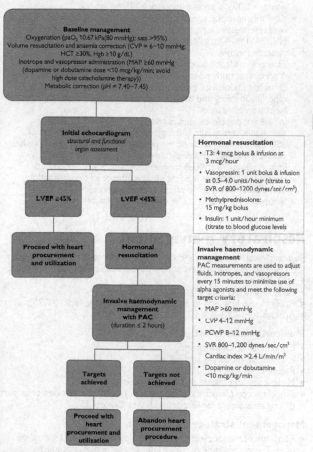

Fig. 13.1 Crystal City algorithm for cardiac donor optimization.

Reproduced from Zaroff JG, Rosenard BR, Armstrong WF, et al. Consensus conference report: maximizing use of organs recovered from the cadaver donor: cardiac recommendations, March 28–29, 2001, Crystal City, Va. Circulation. 2002 Aug 13;106(7):836–41. doi: 10.1161/01.cir.0000025587.40373.75 with permission from Wolters Kluwer.

- *Identification and management of diabetes insipidus:*
  - Diabetes insipidus should be identified and treated early.
  - Dramatic unprovoked rises in urine output should be treated as suspected diabetes insipidus even before confirmatory urine and plasma electrolytes levels and osmolalities are obtained.
  - Confirmatory tests include a rising serum sodium level, urine specific gravity <1.005, a urine osmolality >295 mOsm/kg.
  - If >4 mL/kg/hour, consider diabetes insipidus and treat promptly with vasopressin/terlipressin and/or desmopressin (DDAVP). Dose of DDAVP 1–4 mcg IV titrated to effect.
- *Simvastatin therapy:*
  - Emerging evidence supporting its use in donor optimization.
  - A preclinical study revealed that donor simvastatin treatment enhanced endothelial-pericyte integrity, and inhibited ischaemia-reperfusion injury and the development of allograft vasculopathy after heart transplantation.
  - In a recent double-blinded randomized controlled trial, donor nasogastric simvastatin (80 mg) administration within 2 hours of BSD confirmation reduced the number of treatments with IV pulsed steroids, plasmapheresis, antithymocyte globulin, or intravenous immunoglobulins (IVIGs) for haemodynamically compromised rejection episodes in the first 30 days after heart transplantation. There was, however, no effect on the incidence, or severity, of biopsy-proven acute cellular or antibody-mediated rejections.

Respiratory management

Regular clinical assessment and monitoring response to treatment is essential. The following parameters should be monitored and targets achieved:
- SpO_2 >95%.
- PaO_2 10.0 kPa (75 mmHg) (FiO_2 <0.4 as able).
- $PaCO_2$ 5–6.5 kPa (35–45 mmHg) (or higher as long as pH >7.25).
- Acidosis (pH 7.40–7.45).

Monitoring and investigations

- Continuous SpO_2 monitoring.
- Intermittent blood gas analysis.
- Recent CXR.
- Microscopy and culture of airway secretions.
- Bronchoscopy (diagnostic or therapeutic) if clinically indicated or as part of lung assessment for lung retrieval (see Chapter 25).

Management strategy

- Recruitment manoeuvres normally employed at each ICU should be used. These should be repeated after any suctioning procedure.
- Tidal volumes should be 4–8 mL/kg of ideal body weight.
- Peak inspiratory pressures should be limited to <30 cmH_2O.
- Positive end-expiratory pressure (PEEP) should be maintained at 5–10 cmH_2O to reduce airway collapse and improve alveolar recruitment.

- FiO_2 should be adjusted to maintain PaO_2 of >8.0 kPa and maintain an SpO_2 of 92–95%. The minimum amount of FiO_2 should be used to reduce absorption atelectasis and risk of oxygen toxicity.
- Alter minute ventilation (respiratory rate and tidal volume) to allow permissive hypercarbia while achieving a pH of >7.25. This minimizes ventilator-associated lung injury.
- Measures to improve airway clearance and reduce risk of aspiration include:
  - Monitoring endotracheal tube position and cuff pressures. Remember cuff leaks lead to lung de-recruitment and increased risk of aspiration. High pressures can lead to mucosal injury.
  - Raised head-up position (30–45°)—also improves functional residual capacity.
  - Turning, suctioning, and regular physiotherapy.
- If secretions are viscous or purulent, consider regular nebulized hypertonic saline and/or bronchoscopy Antibiotics should be administered if clinically indicated (purulent secretions).

General critical care

- Regular turning to minimize the pressure sores.
- Review all drugs being administered and discontinue those that are not required.

Nutrition

- Start enteral feeding unless otherwise instructed by the procurement team:
  - Improves electrolyte balance, glycaemic control, and splanchnic perfusion.

Thromboembolic prevention

- Heparin or low-molecular-weight heparin.
- Thromboembolic deterrent (TED) stockings.
- With or without calf compressors.

Haematological management

- Target haematocrit ≥30% and haemoglobin ≥10 g/dL.
- If haemoglobin levels are <10 g/dL, blood transfusion can be considered. There is, however, evidence suggesting that blood transfusions can adversely affect organ function post transplantation.
- Adequate group and save sample should be present prior to any procurement procedure.
- Any coagulation derangement should be treated particularly if there is ongoing bleeding. Fresh frozen plasma and platelets should be used. Antifibrinolytics may cause microvascular thrombi and should generally be avoided.

Temperature management

- Aim for a core body temperature between 36°C and 37.5°C.
- Hypothermia is commoner than hyperthermia and can be managed by:

- Using active warming blankets.
- Warming administered fluids.
- Heating and humidifying inspired gases.
- Increasing ambient temperatures.

Donor risk scoring systems

- Key determinant of success has more to do with the health of the recipient than the donor.
- As highlighted previously, there are multiple donor factors that increase the risk of post-transplant mortality.
- Multivariate donor risk scores are routinely used in kidney transplantation (Kidney Donor Profile Index (KDPI) to improve donor selection, reduce discard rates, and improve outcomes).
- Although in the context of cardiac donor assessment and selection, the formal use of donor risk scores is not yet routine, their components highlight the important donor determinants of outcomes and have been shown to be predictive.

Mortality risk scores

There are multiple mortality risk scoring systems that have been devised. The most detailed is the Eurotransplant Heart Donor Score (HDS) (Table 13.2):

- Consists of ten variables—age, cause of death, history of malignancy, sepsis, drug abuse, meningitis, or positive virology, hypertension, cardiac arrest, LV function, valvular function, LVH, coronary angiogram, serum sodium, norepinephrine therapy, and dopamine/dobutamine therapy.
- Predicts 3-year mortality.
- Scores above the median were associated with a higher organ non-use (35%) versus lower scores (7%).
- Each HDS point above 17 increased the predicted 3-year mortality by 4%.
- Only donor age and LVH, as individual donor variables, were statistically significant predictors of mortality at 3 years after heart transplantation.

Deficiencies with using risk scores

- Not widely used.
- Do not take into account the enlarging patient population with long-term LVAD as a BTT.
- They do not combine recipient factors, including expected waiting list mortality, and donor-related factors, including risk of primary graft dysfunction.

Table 13.2 Eurotransplant Heart Donor Score (score ≥17 = high risk)

Donor characteristics	Range of points
Age	1 (age <45 years) to 11 (age ≥60 years)
Cause of death	1 (drugs, sepsis, subarachnoid bleeding, meningitis, head trauma) to 7 (carbon monoxide intoxication)
History of malignancy, sepsis, drug abuse, meningitis, or positive virology	1 (no) vs 19 (yes)
Hypertension	1 (no) vs 2 (yes)
Cardiac arrest	1 (no) vs 2 (yes)
Left ventricular function	1 (EF >55%) to 22 (EF <45%)
Valvular function	1 (normal) to 7 (abnormal)
Left ventricular hypertrophy	1 (10 mm) to 4 (>14 mm)
Coronary angiogram	1 (no stenosis) to 70 (>1-vessel stenosis)
Serum sodium	1 (<130 mmol/litre) to 3 (≥170 mmol/litre)
Norepinephrine therapy	1 (<0.1 mcg/kg/min) to 5 (>0.8 mcg/kg/min)
Dopamine/dobutamine therapy	1 (<5 mcg/kg/min) to 2 (>10 mcg/kg/min)

Reproduced from Kransdorf EP, Stehlik J. Donor evaluation in heart transplantation: The end of the beginning. J Heart Lung Transplant. 2014 Nov;33(11):1105–13. doi: 10.1016/j.healun.2014.05.002 with permission from Elsevier.

Effect of donor risk factors on outcomes of transplantation in recipients supported with long-term LVADs

- Paucity of data on the impact of donor-related variables on outcomes post transplantation in patients bridged with durable LVADs.
- In a prospective cohort study, LVAD recipients, whether transplanted with high- or low-risk donors (on the basis of age >50 years, history of diabetes, three or more inotropic agents at the time of incision, and BUN >25 mg/dL), exhibited worse early (but not late) survival and higher early complication rates than standard recipients.
- Adverse donor characteristics were less predictive outcomes than in standard recipients.

Effect of donor risk factors on outcomes of transplantation in recipients supported with long-term LVAD

Extended criteria heart donors and perfusion storage

Introduction

As the pool of cardiac donors is limited and the number of patients suffering from HF is increasing, there is an ever-growing imbalance between the demand and supply of donor hearts available for transplantation. Thus, there is mounting pressure to consider donors who are suboptimal. Over the years, a distinction has emerged between the term 'high-risk donors', for example, people with HCV or drug users who may be infected with contagious viral infections such as HIV, and the term 'marginal donors' that reflects either the donor characteristics or the cardiac parameters. As a consequence, we are constantly revising what should be considered as 'good enough' to transplant rather than waiting for the 'ideal' organ.

Donor selection is probably one of the most complex decisions that has to be taken in the transplantation process, reflecting both the recipient medical condition and urgency, how good or marginal the donor organ is, and the institutional risk tolerance. Furthermore, a known association exists between time spent on the waiting list and mortality, thus contributing to the complexity of matching donors to recipients. Although early experience of using marginal donors for marginal recipients on an 'alternate list' resulted in reduced post-transplant survival, studies from the last 5–10 years examining the use of marginal organs demonstrated results which are noninferior to using 'ideal organs'. In this chapter, we will review the current definition of a marginal donor heart and the outcomes of transplanting such hearts. We shall also discuss the latest technology available to try and mitigate some of the risks associated with the use of these organs.

Marginal donors: definition and outcomes

Throughout the 1980s when heart transplantation was increasingly adopted, there was consensus on the required quality of donor hearts for optimal outcomes. Over the subsequent decade, the demand on heart transplantation continued to rise due to the increasing number of HF patients, forcing HF teams to consider what was termed 'marginal donor' hearts, for example:

- LVH.
- Reduced LV function.
- Prolonged CPR.
- Advanced age.

Recent reports on studies analysing the UNOS database were able to mitigate some of the original concerns about these donors. For example, recipients of donor hearts without LVH (<1.1 cm), with mild LVH (1.1–1.3 cm), and moderate–severe LVH (≥1.4 cm) had equivalent 30-day to 3-year survival. However, subgroup analyses showed an increased risk of death in recipients of allografts with LVH and donor age >55 years or ischaemic time ≥4 hours, attesting in favour of the 'one hit' theory and pointing out the need for something else in order to mitigate the risk completely (e.g. perfusion systems).

Sibona and colleagues examined the impact of LV dysfunction using the UNOS database between January 2000 and March 2016. Among 31,712 heart transplant recipients, no significant differences were found in post-transplant survival up to 15 years of follow-up between those receiving donor hearts with or without LV dysfunction. When using Cox regression analysis with adjustment for propensity variation, EF was not found to have any significant impact on mortality when analysed as a categoric or continuous variable and LVEF normalized 1-year post transplantation. These findings support the notion of the neurogenic stunned myocardium, triggered by the high catecholamine release that is typical after brain death, hence causing reversible LV dysfunction. For recipients receiving donor hearts with a history of CPR (even exceeding 30 minutes), post-transplant outcomes were not found to be inferior.

Older donor age used to be a common reason for concern in the past. However, a recent study reported that there is no survival disadvantage in recipients of older donor hearts (age ≥50 years), albeit with a higher incidence of cardiac allograft vasculopathy at 5 years post transplantation.

In order to facilitate the use of marginal hearts and reduce the related risk, perfusion systems may have a role in their retrieval. This will be reviewed later in the chapter.

Ex vivo organ perfusion

Ex vivo perfusion of isolated hearts has been under investigation for >150 years. Following the pioneering experimental works of Ludwig and Cyon with frog hearts in 1866, Langendorff and Martin independently developed methods to perfuse mammalian hearts at the end of the nineteenth century. However, it wasn't until the middle of the last century that Morgan and Neely converted Langendorff's model into a working heart model.

From a transplant perspective, *ex vivo* heart perfusion with oxygenated and nutrient enriched blood has been developed during the past 20 years with the aim to reduce the cold ischaemic time and to evaluate metabolism and function of preserved grafts prior to transplantation. In times of donor organ shortage, the possibility of organ procurements at geographically distant areas and assessment of hearts from extended criteria donors and donation after circulatory determined death (DCD) are essential to increase organ availability for patients on the heart transplant waiting list. A major difference compared to standard cold storage is that ex vivo perfusion is performed using normothermic donor blood and thus minimizes the cold ischaemic time and avoids another 'hit' on the retrieved heart. This may be of potential benefit when marginal donor hearts are being considered.

Currently, the only system commercially available with the largest clinical experience is the Organ Care System (OCS) Heart (TransMedics, Andover, MA, USA) (see following section). It is hypothesized that using such a system for marginal donor hearts may reduce the risk associated by abiding to the 'one-hit theory' and taking the cold ischaemic time out of the equation.

OCS Heart

The OCS Heart is a portable *ex vivo* perfusion platform for retrieved donor hearts in which the heart is beating and metabolically active. While there have been two reports of out-of-the-body times exceeding 10 hours, the median duration for OCS Heart perfusion is 4–5 hours. The system consists of a durable console with a wireless monitor and a disposable perfusion module (Fig. 14.1). The latter includes an organ chamber, a perfusion circuit, a gas exchanger, a heater, a blood reservoir, and a pulsatile pump (Fig. 14.2).

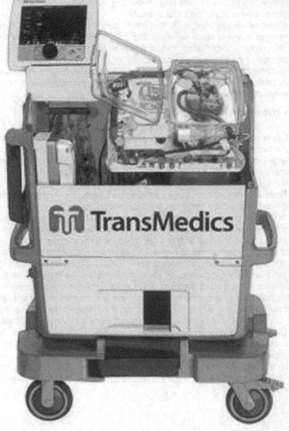

Fig. 14.1 Portable OCS Heart console with the disposable module.

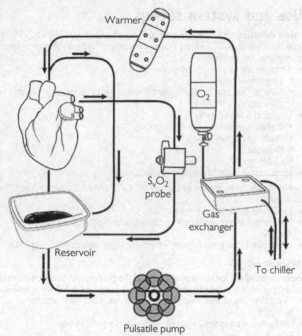

Fig. 14.2 Schematic of the OCS Heart module components.

The OCS Heart system basically represents a modified non-working heart Langendorff perfusion model. In other words, the heart is beating but the LV is not volume loaded. Blood from the OCS reservoir is pumped through an oxygenator and heater in a pulsatile manner into the ascending aorta of the retrieved donor heart via an aortic cannula. The competent aortic valve remains closed and the oxygenated blood is directed into the coronary arteries to perfuse the myocardium. Venous effluent from the coronary sinus collecting in the RA (IVC and SVC are temporarily closed for OCS perfusion), fills the RV during diastole and is ejected across the pulmonary valve into the PA. A cannula in pulmonary trunk directs the venous blood back to the reservoir.

There is a line that connects the aortic cannula with the reservoir for de-airing and a port for administration of cardioplegia administration just prior to removing the heart from the OCS Heart. A vent is placed across the MV into the LV to ensure that it remains unloaded. The vent is allowed to drain passively into the organ chamber of the OCS Heart and then back to the blood reservoir.

Use and system set-up

While evaluating the donor, a decision should be made if the OCS Heart is to be used. The OCS Heart system may be considered in high-risk heart transplants, for example:

- An expected longed ischaemic time:
  - Long travel time.
  - Surgical preparation of recipient is expected to be long, usually due to previous operation(s).
- Extended donor criteria:
  - Presence of ventricular hypertrophy.
  - Prolonged down-time.
  - Reduced EF.
  - Older age.
- Special procurement conditions—DCD.

Nevertheless, in some circumstances the OCS system cannot be used, for example:

- Moderate aortic valve regurgitation.
- Myocardial contusion (often associated with thoracic trauma of the donor).
- Unrepaired interatrial or interventricular septal defects including PFO.

System set-up

Before setting off for the donor hospital, the procurement team is advised to discuss with the coordinator at the donor hospital the following issues:

- Transfuse packed red blood cell to the donor if the haematocrit is < 25%.
- Verify the latest inotropic doses and donor arterial lactate.

Since three different proprietary solutions are required to perfuse a donor heart with the OCS Heart and other additives have to be prepared and added to the fluids, it is advisable for the procurement team to use the checklist that is provided by TransMedics before leaving the base hospital:

1. The priming solution has to be supplemented with 20 mEq of sodium bicarbonate.
2. The maintenance solution containing adenosine requires the addition of 50 IU of regular insulin.
3. The epinephrine solution is made up of 0.25 mg epinephrine and 30 IU of regular insulin in 500 mL of 5% dextrose.
   Other additions to the reservoir include:

- Ciprofloxacin: 100 mg.
- Cefazolin: 1 g.
- Methylprednisolone: 250 mg.
- Heparin: 10,000 units (required for the blood collection bag).
- Multivitamin: 1 unit.
- 25% albumin: 100 mL (especially recommended for longer OCS Heart runs).

Two lots of cardioplegia solution are also required, one for flushing of the donor heart before explant and one before removing the donor heart from the OCS Heart. The type of cardioplegia that is used differs regionally. Whereas the US experience was initially based on a variety of different solutions, during the past 5 years most centres have been using the crystalloid portion of del Nido's cardioplegia. Most European centres rely either on histidine–tryptophan–ketoglutarate solution (HTK, Custodiol) or St. Thomas formulations (Sterile Concentrate for Cardioplegia Infusion, Martindale Pharma, UK).

The following checklists should be reviewed before setting off for the donor hospital:
- Equipment checklist:
  - The batteries are charged.
  - The gas cylinder is sufficiently full.
  - The data card is inserted properly.
  - The defibrillator is operational.
  - Handheld lactate analyser and cartridge available.
  - External pacing box and pacing lead available.
- Medication checklist:
  - Sodium bicarbonate (2 × 20 mEq).
  - Methylprednisolone (250 mg).
  - Adult multivitamin.
  - Regular insulin (80 IU).
  - Epinephrine (0.25 mg).
  - 5% dextrose in water (500 mL).
  - Heparin (10,000 IU).
  - Calcium gluconate.
  - 50% dextrose.
  - Potassium chloride.
  - Sterile water for injection.
- Disposable checklist:
  - BGA syringes.
  - Needles.
  - Alcohol wipes.
  - Gloves.
  - Disposal bag.
  - 9 V batteries.
  - LV vent cannula.
- Organize proper transportation vehicles according to the material (running bag, OCS module box, OCS console).

It is advisable to prepare the priming, the maintenance, and the epinephrine solutions before setting off for the donor hospital. However, the OCS module should be kept sterile until after donor heart inspection and the final decision has been made to retrieve the heart for OCS perfusion and transplantation.

At the procurement site

The donor heart should be assessed as described in Chapter 16. Briefly, this should include the four Cs:
- Conduction.
- Contraction.
- Contusion.
- Coronaries.

Once the decision has been made to accept the donor heart for OCS perfusion, preparation is made for donor blood collection. It is crucial to refrain from intensified vasopressor therapy immediately before and during blood collection because this could lead to graft failure during OCS perfusion. When all the procurement teams are ready to proceed with organ preservation, a two-staged venous cannula is placed into the RA. Alternatively, a 24 Fr cannula is placed into the proximal aortic arch. The canula is connected to the blood collection bag placed at floor level for passive blood drainage. All retrieval teams are reminded not to commence perfusion of their respective organs until donor blood collection is complete. A minimum of 1.2 L of donor blood is required and this process can take up to 90 seconds. In some cases, the Trendelenburg position is required to collect the required amount of donor blood. The arterial blood pressure will inevitably decrease during blood collection and it is paramount that the donor is not given boluses of vasoconstrictors during this time. Once blood collection is complete, the vascular cannula is removed, the ascending aorta is clamped, and cardioplegia infusion is started as usual (0.5–1 L for the heart).

Priming of the OCS module should be performed simultaneously with donor blood collection.

Preparing the heart for the OCS Heart chamber

After the donor heart has been explanted, it is placed in a bowl of cold cardioplegia solution for back table preparation. The SVC is tied and the IVC (and PFO if present) is oversewn. This step can also be performed after OCS perfusion is initiated in order to reduce ischaemia time.

The aorta is transected just below the cardioplegia cannula site and four double pledgetted sutures are inserted along the cut edge. There are four different sizes of aortic cannulas. After inserting the optimal sized cannula, a cable tie is tightened below the pledgetted sutures and the excess sutures are trimmed (Fig. 14.3 and Fig. 14.4).

Donor heart perfusion in the OCS Heart

1. The donor heart is positioned in the perfusion chamber with the back of the LA facing the surgeon. The aorta is positioned at 12 o'clock, the SVC at 1 o'clock, the IVC at 5 o'clock, and the PA at 11 o'clock.
2. As the aortic cannula is approximated with the perfusion port of the heart chamber, the OCS Heart is set to an aortic flow rate of 0.25 L/min, taking care to de-air the aorta before completing the connection. The winged nut is tightened to secure this connection and the aortic flow can be increased back to the target flow rate of 1 L/min.
3. At this point, the donor heart is perfused and the perfusion clock has to be started on the OCS monitor.
4. A vent cannula is placed across the MV into the LV and suture secure along the LA edge.
5. To prevent distension of the perfused donor heart, it is necessary to perform manual massage before the heart starts to beat.
6. The electrode pads in the organ chamber are positioned behind the RA and LV. The external defibrillator is connected and when the ECG is detected, DC cardioversion can be performed if required starting with 10 J.

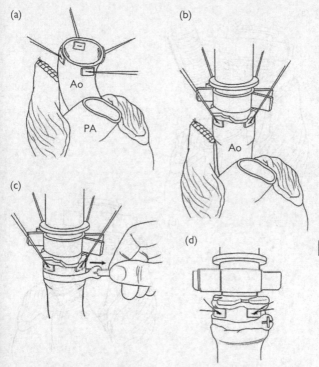

Fig. 14.3 Aortic cannulation for OCS perfusion. There is only one size for the pulmonary cannula. A purse string and umbilical tape secure the cannula position (Fig. 14.4).

7. The donor heart can be paced with the electrode pads or separately inserted epicardial pacing wires if the native heart rate is <80 bpm.
8. After the heart starts beating, the maintenance solution should be delivered in 'AUTO AOP' (aortic pressure) mode with a target AOP of 75–80 mmHg.
9. The PA cannula is connected to a port in the lower right corner of the OCS Heart chamber; the LV vent is secured on the left-hand border of the perfusion chamber.
10. The OCS temperature is set up to 34°C.
11. The positions of the electrode pads are adjusted to ensure good tissue contact in case further DC shocks are required during transportation. These pads can be sutured to the foam backing of the organ chamber if required.

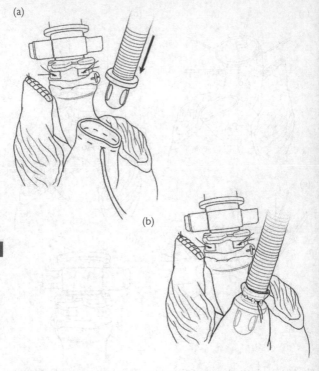

Fig. 14.4 PA cannulation.

Initial stabilization is normally accomplished by the following configuration:
- Pump flow: 1 L/min.
- Coronary flow: 700–800 mL/min.
- Mean AOP: 75–80 mmHg in AUTO AOP mode.

In order to ensure adequate OCS perfusion in DBD donor hearts, paired arterial and venous blood samples should be taken at repeated intervals for lactate evaluation at the following time points:
- Baseline is the first OCS arterial lactate after priming with donor blood but before insertion of the donor heart into the perfusion module.
- Ten minutes after perfusion initiation.
- Every 30–60 minutes of OCS perfusion or 10 minutes after any manual changes to the OCS setting.

For the myocardium, a variety of substrates can provide energy including free fatty acids, glucose, and lactate. As fatty acids are not provided during OCS perfusion, the donor heart would take up and metabolize lactate instead. Thus, if perfusion is adequate, there will be a fall between the arterial and venous lactates (i.e. arterial > venous) (Fig. 14.5). This phenomenon is called 'absorbing lactate' and the lactate level would trend downwards over time. On the other hand, if myocardial perfusion is inadequate, the venous lactate would become higher than the arterial lactate and the heart is said to 'secrete lactate'. If left uncorrected, the lactate level would trend upwards over time.

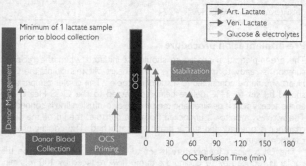

Fig. 14.5 Lactate evaluation scheme in the context of OCS heart perfusion and 'trending down' over time.

It is expected that the first lactate measurement after initiation of OCS perfusion will be higher than the donor arterial lactate just before blood collection. However, if heart perfusion is adequate, the lactate level should trend down over time. For prolonged OCS runs, lactate levels may slightly increase but without relevance for graft performance.

Pearls of OCS Heart perfusion

- Lactate values should always be analysed in the context of the latest donor lactates. In DCD donors, interpretation of lactate levels (high levels) is different from DBD donors.
- Lower venous lactates, compared to arterial samples, as well as stable or decreasing lactate trend are indicative of adequate heart perfusion.
- The OCS Heart aortic flow and the adenosine-rich maintenance solution infusion rate are the main regulators for AOP and coronary flow.
- If AUTO AOP mode is not achieving targeted AOP, the mode should be switched to manual. This can become necessary when the maintenance solution infusion rate of >30 mL/hour is required.
- Venous and arterial lactates should be assessed after no more than 10 minutes following any perfusion adjustments.
- A rapid decrease in the lactate level can be indicative of 'over perfusion'. The aortic flow should be reduced in order to avoid myocardial oedema but maintaining perfusion pressure.
- By applying the ECG synchronization mode, adequate coronary flow can be achieved with lower mean AOP. The circulatory pump is synchronized with the ECG R wave. This mode is recommended for longer OCS Heart runs.
- The decision to begin the patient explant operation should be based on communication between the organ retrieval team and the implanting surgeon regarding the perfusion status of the donor heart on the OCS.

Table 14.1 Summarizers correlation between pump and maintenances solution flow rates with aortic pressure and coronary flows

	Aortic pressure (AOP)	Coronary flow
Pump flow ↓/↑	↓/↑	↓/↑
Maintenance solution rate ↓/↑	↑/↓	↓/↑

Pre-implantation procedure

The pre-implantation procedure should be initiated when the recipient surgeon is ready to transplant the donor heart. At this point, the OCS Heart should be connected to a standard cooler. The cooler temperature should be set to 34°C before being connected to the OCS Heart. The aortic access port is de-aired and the cardioplegic infusion line is connected. The wireless monitor is undocked from the console, the lid of the organ chamber is opened, and sterile drapes are attached. The cooling process can then begin.

The OCS Heart temperature is set to OFF, the temperature on the cooler is reduced by 10°C, and the pump flow reduced by 100 mL/min. This step has to be repeated once the monitor temperature is 2°C higher than the cooler temperature. As the temperature decreases, heart action will decline. Final arrest is induced at 14°C. The aortic vent has to be closed, the aortic line is clamped, the OCS pump is stopped and the cardioplegia infusion is started. The PA cannula is then disconnected to allow the right heart to vent.

Clinical trials

The clinical trials that were performed thus far have established safety of the OCS Heart. The Ex-Vivo Perfusion of Donor Hearts for Human Heart Transplantation (PROCEED II) study was a multicentre randomized study comparing patients who were transplanted with donor hearts preserved on ice and those who were transplanted with donor hearts using the OCS Heart. This showed equivalent outcomes regarding patient and graft survival. However, significant differences in the OCS Heart group included longer total preservation time and shorter cold ischaemic time, demonstrating that the OCS Heart system enabled longer out-of-the-body time without any impact on cardiac function and survival. PROCEED II demonstrated non-inferiority of the OCS Heart compared with cold static storage for standard donor hearts.

The International EXPAND Heart Pivotal Trial was a single-arm study designed to evaluate the effectiveness of the OCS Heart to recruit, preserve, and assess donor hearts that may not meet current standard donor heart acceptance criteria for transplantation to potentially improve donor heart utilization for transplantation. Of the 93 donor hearts placed on the OCS Heart, 75 (81%) were transplanted with 95% recipient survival at 30 days after transplantation. At 6 months, survival was not statistically different when compared to UNOS national average (87.9% vs 92.8%). The incidence of ISHLT-defined moderate or severe PGD was low (14.7%) for this extended criteria donor population.

Conclusion

The ever-growing HF population has driven heart transplant specialists to embrace marginal donor organs and gain experience to achieve optimal post-transplant outcome. Restrictions on age, 'down' time, LVH, comorbidities, as well as reversible LV dysfunction have all been relaxed. Several recent registry database analyses have consistently shown non-inferiority for most of the extended criteria which is reassuring. Although, this chapter does not cover 'high-risk' donors, similar non-inferior outcomes have been reported.

Going forward, more experience will be gained using novel perfusion systems for retrieved donor hearts and subgroups of marginal organs that can truly benefit from these systems will be defined. Other subgroups of marginal donor hearts that do not require the use of these systems will also be explored. One should remember that as these systems are new, the limitations attached to their use (e.g. organ oedema) are still under evaluation and longer follow-up will shed light on their efficacy and cost-effectiveness.

Donor heart procurement: donation after brain death and donation after circulatory determined death

Introduction

The world's first successful heart transplant performed by Christiaan Barnard at the Groote Schuur Hospital, Cape Town, South Africa, in 1967 was from a DCD donor as brain death was not legally recognized at the time. Even though criteria for defining brain death were proposed as early as 1968, it was not until the late 1970s that the definition became widely accepted. In 1967, Barnard placed the asystolic donor on CPB following declaration of death and cooled the heart down to 16°C before transplanting it into the recipient in an adjoining operating theatre. Accordingly, the ischaemic times were minimal in comparison to today's practice. Although there was an initial flurry of heart transplant activity worldwide following Barnard's success, the outcomes were poor with a 1-year survival rate of 15%. It was not until Stanford trialled the use of ciclosporin in 1980 that 1-year survival following heart transplantation became acceptable. By the arrival of ciclosporin, brain death criteria had become universally accepted and controlled DBD heart donation with cold static storage became widely practised with excellent results. Cold static storage with its simplicity and relative reliability remains the universal technique practised today, with >100,000 DBD hearts globally procured and transported this way.

Over the last two decades, as the demand for donor hearts increased, the acceptance criteria for DBD hearts have been relaxed and there has been a resurgence of using DCD hearts for transplantation. With these donor hearts, the limitations of cold static storage have become apparent. In order to overcome the challenges that these particular organs pose and transplant them safely, strategies involving *in situ* and *ex situ* donor heart perfusion have been embraced with the aim of minimizing ischaemic time and reconditioning donor organs in order that successful outcomes can be achieved.

Donation after brain death heart procurement with cold storage

Donor assessment

The donor demographics, history, consent, blood group, virology status, brain death confirmation, ECG, CXR, and echocardiogram must be reviewed and confirmed prior to starting the procurement.

Ideally, a TOE should be undertaken to assess valvular pathology, LV and RV function, and presence of congenital heart disease.

In some countries, a coronary angiogram will be undertaken in donors >40 years old or those with risk factors.

If the donor has not undergone formal right heart catheterization, a PAC can be inserted to assess RA pressure, PA pressures, PCWP, and cardiac output.

Inotropes and filling status should be adjusted to achieve the following parameters while minimizing the vasoconstrictor requirement:
• Mean systemic arterial blood pressure >60 mmHg.
• RA pressure <12 mmHg.
• PCWP <12 mmHg.
• CI >2.5 L/min/m².
• EF >50%.

Team brief and communication

Introductions and a team brief with members of staff from the donor hospital, donor coordinator, and abdominal procurement team should be undertaken. If separate cardiac and pulmonary teams are involved, a clear strategy should be discussed. If machine perfusion technology is involved, for either heart or lungs, measures should be taken in order to ensure length of PA, and/or the need of reconstruction with thoracic aorta. The cardiac retrieval team should be aware of potential specific considerations related to donor, that is, redo surgery which will impact potential cross-clamp time, and need for long vascular structures (SVC, aorta, PA). The WHO surgical checklist should be followed, giving particular importance to preoperative broad-spectrum antibiotics, methyl prednisolone administration, and availability of blood products should they be required. Whether the abdominal procurement team requires the thoracic team to place a cross-clamp on the descending thoracic aorta during abdominal organ perfusion should be established in advance, and a clear strategy for venting of abdominal organ preservation fluid should be agreed upon.

Surgical preparation

- A median sternotomy is undertaken with meticulous attention to haemostasis as it may be 4–6 hours before the donor aorta is cross-clamped to allow for dissection time in complicated recipients.
- The thymus is either removed or divided in the midline. The innominate vein is identified and divided between ligatures to allow the sternum to be retracted fully without stretch on the vessel.
- The pericardium is opened with an inverted T incision and the pericardial edges hitched up.
- An intraoperative assessment of the heart is made. During assessment the heart can become irritable. Manipulation should be undertaken carefully with minimal disturbance to the heart. Internal defibrillation paddles should be available.

Visual inspection

- Overall heart size is assessed to determine the presence of cardiomegaly or LVH.
- Size of LA and RA are assessed determining filling status and evidence of poor cardiac function.
- The LV and RV are assessed for corkscrew-like contraction. A gentle lift of the apex with the palm of the right hand or swab enables this.
- Look for evidence of myocardial contusion or prior infarct.
- Rule out congenital abnormalities, such as left-sided SVC, partial anomalous left-sided drainage, etc.
- Assess the size of the ascending aorta.

Palpation

- CAD: palpation of the entire coronary artery tree should be made in order to assess CAD paying particular attention to the left main stem. This is good practice, even if coronary angiography was performed.
- Aorta: the ascending aorta and aortic root should be palpated to exclude calcification and to detect for palpable thrills which should alert the surgeon to the possibility of aortic stenosis.

- If it has not been possible to insert a PAC, a transduced needle can be placed directly to measure LA and RA filling pressures as well as the PA pressure.
- If right side chambers are unusual enlarged and there is a suspicion of right-to-left shunt, a direct blood gas sample should be taken from the SVC and PA, looking for step-up oxygenation. Ensure ventilation of FiO_2 <50%.

Once the assessment has been made, findings should be relayed to the accepting transplant centre and a provisional cross-clamp time agreed upon.

Preparation for cross clamp

- The distal ascending aorta is dissected from the PA and encircled with a nylon tape.
- Traction of the nylon tape towards the left facilitates access to the SVC and azygos vein.
- The pericardium over the anteromedial aspect of the SVC is incised to the level of the divided innominate vein.
- The SVC is dissected free circumferentially, separating it from the right PA which is directly posterior.
- The azygos vein can then be found draining into the posterior aspect of the SVC cranial to the right PA—this can be divided between heavy ligatures although others may wish to divide it immediately prior to cross-clamping as it can tear easily and be difficult to control.
- The SVC is encircled with a silk tie at the level of the right subclavian vein to be snared down upon later.
- The IVC should be dissected out and encircled with a nylon tape. The diaphragmatic pericardial reflection should be carefully dissected from the IVC freeing up additional length.
- If the heart–lung block needs to be split, Sondergaard's groove should be incised to extend the length of the right-sided pulmonary vein cuff.

Cross-clamp

Permission should be sought to proceed to cross-clamp from the accepting recipient transplant centre, and ensure that the abdominal team and donor coordinator are aware and happy to proceed.

- Administer 300 IU/kg of heparin IV and allowed to circulate for 5 minutes. The Swan–Ganz catheter should be removed and the sheath and the central venous line pulled back out with the intrapericardial SVC.
- An infusion cannula should be placed into the ascending aorta as cranially as possible and secured (some surgeons advocate division of the innominate artery to facilitate more length on the ascending aorta). The cardiac preservation fluid should be primed, de-aired, and connected up to the cannula.
- Once the abdominal team have cannulated and agreed to proceed to cross-clamp, the SVC should be occluded by snugging down on the SVC silk tie.
- The intrapericardial IVC is clamped and almost completely transected on the heart side of the clamp, enabling right-sided venting of the IVC. Alternatively, the IVC can be divided and a sucker placed in the right pleura to vent the abdominal flush and also vent the right side of the heart. Whichever method is adopted, care must be taken to ensure that enough IVC is left to provide adequate margin from the coronary sinus.

- After 5–10 beats to facilitate emptying of the heart, a clamp is applied across the distal ascending aorta and the cardiac preservation fluid is infused into the isolated aortic root (Fig. 15.1).
- The heart is lifted out of the pericardium and the left inferior pulmonary veins are divided (if heart retrieval alone) or the LA appendage tip is divided (if retrieving the heart–lung block) to vent the left heart. It must be stressed that the venting site needs to be large enough so that the heart does not distend when flushing with heart (and lung) preservation solution(s).

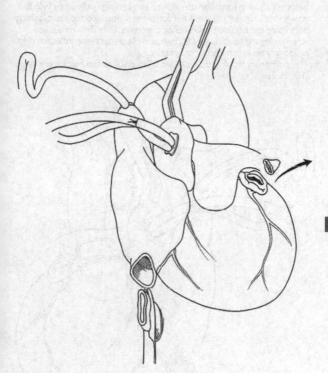

Fig. 15.1 Cannulation of the ascending aorta and venting sites of the DBD donor heart.

- Vigilance must be maintained to ensure that the aortic root is pressurized while being alert to avoiding ventricular distention. The retrieval surgeon may choose to increase preservation fluid volume pending heart size and predicted prolonged ischaemic time. Cold saline is applied for topical cooling of the heart.

- Following completion of the cardiac preservation fluid infusion, the IVC is transected fully. For heart-only retrieval, the four pulmonary veins and the two PAs are individually divided at the level of the pericardial edges.
- If the heart and lung block is to be split, the heart is lifted from the pericardial well following division of the IVC and an incision made in the LA 10 mm medial to the confluence of the left superior and inferior pulmonary veins. An identical incision is then made in the LA 10 mm medial to the confluence of the right superior and inferior pulmonary veins. These two incisions are the joined in a circular fashion giving rise to the LA cuff to the heart while paying particular attention to allow enough pulmonary vein to go with the lungs. Ensure the dissection plane is visualized and clear, looking both inside and outside the LA during dissection. Care should be taken when pulling the heart up, as the dissection plane might jeopardize the right pulmonary veins, in particular the inferior.
- The pulmonary trunk is then divided 2 cm distal to the pulmonary valve (Fig. 15.2).

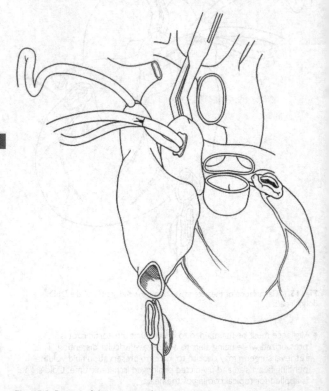

Fig. 15.2 Division of the major vascular structures.

- The aortic clamp is removed and the proximal aortic arch is divided (some surgeons will divide the arch vessels individually and take the aortic arch with the donor heart).
- Finally, the SVC snugger is removed, and the vessel is palpated to ensure it is free from catheters before it is divided as cranially as possible and beyond the divided azygos vein.

Inspection and packing for cold storage

- The heart is placed in a bowl of cold saline solution on the back table and examined for abnormalities or damage. The IVC cuff is assessed to ensure that there is no de-roofing of the coronary sinus and to exclude a left-sided SVC. The SVC is inspected to confirm that there is sufficient length while the fossa ovalis is probed to look for a PFO. The aortic valve is inspected through the ascending aorta to ensure it is trileaflet and free of calcification and vegetation.
- The heart is then triple bagged with 2 L of sterile cold saline or cardiac preservation fluid in each bag being placed in the ice box. The documentation is then signed, and lymph nodes and spleen obtained before the heart is sent.

Normothermic machine perfusion

The Organ Care System (OCS) Heart (TransMedics, Andover, MA, USA) is currently the only device commercially available for isolated donor heart perfusion, receiving its CE mark in 2006 (Fig. 15.3).

The OCS Heart has been assessed in four clinical trials to date, with the ongoing US EXPAND trial for extended criteria donors. The most notable study was the PROCEED II trial where standard DBD hearts were randomized to either the OCS Heart device or cold static storage. Although there was no proven advantage in clinical outcomes, it revealed that the preservation time could be extended by an additional 2 hours compared to cold storage alone. This significant advantage has been reinforced by case reports of successful DBD heart transplantation when the heart has been perfused on the device for >10 hours. The early EXPAND trial results reveal that in a cohort of high-risk donors, OCS Heart-perfused hearts resulted in a rate of primary graft dysfunction which was reduced relative to a predetermined performance standard.

In the current configuration, the OCS Heart perfuses the retrieved donor heart with oxygenated donor blood enriched with nutrients at normothermia. Although the donor heart is beating, the LV is not volume loaded and, therefore, it is not ejecting. This is an important limitation as it is not possible to assess donor heart contractility (Fig. 15.4).

Technique of normothermic machine perfusion

- Following systemic heparinization, 1.2–1.5 L of donor blood is rapidly drained from the donor via a cannula in the RA or aorta in order to prime the device.
- Care is taken to avoid administration of vasopressors to donors during this time period (as this may subsequently affect perfusion of the graft).

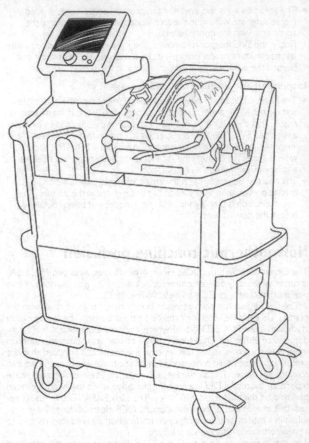

Fig. 15.3 TransMedics OCS Heart device.

- This blood is passed through a leucocyte filter and added to the OCS reservoir pre-primed with 500 mL of the proprietary priming solution. This perfusate is then circulated, oxygenated, and warmed with the addition of the TransMedics maintenance solution containing amino acids with added adenosine.
- Following procurement of the donor heart, the aorta is cannulated with an interfacing aortic connector and secured by a cable tie. This connector is then attached to the organ chamber while carefully de-airing the aortic root.

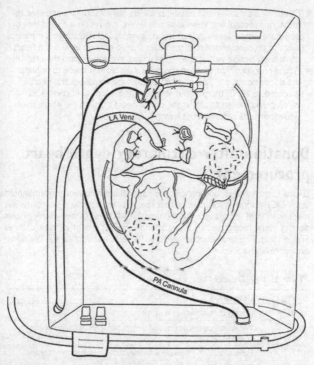

Fig. 15.4 Cannulation of the donor heart on the OCS Heart device.

- After perfusion is restored to the heart and cardiac rhythm is restored, the IVC and SVC are sutured closed to channel the coronary sinus blood through the main PA.
- A vent is placed in the LV to prevent air from being ejected into the aortic root.
- The PA is cannulated and connected to the organ chamber where coronary flow, haemoglobin, haematocrit, and oxygen saturations are measured.
- If the heart fails to restore sinus rhythm, the integrated ECG pad can be used to defibrillate the heart. Pacing wires can be placed in the event of bradycardia.
- Heart perfusion is regulated by ensuring that the aortic root pressure is maintained between 65 and 90 mmHg and coronary flow between 650 and 850 mL/min. This can be controlled by altering the infusion of the vasodilatory maintenance solution as well as varying the pump speed. An automatic perfusion mode is now available to reduce operator interaction and a synchronization mode aimed at reducing oedema by timing pulsatile perfusion with the ECG.

- Donor heart viability and suitability for transplantation are assessed by measuring arterial and venous lactate levels. It is recommended that the perfusate lactate levels do not trend upwards and rise above 5 mmol/L. It is also recommended that the heart should only be used if the heart is consuming lactate with the venous lactate level lower than the arterial.
- At the recipient centre, when the transplant team is ready to implant the donor heart, the SVC and IVC sutures are removed, the heart is cooled to 18°C, the pump is stopped, and 1 L of cold crystalloid cardioplegia is used to arrest the donor heart through the aortic root while the vents remain in the heart.

Donation after circulatory death heart procurement

Livers, lungs, kidneys, and pancreases have all been routinely transplanted from DCD donors for over a decade. At an international consensus meeting in 1994 (Maastricht, Netherlands), four types of non-beating heart donors were recognized in a cascade of shorter warm ischaemic times (Table 15.1). The terms uncontrolled (I, II) versus controlled (III, IV) donation were later added.

Table 15.1 DCD donor Maastricht criteria

Category	Description
I	Declared dead outside hospital
II	Witnessed cardiac arrest and unsuccessful resuscitation within hospital
III	Expected death following withdrawal of life supportive therapy
IV	Brain-dead donors who have undergone cardiac arrest

One of the main challenges facing DCD heart transplantation is the widespread variation that exists across the globe relating to what is acceptable ethical practice, such as antemortem drug administration, interventions, and the duration of the observation period from mechanical asystole to declaration of death, which can vary from 5 to 20 minutes across different European countries. Although all other solid organs from category III DCD donors are routinely retrieved using cold static storage, there had been considerable reservations to transplant DCD hearts due to the associated prolonged obligatory warm ischaemic time which is not well tolerated by the heart. In order to overcome these challenges, pioneers in DCD heart transplantation have adopted techniques aimed at minimizing the warm and cold ischaemic periods, while also allowing a quality check of the heart prior to transplantation, all obstacles to previous successful DCD heart transplant attempts.

There are currently four techniques or combination of techniques that have been used globally for DCD heart procurement leading to successful clinical transplantation in the modern era.

1. Direct procurement after flushing with cold cardiac preservation fluid and cold static storage (DP-CS).
2. Direct procurement and normothermic machine perfusion (DP-MP).
3. Normothermic regional perfusion followed by machine perfusion (NRP-MP).
4. Normothermic regional perfusion followed by cold static storage (NRP-CS).

1. DP-CS

This technique, reported in 2008 by the Denver (CO, USA) group, used cold static storage to preserve three paediatric hearts from DCD donors with a mean donor age of 3.7 days. In order to be successful, they co-located the donor and recipient, employed antemortem cannulation of the femoral vessels, antemortem heparinization, and reduced the observation period from 3 minutes down to 75 seconds to minimize ischaemia. Following declaration of death, an intra-aortic endo-balloon was inflated and cold cardiac preservation fluid was administered into the aortic root before the heart was removed and cold stored. The average total cold ischaemic time was 106 minutes. One recipient required ECMO post transplantation but all were discharged home on average at 20 days post transplantation and all were alive 6 months later.

2. DP-MP

In 2015, the Sydney (Australia) group reported the first three successful adult DCD heart transplants using the DP-MP technique for distantly procured DCD hearts using the OCS Heart device. The protocol is based on donors <40 years old and a donation withdrawal ischaemic period of <30 minutes (time from withdrawal of life-sustaining therapy to starting the infusion of the cardiac preservation fluid). The observation period from asystole to the declaration of death varied from 2 to 5 minutes depending on which Australian state the donor was located in. Following declaration of death, a rapid sternotomy was performed and the donor was exsanguinated. The collected donor blood was leucocyte depleted and added to the pre-primed OCS Heart device. One litre of cold St. Thomas cardioplegia supplemented with erythropoietin and glycerol trinitrate (GTN) was given to the asystolic heart to minimize reperfusion injury. The heart was then explanted and instrumented for OCS perfusion before being transported to the recipient centre. Of the three DCD heart recipients, all survived to discharge with one requiring ECMO support post transplantation.

A recent update on the Sydney experience reported 23 DCD heart transplants using this technique with a 96% overall survival, a 35% reliance on ECMO post transplantation, and an overall increase of heart transplant activity of 15%.

3. NRP-MP

DCD heart transplantation using the NRP technique was first reported by Papworth Hospital (Cambridge, UK) in 2016 following nine successful clinical adult DCD heart transplants. The technique evolved to minimize the risk of primary graft failure in the recipient as previous attempts at DCD heart transplantation had never involved a functional assessment of the DCD donor heart prior to transplantation with primary graft failure requiring ECMO reported at 30%. No antemortem interventions or drugs are permitted in the UK and the observation period is set at 5 minutes. The protocol consisted of donor age <50 years old, a donor warm ischemic time of <4 hours, and a functional warm ischaemic time (systolic <50 mmHg to onset of *in situ* blood reperfusion) <30 minutes. Following declaration of death, the donor is transferred to the operating room where a rapid sternotomy is undertaken. The pericardium is opened and 30,000 IU of heparin is injected into the RA and 20,000 IU into the main PA. The cerebral circulation is excluded by clamps or staple ligation of the three aortic arch branches. The donor then undergoes arterial and venous cannulation before reperfusing the thoraco-abdominal compartments (Fig. 15.5). Recently the technique has been refined to open the distal stumps of the arch vessels to allow active drainage, preventing any pressure build-up through collateral blood flow throughout the NRP period, which can last up to 2 hours.

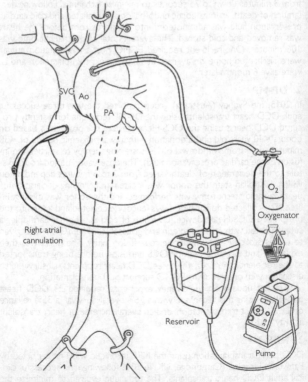

Fig. 15.5 Normothermic regional perfusion circuit configuration.

Following reperfusion, a dopamine infusion is started and the donor is re-intubated and ventilated before weaning the reanimated donor heart from circulatory support. A full functional assessment is undertaken using TOE and thermodilution cardiac outputs by inserting a PAC. Following satisfactory assessment, for distantly procured DCD hearts the TransMedics OCS Heart device is primed with donor blood. The DCD heart is re-arrested with 500 mL of St. Thomas No. 2 cardioplegic solution supplemented with erythropoietin and GTN, explanted from the donor and instrumented for the OCS Heart device. To date, of the 18 DCD heart transplants undertaken at Papworth using NRP-MP, there remains a 100% survival with a 5% reliance on ECMO post transplantation. The main drawback of the practice is that in some countries, restoring heart function in a donor declared dead from circulatory arrest has raised ethical objections.

4. NRP-CS

If the DCD NRP heart donor and the heart transplant recipient happen to be co-located in the same or adjoining hospitals, the recipient operation begins following the satisfactory functional assessment of the DCD heart after NRP has been weaned off. When the recipient surgeon is ready to implant the DCD heart, it can be retrieved in a similar way to a standard DBD heart retrieval with the exception that the DCD heart is arrested with 1 L of cold crystalloid cardioplegia supplemented with erythropoietin and GTN. The heart is then explanted, packaged, and expedited to the awaiting recipient surgeon. The Papworth Hospital team have undertaken three DCD heart transplants using this technique with all surviving to discharge with one requiring ECMO for 12 hours in the early post-transplant period (who was on ECMO as a bridge to heart transplantation). There have been subsequent reports of two successful DCD heart transplants using this technique from Liege in Belgium. The benefit of this technique is a full functional assessment while saving on the financial expense of an ex situ perfusion device.

Technical aspects of heart transplantation

Introduction

The first successful cardiac transplantation was performed by Christiaan Barnard in 1967. However, this was preceded by years of methodological development conducted by Norman Shumway. Heart transplantation has since become the treatment of choice for eligible patients with advanced HF, and >112,000 heart transplants have been reported to the International Heart and Lung Transplant Registry thus far. Despite adverse changes in the donor and recipient populations, post-transplant outcomes continue to improve with a median survival of >12 years.

The most common method for cardiac transplantation is implantation in the orthotopic position using the bicaval technique. In the following chapter we will describe this approach: OHT using hearts from brain-dead donors.

Recipient operation

Preparation and timeline

Recipient 'go-call' is usually made approximately 2.5 hours before the anticipated start time, in order to provide adequate time for the recipient to be transported to the operating room and anaesthesia induction prior to final acceptance of the organ in the donor hospital. Recipient skin incision usually takes place 30 minutes after the designated donor operation begins, once the procuring surgeon has evaluated the donor heart and given the final approval.

Occasionally, there are considerable concerns regarding the viability of the donor heart. In this scenario, the recipient will not be anaesthetized (though some peripheral lines may be placed) until the procuring surgeon has accepted the organ.

The recipient operation is performed under general anaesthetic with orotracheal intubation. Large-bore peripheral and central venous lines and an arterial line are placed. A PAC with continuous cardiac output monitoring and TOE are utilized in all patients. If the INR is elevated, vitamin K and/ or prothrombin complex concentrate may be administered preoperatively. Methylprednisolone (1000 mg) and appropriate antibiotic prophylaxis are administered after the donor heart has been accepted. If the recipient has an ICD, it should be deactivated and external defibrillator pads should be placed on the patient.

Any foreign bodies that will be removed following completion of the transplant (ICD, IABP, LVAD driveline), both groins, and axillary regions should be prepped into the surgical field. Foreign bodies should be covered with a surgical towel and exposed only at the end of the case to minimize the chance of mediastinal contamination.

The timing of the donor cross-clamp is set following communication between the procuring and implanting surgeons, considering anticipated delays in both the donor and recipient operating rooms. If the recipient is a primary sternotomy, skin incision is made 60–90 minutes before the anticipated organ arrival time in the operating room, and CPB is commenced 30–45 minutes before the anticipated arrival time. After confirmation has been received that the air transportation has touched down, the recipient aortic cross-clamp is placed and the cardiectomy is performed. The goal is to coordinate donor heart arrival in the recipient operating room with completion of the recipient cardiectomy, in order to minimize ischaemic time for the donor heart while minimizing the necessary CPB time to complete the cardiectomy. The aim is to limit the total ischaemic time to <4 hours in adult recipients.

Cardiac explanation

See Fig. 16.1.

Cardiac explanation is performed in the following sequence:
1. Median sternotomy and IV heparin.
2. Separate the aorta and PA.
3. Aorto-bicaval cannulation and place umbilical tapes around the IVC and SVC.
4. Place a purse-string in the right superior pulmonary vein.
5. Initiate CPB and cool to 28°C.
6. Place the aortic cross-clamp.
7. Snare the IVC and SVC, and open the free wall of the RA from the right atrial appendage (RAA) parallel with the tricuspid annulus inferiorly into the coronary sinus.
8. If pacemaker or defibrillator leads are present, they are pulled down and out of the SVC as much as possible and then amputated flush with the SVC.
9. With a No. 11 blade, make an incision in the medial aspect of the foramen ovale medially and superiorly towards the dome of the LA and aortic valve.
10. Divide the aorta at the aortic valve (you may place a 2-0 silk suture on the anterior aspect of the remaining aorta for retraction and orientation).
11. Divide the PA at the pulmonic valve (you may place a 2-0 silk suture on the anterior aspect of the remaining PA for retraction and orientation).
12. Extend to the left the incision previously made onto the foramen ovale and the dome of the LA, along the posterior MV annulus and connect it to the previous incision made in the fossa ovalis from the right side, and extract the heart.
13. Create the IVC cuff (2–3 cm away from the cannula) by separating it from the remaining LA tissue, being careful not enter the LA and keep the plane of dissection inferior to the right inferior pulmonary vein (you may place a 2-0 silk suture in the anterior aspect of the remaining atrial tissue for retraction and orientation).
14. Create the SVC cuff by transecting it cranial to the cavoatrial junction with scissors and then separating it from the right PA posteriorly (you may place a 2-0 silk suture in the anterior aspect of the remaining atrial tissue for retraction and orientation).
15. Tailor the remaining LA tissue to create a symmetrical cuff. Be sure to excise any remaining coronary sinus and the LAA, but leave adequate LA tissue to ensure a generous cuff.

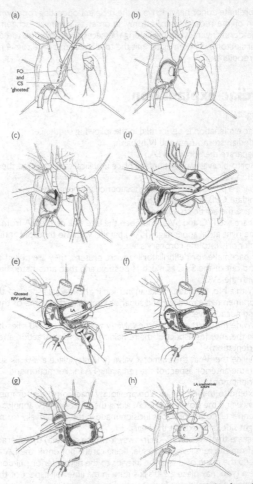

Fig. 16.1 Recipient cardiotomy. (a) Right atriotomy is made extending from the RAA caudally. (b) The right atriotomy is extended parallel to the AV groove from the RAA into the coronary sinus. (c) The medial aspect of the fossa ovalis (FO) is incised and extended superiorly onto the roof of the LA between the SVC and the aorta. (d) The aorta and PA are divided at the level of the semilunar valves. (e) The left atriotomy is extended across the roof of the LA towards the posterior margin of the LAA and the left atriotomy is then extended along the posterior mitral valve annulus. (f) The remnant of the RA is divided and the cavae are mobilized. (g) The SVC and IVC cuffs are completed by separating the posterior aspect of the caval vessels from the anterior aspect of the LA. The redundant tissue between the two marked incisions can be excised. (h) Completed recipient cardiotomy.

16. Place a 3-0 SH polypropylene suture in the LA cuff that corresponds to a point under the middle of the PA (where the LAA was previously). This suture will be used for the LA anastomosis.
17. Quadrangulate the remaining LA cuff with three 4-0 polypropylene sutures to optimize exposure during the LA anastomosis.
18. Mobilize the posterior aspect of the aorta, PA, and SVC.
19. Obtain haemostasis of the posterior pericardial contents.
20. Place a LV vent through the previously placed purse string in the right superior pulmonary vein.

Special situations

Redo sternotomy

The additional time required to complete dissection of the recipient heart and cannulate for CPB in the redo scenario may necessitate delaying of the donor cross-clamp time. When the recipient operation has progressed to a point such that the estimated surgical time remaining until recipient cardiectomy will be completed is equivalent with the estimated organ transport time from the donor hospital, it is safe to proceed with donor cross-clamp.

A number of additional precautions are taken prior to initiating the recipient operation in a patient with prior sternotomies:

1. The CT scan is reviewed to identify the proximity of vital structures to the posterior sternal table (outflow graft, aorta, innominate vein, RV, driveline).
2. External defibrillator pads are placed on the patient.
3. Micropuncture catheters (5 Fr) are placed in the femoral artery and vein in case the need for emergency cannulation arises.
4. Peripheral CPB cannulas and a minimum of 4 units of red blood cells should be readily available prior to sternotomy.
5. If the redo sternotomy is deemed to be particularly high risk based on preoperative imaging, right axillary artery and femoral venous cannulation are performed and the patient is placed on CPB prior to sternotomy.

LVAD explanation

Preoperative precautions are taken as described above for patients with previous sternotomies.

1. Following redo sternotomy, appropriate sites for aortic and venous cannulation are dissected out. The remainder of the heart and LVAD are mobilized, paying particular attention to not damage the outflow graft or LVAD driveline. As much of this dissection as possible is performed prior to initiation of CPB; however, complete dissection typically requires initiation of bypass.
2. Following initiation of CPB, the speed on the LVAD should be reduced such that the LV is adequately decompressed but not completely collapsed.
3. More time may be required to complete the recipient cardiotomy and obtain haemostasis following placement of the aortic cross-clamp in

the redo scenario. Consequently, the aortic cross-clamp may need to be placed prior to touchdown of air transportation in some scenarios in order to minimize donor organ ischaemic time.

4. Following placement of the aortic cross-clamp, the outflow graft is ligated and divided, and the LVAD is turned off (the driveline can be divided later).

5. Meticulous haemostasis of the posterior pericardium should be obtained following recipient cardiectomy.

6. If the dissection is particularly difficult and the heart has arrived in the recipient operating room before the cardiectomy has been completed, the LV apex can be amputated to facilitate cardiectomy and minimize ischaemic time. The LVAD can be removed after the cardiectomy has been completed or even after the heart has been implanted.

Heart transplantation following a congenital operation

1. The procuring surgeon should discuss with the implanting surgeon what additional tissue should be procured. This may include the entire aortic arch and a portion of the descending thoracic aorta, the PAs out into the lung hilum, and the entire SVC and innominate vein complex.

2. The procuring team should ensure an appropriately sized cardioplegia cannula and sternal retractor are available.

3. Appropriate recipient imaging should be obtained to determine the patency of upper and lower extremity vasculature, and to investigate the proximity of vital structures to the posterior sternal table.

4. The implanting surgeon should:
   a. Take appropriate precautions as for any redo sternotomy.
   b. Be prepared to address the significant aortopulmonary collaterals that are common in this patient population.
   c. Be prepared for the need for complex reconstruction of the IVC and SVC, the innominate vein, the PAs, and the aortic arch, depending on the patient's HF aetiology and the nature of the previous surgical procedures. As much of the reconstruction as possible should be performed prior to donor heart arrival.

Allograft implantation

Back-table preparation

1. Place the donor heart in a basin of cold saline.
2. Verify the integrity of all cardiac valves and the coronary sinus.
3. Close the foramen ovale if patent.
4. Create a common LA cuff by connecting the pulmonary veins. Tailor the LA cuff by resecting excess tissue.
5. Separate the aorta and the PA (exercise caution so as to not injure the left main coronary artery as it courses posterior to the main PA).

Heart transplantation

See Fig. 16.2.

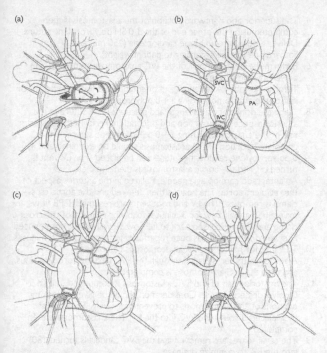

Fig. 16.2 Allograft implantation. (a) Pericardial well prepared for the new heart. A right superior pulmonary vein (RSPV) vent placed in the LA well. (b) LA anastomosis. RSPV vent will be placed through the MV into the LV before tie-down. (c) IVC, aorta, and PA back-wall anastomosis. (d) Completed aorta anastomosis. (e) IVC and PA anterior wall anastomosis as well as SVC anastomosis.

1. Deliver a dose of cold blood cardioplegia to the donor heart following completion of the back-table dissection (300 mL).
2. Place the heart on the recipient left chest wall, such that the LA cuff is facing the implanting surgeon. Using the 3-0 SH polypropylene suture previously placed under the recipient PA, begin the LA anastomosis starting at the donor LAA. The heart is parachuted down on top of an icy sponge in the left lateral pericardial space and covered in ice.
3. The leftward and then inferior portions of the anastomosis are performed in an everting and running fashion. The IVC marks the half-way point. The right superior pulmonary vein vent should be placed across the mitral valve. The completed portion of the anastomosis should be examined and 4-0 polypropylene reinforcing sutures can be placed on the back wall if needed.

4. The superior and rightward portion of the anastomosis is then completed using the other end of the 3-0 SH polypropylene suture.
5. Deliver a dose of cold blood cardioplegia (250 mL) and IV liothyronine (dosed according to patient weight).
6. Perform the posterior half of the IVC anastomosis using a 4-0 SH polypropylene suture.
7. Tailor the donor PA to length and orientation. Perform the posterior half of the anastomosis using a 4-0 polypropylene suture.
8. Tailor the donor aorta to length and place a 2-0 silk suture at the anterior aspect for retraction and orientation. Perform the posterior half of the anastomosis using a 4-0 polypropylene suture. The completed portion of the anastomosis should be examined and 4-0 polypropylene reinforcing sutures can be placed. The LV vent is turned off and the aortic anastomosis is then completed.
9. An antegrade cardioplegia needle is placed in the anterior aspect of the recipient aorta. The heart is then de-aired and the aortic cross-clamp is removed. The LV and root vents are resumed. CPB flows are maintained at half-flow for 3 minutes following removal of the cross-clamp and then increased back to full flow. Rewarming is commenced after the donor heart has been reperfused for a period of 15 minutes.
10. The anterior half of the PA anastomosis is completed.
11. A suction catheter is placed through the SVC into the coronary sinus, and then the IVC anastomosis is completed.
12. The posterior half of the SVC anastomosis is completed using a 5-0 polypropylene suture. Consideration should be given to locking portions of this anastomosis to prevent narrowing. The PAC is then placed through the SVC into the RV. The anastomosis is then completed.
13. The caval snares are removed and the SVC cannula is turned 180° into the RA to optimize drainage.
14. An epinephrine infusion is started at 0.04 mcg/kg/min after the patient is rewarmed.
15. All anastomoses are inspected for bleeding sites that require additional sutures. Atrial and ventricular pacing wires are placed and the heart is paced sequentially at 90 bpm.
16. The patient is ventilated with an inhaled pulmonary vasodilator (e.g. nitric oxide (NO)) and any necessary corrections to the arterial blood gas are made.
17. Wean from CPB and begin collecting continuous cardiac output data.
18. Assess cardiac function using TOE.
19. Optimize haemoglobin concentration, ventilation, oxygenation, heart rate and rhythm, preload, afterload, and inotropic support.
20. Evaluate the need for delayed chest closure, or mechanical support.
21. If clinical stability is achieved and there is no need to return to CPB, basiliximab (20 mg) is administered.
22. After the sternal incision has been closed and dressed, remove the ICD and the remainder of the driveline (if present) and pack the wound with gauze.

Primary graft dysfunction (PGD)

A successful cardiac transplantation requires thoughtful donor–recipient matching, minimized donor ischaemic time, diligent myocardial protection during implantation, and meticulous surgical technique. Weaning from CPB is facilitated through optimization of haemoglobin concentration, oxygenation, and ventilation with a pulmonary vasodilator. The heart is paced at a rate of 90–100 bpm (AAI or DDD), the CVP is maintained at 8–12 mmHg, and the MAP at 80–90 mmHg. Inotropic support is optimized (e.g. epinephrine, norepinephrine, and dopamine for the LV and milrinone and NO for the RV, if needed) and adequacy of the systemic circulation is evaluated.

However, regardless of the above-mentioned points, PGD may develop in patients undergoing heart transplantation, and is associated with 30% mortality at 30 days. PGD may result from LV failure, RV failure, or biventricular failure and is graded as mild, moderate, or severe LV PGD and as RV PGD as described by Kobashigawa.

If high-dose inotropic support is required to maintain an adequate CI, there should be a low threshold to insert an intra-aortic balloon and/or more advanced MCS devices. In the situation of isolated RV failure, central RVAD support can be considered. In this situation, it is advisable to tunnel the cannulas through the epigastrium to allow closure of the sternotomy incision. A 34–36 Fr angled cannula is placed in the RA, and a 19–21 Fr percutaneous femoral cannula (the additional length of this cannula can be helpful) is placed in the PA. A 2-0 Ethibond suture is used to place one purse string in the RA and two purse strings in the PA. Multiple intervening pledgets are placed on each purse string. The tip of the PA cannula can be trimmed back, and care is taken when inserting this cannula so that only 2 cm of cannula is in the PA past the last infusion port of the cannula. This ensures that the tip of the cannula is proximal to the PA bifurcation and prevents streaming of the RVAD outflow into one PA. The cannulas are de-aired and connected to the temporary pump (e.g. RotaFlow, CentriMag, etc.). Flow is increased slowly and typically in order to adequately fill the LV and facilitate weaning of inotropic support.

If there is any concern regarding LV or pulmonary function, central VA ECMO should be instituted. If the duration of support is expected to be short (24–48 hours), then the CPB cannulas can be used and brought out through an open chest. However, tunnelling new cannulas through the epigastrium is preferred as this would facilitate chest closure, early extubation, and mobilization until myocardial recovery occurs. Cannulation (34–36 Fr angled cannula in the RA and 19–21 Fr percutaneous femoral cannula in the ascending aorta) proceeds in the same manner as described for insertion of the RVAD. If myocardial recovery does not occur, the patient should be considered for relisting for retransplantation. That being said, one should take into consideration that acute heart retransplantation has very poor outcomes and there is much ethical debate about its appropriateness.

Conclusion

Since the first heart transplantation performed in 1967, improvements in surgical techniques, preservation methods, and immunosuppression have enabled outstanding 1-year survival and graft half-life of >12 years.

The current era of heart transplantation is evolving around preservation machines, which will enable substantial increases in transport time, minimizing the cold ischaemic time and enabling the use of marginal/DCD donors, thus increasing the donor pool and as a consequence increasing the number of transplants being performed all around the world substantially. Furthermore, it may enable organ sharing between countries that previously were not able to do so owing to transport time.

Future research efforts should be directed to minimize cardiac allograft vasculopathy (10%) and malignancy (20%) that account for most cardiac recipient deaths. These numbers highlight that regardless of the progress that has been accomplished over the years in all aspects of cardiac transplantation, the consequences of chronic administration of immunosuppression on long-term survival is pronounced. Thus, the need to develop new drugs or tolerance strategies that achieve better long-term graft survival is genuine.

Hence, standardizing the surgical technique as explained in this chapter is a crucial step, but merely one of many steps needed.

Critical care management and primary graft dysfunction following cardiac transplantation

Monitoring and investigations

The patient should arrive from theatre with full monitoring in place. The ISHLT recommends the following:

1. Peripheral oxygen saturation.
2. ECG (telemetry).
3. Invasive arterial blood pressure.
4. CVP/RA pressure.
5. PA pressure.
6. PCWP/LA pressure.
7. Cardiac output.
8. Urinary output.

Baseline investigations should be performed on arrival and thereafter as clinically indicated.

Arterial blood gases provide an early assessment of gas exchange, oxygen delivery, acid–base status, and important serum electrolyte levels including potassium and ionized calcium. Bedside tests of coagulation including heparinase ACT plus thromboelastometry may be repeated following blood products or if there is ongoing blood loss.

Haematology tests including full blood count and coagulation screen are used to guide transfusion of blood products. Biochemistry tests including urea and electrolytes allow diagnosis of common electrolyte imbalances such as hypokalaemia, hypomagnesaemia, and hypocalcaemia.

CXR should be performed to confirm correct positioning of endotracheal tube, invasive monitoring lines, and mediastinal/intercostal drains.

Lung ultrasonography in the ICU setting has increased in the past decade and can be invaluable for the assessment of lung function in the postoperative period. A consensus document by the International Liaison Committee on Lung Ultrasound provides recommendations for the identification and follow-up of common complications such as pulmonary oedema, consolidation, and pleural effusions.

Echocardiography plays a crucial role in the postoperative period, guiding cardiovascular management and identifying cardiac complications such as tamponade. Filling status, ventricular function, and pericardial collections can all be assessed and monitored at the bedside.

Cardiovascular management

Haemodynamic management starts in theatre and continues into the postoperative period in the ICU. Common haemodynamic goals include an adequate CI and systemic blood pressure to maintain organ perfusion while avoiding excessive myocardial oxygen demand and promoting recovery of graft function.

Chronotropic medications and/or AV pacing continue to achieve heart rate of 90–110 bpm with AV synchrony. Fluid or diuretics are titrated according to filling pressures and appearances on echocardiography noting that diastolic dysfunction may be a prominent feature of the first 12–24 hours. A CVP <10 mmHg is desirable to promote RV recovery. Pulmonary vasodilators continue in the context of elevated pulmonary pressures and RV failure to promote left-sided filling. Inotropes are titrated according to ventricular function on echocardiography to achieve a CI of 2–2.5 L/min/m². IABPs implanted in theatre are generally continued for 48–72 hours with careful attention to lower limb perfusion. Vasopressors are titrated to achieve a MAP of 65–70 mmHg. Packed red blood cells are transfused to maintain haemoglobin >7.5 g/dL. Higher levels (e.g. haemoglobin 10 g/dL) may be targeted if SvO_2 is <60%.

Commonly used inotropes/vasopressors are summarized in Table 17.1.

Table 17.1 Commonly used inotropes/vasopressors

Agent	Dosage	Half-life	Peripheral vasocon-striction	Cardiac con-tractility	Peripheral vasodi-lation	Chrono tropic effect
Dopamine	1–10 mcg/kg/min	1 minute	+ +	+ + +	+	+
Dobutamine	1–10 mcg/kg/min	4 minutes	0	+ + +	+ +	+
Epinephrine	0.01–0.2 mcg/kg/min	2–3 minutes	+ + +	+ + + +	+	+ +
Milrinone	0.1–0.5 mcg/kg/min	2–4 hours	0	+ + +	+	+ +
Norepinephrine	0.01–0.2 mcg/kg/min	2–2.5 minutes	+ + + +	+ + +	0	+
Vaso pressin	0.018–0.12 IU/kg/min	10–35 minutes	+ + + +	0	0	0
Levosimendan	Loading dose: 6–24 mcg/kg over 10 minutes Infusion: 0.05–0.2 mcg/kg/min	70–80 hours	0	+ + +	+ +	+

Mechanical circulatory support

MCS is generally reserved for patients with persisting graft dysfunction and compromised organ perfusion despite the above-discussed measures. Ideally, MCS should be instituted in theatre but may also be required in the postoperative period in the context of escalating pharmacological support. Commonly used devices include VA ECMO for biventricular failure and short-term RVAD for isolated RV failure. These devices support cardiac output and maintain organ perfusion while allowing weaning of inotropes and recovery of the injured ventricle. Ongoing management requires regular input from the multidisciplinary team including surgery, ICU, nursing, and perfusion to avoid device-related complications for the duration of the support.

Weaning support

Pharmacological support commenced in theatre should be continued for 48–72 hours postoperatively. Following a period of haemodynamic stability, support is weaned as cardiac function recovers and vascular tone returns. Inhaled pulmonary vasodilators are weaned first to facilitate extubation. Nebulized iloprost or nasogastric sildenafil may be used to avoid rebound PH. Inotropes are weaned slowly in the context of adequate CI and ventricular function on echocardiography. Vasopressors are weaned in the context of an adequate MAP for organ perfusion (usually 65–70 mmHg). IABP may be explanted once inotropes are weaned to moderate levels (e.g. dobutamine 5–10 mcg/kg/min) facilitating mobilization.

Hypertension may become a prominent feature following myocardial recovery reflecting the patient's vasculature adapted to a low cardiac output. Commonly used antihypertensive agents include GTN, hydralazine, and calcium channel blockers. BBs and ACEis are best avoided in the immediate postoperative period.

Fluid management

The patient may be subject to large fluid shifts intraoperatively due to increased capillary permeability secondary to CPB, on-pump ultrafiltration, bleeding (especially in re-sternotomies), and blood product transfusion. The goals of fluid management in ICU are to maintain preload while avoiding RV distension and ultimately achieving euvolaemia. Invasive monitoring including CVP/PCWP and echocardiography should be used to guide management including cautious fluid resuscitation or IV diuretics by bolus or infusion (e.g. furosemide 10–40 mg/hour) as required. A positive fluid balance may be necessary for 24–48 hours postoperatively before diuresis can be used to achieve a daily negative fluid balance targeting euvolaemia. Continuous renal replacement therapy should be considered early in the context of fluid overload and inadequate urine output despite diuretic infusion/acute kidney injury.

Respiratory management

The goals of respiratory management after transplantation are to avoid physiological causes of increased PVR such as hypoxia and hypercapnia while minimizing the deleterious effects of positive pressure ventilation on RV function. While the patient remains sedated and intubated, protective ventilation is employed with low tidal volumes and minimum PEEP required to avoid de-recruitment. FiO_2 and respiratory rate are titrated to achieve PO_2 >10 kPa, and CO_2 <5.5 kPa. Following a period of haemodynamic stability, sedation is weaned with a view to spontaneous ventilation and early extubation. In scenarios where extubation is felt likely to be delayed, percutaneous tracheostomy should be considered to facilitate spontaneous ventilation and weaning from the ventilator.

Immunosuppression

Immunosuppression protocols should be well established at each centre and should be easily accessible to all staff. Timing of induction, tailoring of agents, and timing of sampling (CD3 count/tacrolimus/ciclosporin levels) should be clearly outlined, alongside management of the early adverse effects of immunosuppression (renal impairment, thrombocytopaenia, marrow suppression, etc.). A multimodal approach involving the surgeons, transplant physicians, intensivists, and nursing staff is needed with precise handovers to ensure continuity of care. Further details regarding immuno-suppression are discussed in Chapter 20.

Infection management

Perioperative immunosuppression is associated with an increased risk of infection during the intensive care period and beyond. Post-transplant in-fection remains one of the leading causes of death in the first-year after transplantation, accounting for 25–32% of all deaths. The risk of death is highest between 1 month to 1 year post transplantation.

Risk factors for post-transplant infections include age, use of MCS, reoperation, previous bacterial infections, and relapsing viral infections (Table 17.2).

Table 17.2 A list of infections that predominate in the first month post transplantation

Infection type	Early infection (<1 month)
Viral	Herpes simplex virus
Bacterial	Nocardia
	Clostridium difficile
	Pseudomonas
	Vancomycin-resistant enterococci
	Methicillin-resistant Staphylococcus aureus
Fungal	Candida
	Aspergillus

Ideally the post-transplant patient should be cared for in an isolated, positive pressure room with restricted visitor numbers. People entering the room should wear a protective gown and perform hand hygiene prior to interacting with the patient's environment.

Antibiotic prophylaxis commenced in theatre as per local policy and is continued in the ICU for 24–48 hours. Commonly used agents include beta-lactams, cephalosporins, and glycopeptides often requiring level monitoring and/or dose reduction in the context of renal dysfunction.

Early extubation, patient mobilization, and removal of indwelling cath-eters are important steps in reducing the risk of nosocomial infections.

Candida species are common fungal pathogens. Oral nystatin is routinely used to prevent mucocutaneous candidiasis. *Pneumocystis* pneumonia is a common opportunistic infection in immunosuppressed patients. Prophylaxis with antiprotozoals is commenced in the early postoperative period and continued for up to 12 months. CMV-positive donor or recipient are considered at high risk of CMV infection and prophylaxis with ganciclovir/valganciclovir as recommended by the ISHLT is started within 24–48 hours.

Special indications, such as the use of organs from HCV-infected donors, may require administration of antivirals, guided by locally agreed protocols involving discussions with hepatologists and virologists.

The systemic response to sepsis may also be suppressed in the immunocompromised patient, necessitating a high degree of clinical suspicion for diagnosis. Clinicians should have a low threshold for performing cultures and commencing or changing antibiotics based on new positive results and sensitivities. Daily input from a specialist microbiology team is vital. Vigilance is also needed to promptly identify wound or line infections in the immunosuppressed patient. Severe infections often require dose adjustments of immunosuppression, increasing the risk of allograft rejection.

Nutrition

Weight loss may be a feature of chronic HF and may be accelerated pre-operatively with low cardiac output states particularly in patients supported with short-term MCS. Early enteral nutrition is the goal in the postoperative period preferably via the oral route. Nasogastric feeding should be commenced early if delayed extubation appears likely. Attention should be paid to feeding interruptions, such as for invasive procedures, and feeding rates adjusted accordingly to achieve overall nutritional requirements. Glycaemic control may be particularly challenging in the context of steroids and catecholamine infusions and a variable rate insulin infusion is commonly required.

Psychosocial support

Cardiac transplant recipients are often young patients who may have been affected by long-standing illness with multiple hospital admissions and potentially prolonged inpatient care. Patients and their families may be a long way from home, bringing additional challenges around normal life commitments. Perceptions of intensive care can vary. Ideally, the patient and their family should visit the ICU prior to surgery but most will require ongoing education and reorientation in the ICU environment. Emotions in the postoperative period will also vary from patient to patient and can impact their recovery. Patients may benefit from psychology support when dealing with emotions of fear, low mood, and guilt. Ongoing communication with the patient and family is also essential to update them on progress. Donor anonymity should be maintained at all times including during communication within the clinical team and with the patient and family members.

Multidisciplinary team working

Postoperative care for the cardiac transplant patient is delivered by a multi-disciplinary team including the various different medical specialties, specialist nursing groups, and allied health professionals. Management in intensive care is directed by the intensive care consultant with regular input from other members of the team on ward rounds and during regular multidisciplinary team meetings. Each unit should have local cardiac transplant guidelines including protocols on aspects of perioperative care. Daily management plans should be clearly documented in the medical notes with deviations from protocol noted and communicated to the multidisciplinary team.

Early post-transplant complications

Hyperacute rejection

Hyperacute rejection is a relatively rare event in organ transplant recipients. It is an irreversible process due to:

- The previous formation of antibodies to the HLA system present in the transplanted graft, above all antibodies to class I antigens (HLA-A, -B, or -C).
- The existence of preformed ABO antibodies in the graft recipient at the time of transplantation.
- Xenotransplantation between phylogenetically distant species.

It occurs from the time of transplant to 48 hours postoperatively and result in rapid ischaemic and necrotic changes to the graft with polymorphonucleocyte infiltration. It may occur upon allograft reperfusion when the preformed antibodies against the donor are first in contact with the graft. It was relatively more common in the earlier days of transplant-ation, before HLA-matching techniques were well developed. It results in profound haemodynamic instability, for which inotropic and vasopressor support is invariably required alongside MCS. High-dose immunosuppres-sion (corticosteroids, cytolytic induction therapy, antimetabolites) are often administered and plasmapheresis may have a role in removing circulatory antibodies from the blood while on the bypass circuit. IVIG can be adminis-tered to inactivate antibodies. Endomyocardial biopsy can be performed to confirm the diagnosis. Retransplantation may be considered, but the mor-tality remains high.

Bleeding

Risk factors for postoperative bleeding include patient factors such as pre-operative anticoagulation and operative factors such as reoperation and prolonged CPB time. Clinical signs of ongoing blood loss include hypo-tension with low cardiac output and low filling pressures. Invasive moni-toring may show low blood pressure and low cardiac output with low CVP and/or pulmonary diastolic pressure/PCWP. Chest and mediastinal drain monitoring may identify ongoing drain losses. CXR and/or lung US may demonstrate pleural/mediastinal collections. Echocardiography may show underfilled LV and RV with or without pericardial collection.

Hypothermia and hypocalcaemia should be reversed. Heparin excess should be identified with a heparinase ACT and treated with additional protamine. In the context of ongoing bleeding, transfusion of blood products should be guided by point-of-care testing (e.g. TEG, thromboelastometry) along with laboratory tests including full blood count and coagulation screen. Blood products for transfusion should be irradiated for all transplant patients. CMV-negative recipients should only receive CMV-negative blood.

Importantly, coagulopathic bleeding should be medically managed. Bleeding which continues despite correction of coagulation abnormalities should prompt surgical re-exploration to identify a bleeding source.

Tamponade

Diagnosing tamponade in the post-transplant setting may be challenging. Tachycardia is often masked and the triad of hypotension, low cardiac output, and raised CVP may be attributed to RV failure, another common complication following cardiac transplantation. In the presence of clinical suspicion, the team should have a low threshold for further investigation. CXR may demonstrate a widened mediastinum and echocardiography may reveal a local or generalized pericardial effusion with or without chamber compression. Variation in transmitral velocities may not be seen in the ventilated patient. Clinical diagnosis should prompt management including chest drain clot removal and emergent surgical re-exploration. If the patient has been extubated, induction of anaesthesia should be managed with extreme caution given the high vascular tone required to maintain cardiac filling pressures and the potential for additional cardiac dysfunction.

Arrythmias

Conduction abnormalities in the immediate post-transplant setting are multifactorial. Electrolyte disturbance including abnormal potassium, magnesium, and phosphate levels are common following prolonged CPB and predispose to arrhythmias. The denervated heart has a higher resting heart rate due to the loss of vagal stimulation and does not exhibit the expected response to many cardiac medications. The biatrial surgical implantation technique involves the anastomosis of the donor and recipient RA and is associated with a higher rate of sinoatrial node injury, increasing the risk of atrial arrhythmias including bradycardias. It is also associated with a higher incidence of permanent pacemaker implantations compared with the bicaval technique. Rhythm control is desirable in the early postoperative period with stroke volume being particularly dependent on ventricular filling. Temporary epicardial pacing wires are left *in situ* until rhythm has been stable for 48 hours off chronotropic drugs and/or after the first endomyocardial biopsy.

Atrial arrhythmias

Atrial fibrillation, atrial flutter, and supraventricular tachycardia are the most common arrhythmias post transplantation though the frequency of atrial arrhythmias in general is significantly lower than following general cardiac surgery, possibly due to the exclusion of the pulmonary veins. New or sustained atrial tachyarrhythmias should prompt a full workup to rule out acute rejection. Treatment is similar to the general post-cardiac surgical patient including electrolyte replacement, antiarrhythmic drugs, and DC cardioversion if required. Amiodarone is associated with significant drug interaction with ciclosporin or tacrolimus, requiring close monitoring of immunosuppressant levels.

Ventricular arrhythmias

Non-sustained ventricular tachycardia is relatively common in the early postoperative period. It is often benign but may also be associated with acute rejection or early graft failure. Sustained ventricular tachycardia is uncommon and should prompt consideration of hyperacute rejection.

Acute kidney injury

Acute kidney injury in the immediate postoperative period occurs in up to 70% of heart transplant patients. Perioperative renal failure may significantly complicate the management of intravascular volume and ventricular filling pressures.

The incidence of renal replacement therapy in the immediate postoperative period varies (6–25%) which may indicate the heterogeneity of patients and their comorbidities. Previous cardiac surgery, high levels of preoperative creatinine, prolonged CPB time, HF medical therapy, diabetes mellitus, advancing age, low cardiac output, and low serum albumin concentration have all been reported as independent preoperative risk factors for acute kidney injury requiring renal replacement therapy.

Management includes optimization of cardiac output and MAP to maintain renal perfusion with careful attention to fluid balance. Nephrotoxic drugs are discontinued, avoided, or delayed until renal function has recovered including immunosuppressant drugs such as the calcineurin inhibitors.

Renal replacement therapy should be considered early in the context of fluid overload refractory to diuretics or electrolyte disturbance with the increased risk of cardiac arrhythmias. If renal replacement therapy is required, continuous renal replacement is preferred to intermittent haemodialysis aiming to avoid cardiovascular instability and large variations in filling pressures. Care should be taken to monitor drug levels where possible, including antimicrobials and immunosuppression drugs.

Right ventricular dysfunction

RV dysfunction is common following cardiac transplantation and is a cause of major morbidity and mortality. It results from a combination of donor and recipient factors including the ischaemic injury sustained during organ procurement and increased PVR in the recipient. Diagnosis requires clinical and echocardiographic assessments and management includes optimization of filling status, titration of vasoactive medications, and early consideration of MCS. RV dysfunction is covered in detail in Chapter 36.

Primary graft dysfunction

PGD is defined as:
- Severe ventricular dysfunction of the donor graft which fails to meet the circulatory requirements of the recipient despite adequate filling pressures.
- In the immediate post-transplant period.
- Manifest as either single or biventricular dysfunction.

It is differentiated from secondary graft dysfunction, which is when a discernible cause for allograft dysfunction is identified (e.g. hyperacute rejection, PH, or surgical complications).

PGD can be classified into two categories:
- PGD-LV: includes LV dysfunction or biventricular dysfunction.
- PGD-RV: includes RV dysfunction alone.

Both occur within 24 hours of transplantation.

Classification

Classification follows the ISHLT 2014 'Consensus Statement Definition of Severity Scale for Primary Graft Dysfunction (PGD)' (Table 17.3 and Table 17.4).

Incidence

The incidence of PGD has a significant variation in incidence reporting (2.3–32.4%) prior to the ISHLT consensus statement. There is an increasing trend towards utilization of extended criteria donor organs which may have lowered the threshold for initiating MCS in some patients during the initial phase of reperfusion, potentially causing an overestimation of the true incidence of PGD.

Mortality

The 30-day mortality ranges widely from 17% to 80% due to variations in earlier definitions. Early mortality has improved with increased timely initiation of MCS for PGD. To date, treatment for PGD is primarily supportive. Retransplantation may be of benefit in selected individuals; however, mortality from early retransplantation remains high.

Risk factors

Risk factors for PGD can be classified into donor, recipient, and procedural factors (Table 17.5). The RADIAL score (Table 17.6) and PREDICTA score (Table 17.7) are also useful tools for PGD. They are simple additive scores used to predict recipient and donor combinations that may be at a higher risk of PGD. PGD incidence increased significantly as the PREDICTA or RADIAL score increased. Other risk factors described in the literature are as follows:

Management

The management of PGD is primarily supportive, initially with inotropic support and adjuncts such as vasopressors and/or inhaled pulmonary vasodilators. Early escalation to an IABP or temporary MCS (percutaneous/surgical) is warranted for patients who remain haemodynamically unstable. In some instances, retransplantation may be considered following failure to wean from MCS.

Table 17.3 PGD-LV severity is separated into mild, moderate, and severe PGD based on either echocardiographic/invasive cardiac monitoring *and* inotrope score *or* intervention criteria

PGD-LV severity	LVEF by echo cardiography	Invasive cardiac monitoring	Inotrope score[a]	Intervention criteria
Mild	≤40%	1. RA pressure >15 mmHg 2. CI <2.0 L/min/m² 3. PCWP >20 mmHg 4. MAP <70 mmHg *(Lasting >1 hour)*	≤10	n/a
Moderate	≤40%	1. RA pressure >15 mmHg, 2. CI <2.0 L/min/m² 3. PCWP >20 mmHg 4. MAP <70 mmHg *(Lasting >1 hour)*	>10	Newly placed IABP *(regardless of inotrope score)*
Severe	n/a	n/a	n/a	Dependence on left/biventricular MCS (ECMO, BiVAD, LVAD, or percutaneous LVAD) *Excludes IABP*

[a] Inotrope score = dopamine (×1) + dobutamine (×1) + amrinone (×1) + milrinone (×15) + epinephrine/adrenaline (×100) + norepinephrine/noradrenaline (×100) with each drug dosed in mcg/kg/min.

Table 17.4 PGD-RV is diagnosed by either invasive cardiac monitoring or intervention criteria

Invasive cardiac monitoring	Intervention criteria
1. RA pressure >15 mmHg 2. PCWP <15 mmHg 3. CI <2.0 L/min/m² And 1. Transpulmonary pressure gradient <15 mmHg and/or 2. PA systolic pressure <50 mmHg	Need for RVAD

Table 17.5 Risk factors for PGD

Donor factors	Recipient factors	Procedural factors
Advancing age	Advancing age	Prolonged ischaemic time
Donor cause of death	Weight	Donor–recipient sex mismatch
Trauma	MCS	Weight mismatch
Inotropic support	Congenital heart disease as aetiology for HF	Experience of procurement team and centre volume
Comorbidities (diabetes, hypertension)	Multiple reoperations	Increased blood transfusion requirement
Prolonged downtime following cardiac arrest	LVAD explant	Elective vs emergency transplant
LVH	Comorbidities: renal dysfunction, liver dysfunction, diabetes mellitus	Prolonged CPB time
Drug abuse	Infection	
CAD/wall motion abnormalities on TTE	Amiodarone therapy	

Table 17.6 RADIAL score

Variable	Points
Right atrial pressure ≥10 mm Hg	1
Age (recipient) ≥60 years	1
Diabetes mellitus	1
Inotrope dependence	1
Age (donor) ≥30 years	1
Length of ischaemic time ≥240 minutes	1
Total score	__/6

Source data from Segovia et al., 2011.

Vasoplegic syndrome after heart transplantation

Vasoplegic syndrome is characterized by persistent hypotension, reduced SVR, and normal or increased cardiac output. It occurs in up to one-third of patients following cardiac transplantation (depending on definition) and has been shown to be associated with increased morbidity and mortality.

While the exact cause is unknown, several risk factors have been identified following cardiac surgery. These include the use of medications

Table 17.7 PREDICTA score

Variable	Points
Preoperative MCS (ST-VADs and ECMO)	3
Diabetes mellitus (recipient)	3
Cardiopulmonary bypass time >180 minutes	2
Implant **T**ime	
≤45 minutes	0
46–60 minutes	1
61–90 minutes	2
>90 minutes	3
Donor **A**ge	
<21 years	0
21–40 years	1
41–50 years	2
>50 years	3
Total	__/14

Source data from Avtaar Singh et al., 2019.

targeted at the renin–angiotensin system (ACEi, ARBs neprilysin/angio-tensin receptor inhibitors), obesity, male sex, higher serum thyroxine level, preoperative IV heparin usage, aspirin, preoperative vasodilators (e.g. milrinone), prolonged bypass time, prior cardiac surgery, continuous-flow LVADs, and prolonged ischaemic time.

The pathogenesis of vasoplegic syndrome may have several mechanistic pathways which combine and contribute to the evolution of the shock state.

Current management strategies include titration of norepinephrine and vasopressin, with methylene blue, a direct NO synthase inhibitor, used as required for refractory hypotension. Additional treatment options including high-dose hydroxycobalamin and *N*-acetylcysteine have also been described though their role in management is less clear. In cases of refractory organ failure despite maximum dose vasoconstrictors, circulatory support should be considered.

Assessment and management of chronic complications following heart transplantation

Cardiac allograft vasculopathy

Definition

* Cardiac allograft vasculopathy (CAV) is a form of aggressive CAD that occurs following cardiac transplantation.
* Accelerated fibroproliferative disease resulting in pathological smooth muscle proliferation within the intima of the coronary vessels, with accumulation of inflammatory cells and lipid deposition.
* Circumferential intimal thickening—diffuse affecting epicardial and intramural coronary vessels (note contrast to coronary artery atherosclerosis).
* Almost one in three patients develop some form of CAV at 5 years and the condition is said to account for one in eight deaths beyond a year.

Pathophysiology

Involves a combination of immunological and non-immunological factors contributing to vascular inflammation, endothelial injury, and a cascade of vascular cell proliferation, fibrosis, and adverse remodelling (Table 18.1).

Table 18.1 Cardiac allograft vasculopathy pathophysiology

Immunological factors	Non-immunological factors
Histocompatibility mismatch	Age
Presence of HLA antibodies	Sex
Rejection—both cellular/antibody mediated	Obesity
	Dyslipidaemia
	Hypertension
	Smoking
	CMV infection
	Brain death
	Organ preservation
	Ischaemia-reperfusion injury
	Donor native atherosclerosis

Diagnosis

The recognition of early CAV as an adverse prognostic marker has led to awareness of the need for surveillance and early detection. Diagnosis can be challenging:

* Due to the cardiac denervation at the time of transplant, most patients do not experience anginal chest pain.
* Presentation can involve graft dysfunction noted on imaging, clinical HF, dysrhythmia, or even sudden cardiac death.
* Coronary angiography can be an insensitive tool due to the diffuse and concentric nature of CAV—it cannot visualize beyond the arterial lumen or beyond the larger epicardial vessels. Often luminal obstruction is a late phenomenon in CAV.

- Intravascular ultrasound can be employed in addition to routine coronary angiography, providing cross-sectional imaging of the lumen and vessel wall.
- The use of optical coherence tomography can provide high-resolution intravascular imaging that is suited to assess the vessel intimal and consequent plague morphology. However, it is limited by cost, contrast load, and lower tissue penetration.
- Imaging modalities such as dobutamine stress echocardiography, myocardial perfusion imaging, cardiac MRI, and CT coronary angiography may all have a role in detection of occult CAV.

Treatment and prevention

- Clinically, the main focus in treatment of cardiac allograft vasculopathy remains preventative. Primary prevention of CAV in heart transplant recipients should involve strict control of cardiovascular risk factors (hypertension/diabetes/hyperlipidaemia/smoking/obesity) as well as strategies to prevent CMV infection (ISHLT class I, level of evidence C).
- Aspirin: tends to be used empirically in routine post-transplant care, although little evidence to support its use (ISHLT class I, level of evidence C).
- Statin therapy: unfortunately, hyperlipidaemia is often the result of treatment with immunosuppressive regimens including steroids, ciclosporin, and tacrolimus. Statin therapy should be considered for all transplant recipients (ISHLT class I, level of evidence A).
- Mycophenolic acid: reduces progression of intimal thickening as compared to azathioprine and is the most preferred antimetabolite.
- In cardiac transplant recipients with established coronary allograft vasculopathy, the substitution of mycophenolate mofetil (MMF)/ azathioprine with sirolimus or everolimus can be considered (ISHLT class IIa, level C).
- Annual or biannual coronary angiography should be considered to assess the development of CAV (ISHLT class I, level C).
- Treatment options such as coronary angioplasty, PCI, and redo transplantation offer symptom control and palliative solutions once cardiac allograft vasculopathy has been established:
  - PCI may be limited due to the diffuse nature of the disease, distal vessel pruning, presence of diabetes/dyslipidaemia/renal dysfunction, and high rates of in-stent restenosis.
  - Drug-eluting stents are recommended (ISHLT class IIa, level of evidence C) and follow-up coronary angiography is recommended 6 months after a percutaneous intervention (ISHLT class I, level of evidence C).
  - Surgical revascularization is an option in highly selected patients but is associated with a high operative mortality.
  - The option of repeat cardiac transplantation exists, although this is rare in clinical practice and is associated with increased mortality and increased rates of subsequent CAV.

Common general side effects and complications of immunosuppression

Immunosuppression is essential in all heart recipients to prevent allograft rejection. As with all pharmacotherapy, these can be associated with side effects and interactions.

- Calcineurin inhibitors (CNIs) (tacrolimus/ciclosporin).
- Antiproliferative agents (mycophenolate mofetil (MMF)/azathioprine).
- Corticosteroids.
- Mechanistic target of rapamycin (mTOR) inhibitors (sirolimus/everolimus).

A typical immunosuppression regimen following cardiac transplantation includes an antiproliferative agent (e.g. MMF or azathioprine), a CNI (e.g. tacrolimus or ciclosporin), and, initially, a corticosteroid.

Calcineurin inhibitors

CNIs antagonize interleukin-2 (IL-2). The most commonly encountered agents are tacrolimus and ciclosporin. These each have different branded preparations. As different brands have potential diversity in bioavailability, a patient should ideally not be switched between brands or from branded to generic preparations without caution.

Tacrolimus

Complications/side effects

- Nephrotoxicity—care with co-administration of other nephrotoxic agents (e.g. gentamicin/vancomycin, NSAIDs).
- Diabetes mellitus.
- Neurotoxicity (most seriously—posterior reversible encephalopathy syndrome (PRES). Also, peripheral neuropathy, tremor, headache, paraesthesia).
- Electrolyte disturbance: hyperkalaemia (care with co-administration of other drug causing hyperkalaemia, e.g. spironolactone/ACEi, etc.), hypomagnesaemia.
- Nausea.
- Diarrhoea.
- Alopecia.

Ciclosporin

Side effects

- Hypertension.
- Nephrotoxicity—as per tacrolimus.
- Neurotoxicity (headaches, tremors, convulsions).
- Hyperkalaemia and hypomagnesaemia.
- Gingival hyperplasia.
- Hirsutism.
- Hepatic dysfunction.

Antiproliferative agents

Antiproliferative agents are generally required lifelong. The most commonly encountered agents are MMF and azathioprine.

Common side effects

- GI: nausea, anorexia, diarrhoea, oesophagitis, and abdominal pain most common.
- Minimized by taking the dose with food, or a dose reduction may be necessary.
- Changing from twice-daily to four times daily dosing may also help.
- Bone marrow suppression: MMF is less myelosuppressive than azathioprine.
- Adverse effects are usually reversed on discontinuation of MMF.
- Stop or reduce dose if white cell count <4 × 10⁹/L, or thrombocytopenia, cholestatic jaundice, or pancreatitis.
- Teratogenic: counsel young patients (male and female) accordingly as per Medicines and Healthcare products Regulatory Agency (MHRA) guidance.

Azathioprine

Usually given second line when MMF is not tolerated—typically, due to GI side effects.

Caution

Consider withholding in situations where bone marrow suppression is a concern, such as leuco/neutropenia, thrombocytopenia, or if there is evidence of jaundice.

Side effects

- Haematological abnormalities:
  - Bone marrow suppression.
  - Macrocytic anaemia.
- Hepatic abnormalities:
  - Jaundice.
  - Transaminitis.

Corticosteroids

Duration of treatment and dosing

- Corticosteroids are commenced immediately post transplantation, and are converted to an oral steroid tapering regimen (typically prednisolone).
- Corticosteroids are generally commenced at high dose during or immediately post transplantation. Weaning and withdrawal may be considered 3–6 months after transplant in low-risk patients (e.g. no circulating anti-HLA antibodies, non-multiparous women, no history of rejection, older age).

Consider weaning if corticosteroids cause significant side effects and there have been no recent (i.e. within 6 months) episodes of rejection.

Sirolimus

Sirolimus is a mTOR inhibitor. It is not first line but used in certain circumstances:
- Renal-sparing chronic immunosuppressive regimen (>3 months from transplant) in place of CNI.
- Maintenance immunosuppression in place of CNI in post-transplant lymphoproliferative disorder (PTLD).
- Maintenance immunosuppression in addition to CNI in significant CAV.
- Rejection refractory to tacrolimus and MMF.

Side effects

- Lipid disturbances: hyperlipidaemia, hypercholesterolaemia.
- Bone marrow suppression: thrombocytopenia, leucopenia, anaemia.
- Pharyngitis (usually transient).
- GI—diarrhoea, oral aphthous ulceration.
- Acneiform and other skin rashes.
- Significant proteinuria/nephrotic syndrome.
- Impaired wound healing—therefore caution needed in peri-transplant period.
- Drug-induced pneumonitis—rare but potentially serious.

Malignancy

More than 10% of heart transplant recipients developed a *de novo* malignancy 1–5 years post transplantation.

Skin cancers

Compared to the incidence of skin cancer in the general population, in heart transplant recipients, the incidence is approximately 65–250 times more frequent. More than 90% of cases are due to squamous and basal cell carcinomas. Squamous cell carcinoma tends to be more aggressive in the post-transplant patient in comparison to the general population, with greater metastatic potential and more local recurrence noted.

Factors that contribute to the development of skin malignancies:
- Duration of immunosuppression.
- Intensity of the immunosuppressive regimen used.
- Increasing age.
- Male sex.
- Caucasian.
- Smoking.
- Sun exposure.
- The presence of Epstein–Barr virus (EBV), human papillomavirus, herpes simplex virus (HSV), herpes zoster virus, and polyoma.

In clinical practice, yearly review at a specialist dermatology clinic is recommended and patients are counselled regarding reducing sun exposure.

Post-transplant lymphoproliferative disorder

PTLD encompasses disorders ranging from infectious mononucleosis to malignant lymphoma (T-cell/B-cell lymphoma, Hodgkin's lymphoma, and Hodgkin's like PTLD).

- Results from uncontrolled lymphoid growth in the immunosuppressed patient.
- PTLD has been reported in 6.4% of cardiac transplants.
- Over a 10-year period, the risk of a post-transplant patient developing lymphoma is 11.8 times higher than the general population.
- The pathogenesis of PTLD is a combination of immunosuppressive agents, infection by oncogenic viruses such as EBV, and possible genetic and epigenetic mutations.

Presentation

Often non-specific—fever, lymphadenopathy, weight loss, abdominal pain, splenomegaly, etc. Often presents at extranodal sites (e.g. GI tract).

Diagnosis

Excisional biopsies are preferred and fine needle aspiration should be avoided where possible. Staining for EBV is mandatory.

Treatment

- Modification and reduction of immunosuppression regimen wherever possible.
- Surgery for localized disease.
- Localized radiotherapy.
- Targeted chemotherapy (most commonly used regimen CHOP/rituximab).
- More recently, adoptive T-cell immunotherapy (via infusion of EBV-specific cytotoxic T lymphocytes in patients with EBV-positive PTLD) has shown some promise but presently is far from established in clinical practice.

Solid organ malignancies

There is no specific evidence to recommend reduction in immunosuppression in patients with solid tumours unrelated to the lymphoid system. A multidisciplinary team approach involving the transplant team and oncologists to tailor strategies on a case-by-case basis is advised.

Heart transplant recipients should undergo routine screening for breast, colon, and prostate cancer as per the general population recommendations.

Infection

Infection in transplant patients can range from mild to fatal.

General principles

- Infection is one of the leading causes of death in transplant recipients.
- The need for effective lifelong immunosuppression places patients at an increased risk of developing infection.
- Pathogens may be bacterial, viral, fungal, or protozoal.
- The pathophysiological response to infection is altered which can make timely diagnosis challenging.
- Responsible microorganisms can differ from those affecting the general population.
- Common microorganisms include CMV, *Candida* species, Gram-negative bacilli, staphylococci, and *Pneumocystis jirovecii*.

- Common sites of infection include the respiratory tract, mouth, skin, and urinary tract.
- Less common sites such as CNS infection should always be considered.
- Consider temporary suspension of antiproliferative agents in severe infection or leucopenia/neutropenia.
- In all cases, the cardiac transplant recipient with infection should be managed in close discussion with the transplant medicine, infectious diseases, and microbiology team.

Physiological response to infection in the immunosuppressed

- Immunosuppressive medication (particularly antiproliferative agents) attenuate the physiological ability to generate pyrexia and leucocytosis in response to infection.
- Corticosteroids do not appear to have these effects, but may mask clinical signs of infection, allowing the condition to worsen and present late.

CMV infection

- Symptoms can be initially be constitutional and generalized if CMV viraemia with no end-organ involvement.
- Sometimes there may be focal organ involvement and specific related symptoms (e.g. retinitis, pneumonitis, colitis, hepatitis).
- Treatment guided by monitoring blood for CMV by PCR.
- Antimicrobial therapy generally involves ganciclovir first line.

Pneumocystis jirovecii infection

See Fig. 18.1.
- Consider in the patient with shortness of breath or other respiratory tract symptoms.
- Pulse oximetry on exertion should be performed. Classically, this would show an exertional drop in saturations.
- There should be a low threshold for bronchoalveolar lavage if there is a high index of suspicion.
- Management is with respiratory support and aggressive antimicrobial therapy—usually co-trimoxazole (adjusted for renal function).
- Alternatives (e.g. in G6PD deficiency, sulfa allergies) include a combination of dapsone ± trimethoprim or pyrimethamine, atovaquone, or clindamycin and pyrimethamine.
- Consider concurrent steroids and folinic acid.
- Oral prophylaxis should continue indefinitely following recovery.

Infective endocarditis prophylaxis

- Limited evidence to support any particular approach.
- Transplant recipients at increased risk of valvular disease.
- Outcomes in infective endocarditis are extremely poor.
- Reasonable to give antibiotic prophylaxis prior to dental procedures in transplant recipients with valvular heart disease.

(a)

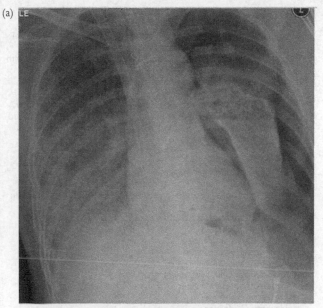

(b)

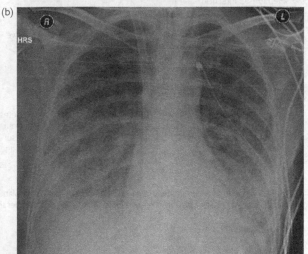

Fig. 18.1 Anteroposterior CXRs demonstrating *Pneumocystis jirovecii* infection. Sternotomy wires from cardiac transplantation, VV ECMO cannula *in situ* (a), and left intercostal chest drain for associated left-sided pneumothorax (b) are also seen. See plate section.

Diabetes mellitus

- Deranged glucose metabolism and development of diabetes mellitus is common following cardiac transplantation.
- The chances of developing diabetes post transplantation increases with time and may occur as late as 15 years post transplantation.
- Some series report rates up to 32% at 5 years following heart transplantation.
- The International Consensus Guidelines for new-onset diabetes after transplantation (NODAT) were published in 2003, and although based on renal transplant patients, they have been adopted in the setting of other solid organ transplants.

Risk factors

- Risk factors for developing diabetes following heart transplantation are not well defined, but higher preoperative blood glucose levels, corticosteroid dose post-transplantation, and family history have been predictive in some populations.
- In liver and kidney transplantation, risk factors are more extensively defined and include:
  - Black/Hispanic ethnicity.
  - Family history of diabetes.
  - Age >40 years.
  - Pre-transplant glucose intolerance.
  - Immunosuppressive agents.
  - Metabolic syndrome.
  - Hepatitis C infection.
  - Cadaveric kidney.
  - Obesity.
- In many cases, diabetes may develop as a result of immunosuppressive medication (e.g. corticosteroids, tacrolimus) which cause hyperglycaemia by increasing insulin resistance.
- Ciclosporin confers less of a risk than tacrolimus.

Consequences of developing diabetes following heart transplantation

Though data are limited to relatively small populations, developing diabetes following heart transplantation appears to be associated with worse outcomes, notably, increased risk of serious infection, reduced long-term survival, increased risk of ischaemic heart disease, cardiovascular mortality, and risk of developing CAV.

Diagnosis

The NODAT guidelines recommend that diabetes in the post-transplant population should be diagnosed by the same criteria as used for the general population, namely:
- Symptoms of diabetes, and:
  - Random glucose ≥11.1 mmol/L or 200 mg/dL or
  - Fasting glucose ≥7 mmol/L or 126 mg/dL or
  - Plasma glucose ≥11.1 mmol/L or 200 mg/dL 2 hours following a 75 g glucose load.

- HbA1c has been adopted as a diagnostic test for diabetes since the publication of the NODAT guidelines in 2003. A threshold of ≥48 mmol/mol or 7.8% is diagnostic of diabetes mellitus in the presence of symptoms.
- In asymptomatic patients, HbA1c should be repeated in 6 months, or sooner if risk of developing diabetes is high.

Management

- Finger-prick glucose should be monitored weekly for the first 4 weeks following transplantation, then at 3 and 6 months, then annually.
- If a patient develops diabetes, assess other risk factors such as serum lipid profile, blood pressure, and evidence of end-organ complications.
- Stepwise management of diabetes will include:
  - Conservative measures: dietary and lifestyle advice.
  - Oral anti-hyperglycaemics.
  - Insulin.
  - Combination of oral anti-hyperglycaemics and insulin.
  - Transplant-specific considerations: modification of immunosuppression (reducing corticosteroid dose, ciclosporin as an alternative to tacrolimus).
- A specialist in diabetes should be involved in the care of the post-transplant patient with new diabetes.
- Disordered lipid profile and hypertension should be treated aggressively to reduce the risk of diabetic complications.

Oral anti-hyperglycaemic agents

- The choice of oral agent should be tailored to the patient based on factors such as weight, renal function, and occupation (i.e. if hypoglycaemic episodes would be dangerous).
- Thiazolidinediones can cause fluid retention and HF. Conversely, sodium-glucose co-transporter 2 (SGLT2) inhibitors reduce adverse events in HF with reduced ejection fraction. No robust data exist examining their use in the post-heart transplant recipient.

Bone mineral density loss and osteoporosis

- Cardiac transplant recipients require prolonged courses of prednisolone or high doses of IV methylprednisolone (in cases of rejection) and are therefore at high risk of developing corticosteroid-related bone disease.
- Prevention strategies should be considered early in a patient's transplantation journey, particularly as rapid bone loss and fractures generally occur during the first 3–12 months post transplantation.

Pre transplantation

All adult heart transplant patients should be screened for pre-existing bone disease prior to placement on the transplant waiting list wherever feasible. Baseline bone mineral density is obtained with a dual-energy X-ray absorptiometry scan of lumbar spine and neck of femur. A bone mineral density score is calculated (T score and Z score).

The presence of pre-existing low bone mineral density should prompt further evaluation and treatment of any correctable causes. Bisphosphonate therapy is recommended where indicated.

All patients are advised on the recommended daily allowance of calcium (1000–1500 mg) and vitamin D (400–1000 IU) to maintain serum 25-hydroxyvitamin D levels >30 ng/mL.

Post transplantation

Patients are encouraged regarding regular weight-bearing and muscle-strengthening exercise.

All patients should begin regular bisphosphonate therapy immediately after transplantation and continue for at least the first post-transplant year (or longer if necessary). IV therapy is an option for patients who are unable to safely swallow tablets in the immediate post-transplant phase.

Bone mineral density is usually reassessed at the 1-year post-transplant mark. It is reasonable to stop the bisphosphonate if corticosteroids have been discontinued and bone mineral density is preserved (T score >1.5).

Chronic kidney disease

Causes

Renal dysfunction can result from a variety of causes including hypertension, immunosuppressive therapy (in particular, CNIs), and recurrence of HF.

Screening

Check an eGFR at least annually, more frequently if <60 mL/min/1.73 m² and/or decline by >4 mL/min/1.73 m² per year.

Management

- Consider referral to specialist renal services if eGFR decreases to <30 mL/min/1.73 m².
- Measures that have been showed to slow progression of chronic kidney disease in the general population should be applied to heart transplant recipients:
  - Aggressively control abnormalities in blood pressure and blood glucose.
  - Consider introducing an ACEi/ARB.
- Check haemoglobin at least annually.
- If low, check iron status and commence erythropoiesis-stimulating agents where appropriate, targeting haemoglobin 110–130 mg/L or 11–13 g/dL.

- End-stage renal failure should be preferentially managed with kidney transplantation in all heart transplant recipients for whom this is appropriate.

Immunosuppression adjustment

- Renal-sparing immunosuppression strategies can be considered in select cases. These can involve either replacement of a CNI with a different agent (e.g. sirolimus) or stopping CNI with subsequent maintenance on a corticosteroid/antiproliferative agent dual-agent regimen. Caution is advised in patients with a history of rejection or those with circulating donor specific antibodies.
- If CNIs are continued, lower the target level to the minimum acceptable to prevent rejection.

Hypertension

- Although there is limited specific evidence pertaining to hypertension in the post-cardiac transplant population, it is generally recognized that the same blood pressure targets should be sought as for the general population.
- Lifestyle factors such as increased exercise, weight loss, and reducing dietary salt and fat should be advocated.
- Medical management should follow established guidance, and will generally involve calcium channel blockers or ACEis/ARBs as first-line therapy.
- Calcium channel blockers are often preferred due to their renal-sparing properties.
- Both dihydropyridine and non-dihydropyridine calcium channel blockers can interfere with metabolism of CNIs, resulting in CNI toxicity.
- As such, close monitoring of therapeutic CNI levels should be considered when commencing a calcium channel blocker.
- Presence of other comorbidities should be taken into account as this may guide choice of an initial agent (e.g. ACEi/ARB in patients with diabetes mellitus).
- Combination of two agents (e.g. ACEi/ARB and calcium channel blocker) may be required to achieve adequate control.
- Screening for additional risk factors such as high cholesterol or diabetes mellitus should be undertaken.
- End-organ damage should be assessed for and treated, such as urine dip for protein/formal urinary protein:creatinine to assess for nephropathy, and fundoscopy to assess for hypertensive retinopathy.

Reproductive health and pregnancy

Pregnancy

- Having children is very important to many patients following cardiac transplantation.
- Clinicians should take a patient-centred approach to discussions surrounding pregnancy and should support patients and their families.

- Ideally, pregnancies should be planned and monitored with involvement from the multidisciplinary team. This would typically include specialists such as an obstetrician specializing in maternal and fetal medicine, a neonatologist, psychologist, clinical geneticist, transplant cardiologist, an anaesthetist, and the patient's primary care doctor and midwife.

Female patients

Pre-conception counselling

- The approach to managing a pregnant transplant recipient should be individualized according to patient factors such as immunosuppressive regimen, graft function, time since transplantation, and the patient's own wishes and preferences.
- Ideally, pregnancy would be delayed until at least 1 year following cardiac transplantation.
- The likely risks of complications such as infection, rejection, cardiac graft vasculopathy, and fetal abnormality, should be considered and communicated to the patient.
- If, despite the best efforts to modify them, the risk of any of the above factors is high enough to preclude a successful pregnancy and birth, the patient should be advised against pregnancy.

Immunosuppression

- Immunosuppressive regimen should be reviewed and modified by reducing/switching any agents likely to be teratogenic or toxic to fetal growth, and graft function assessed on the modified regimen to ensure stability.
- MMF should be discontinued.
- CNIs and corticosteroids can be continued.
- CNI levels may fluctuate due to physiological changes in plasma volume and renal function in pregnancy and should be monitored closely.

Male patients

- Patients hoping to achieve pregnancy with a female partner should have their immunosuppressive regimens reviewed and modified.
- MMF should be discontinued.

Hormonal contraception

As these agents inhibit cytochrome P450, monitor CNI drug levels carefully.

Barrier methods

Barrier methods such as the male or female condom should be advocated as an adjunct to other methods of contraception and to reduce risk of sexually transmitted infection.

Psychological disorders

General principles

- Robust psychological assessment is mandatory prior to cardiac transplantation to ensure candidacy for the procedure.
- A nurse specialist or psychologist should be accessible for all patients following cardiac transplantation for any problems that may arise.

Adherence to therapy

• Review the patient's adherence to therapy at each outpatient visit, being sure to identify and address any barriers to adherence using a patient-centred solution-focused approach.

Depression

• Screen for evidence of depression routinely during follow-up.
• Any patients found to have depression should have input from a psychologist and the wider multidisciplinary team.
• Pharmacotherapy:
  • Selective serotonin reuptake inhibitors do not impact haemodynamics or cardiac conduction so represent a good choice.
  • Avoid cytochrome P450 agents as these may interact with tacrolimus metabolism and alter levels.

Recurrence of heart failure and retransplantation

• May arise from a range of pathologies—valvular failure (e.g. TR arising from damage from right heart procedures such as endomyocardial biopsy), chronic rejection, or ischaemic heart disease from graft vasculopathy.
• Limited evidence base for recurrent cardiac failure following cardiac transplantation, but generally managed as for failure in a native heart with disease-modifying therapies— Angiotensin receptor-neprilysin inhibitor (ARNI)/ACEi/ARB, BB, MRA, SGLT2 inhibitor.
• Retransplantation can be considered in the following circumstances:
  • CAV not amenable to medical therapy, or revascularization either percutaneously or surgically, where there is clinical evidence of HF or myocardial ischaemia.
  • CAV not amenable to medical therapy or revascularization, with asymptomatic moderate to severe LV systolic dysfunction.
  • Allograft dysfunction and clinical manifestations of HF without evidence of acute rejection.
• The decision to list for retransplantation should be made by the wider transplant multidisciplinary team, taking into consideration changes in the patient's comorbidities and biopsychosocial circumstances, as these may affect eligibility.
• The patient's views and wishes should be taken into account in any decision to pursue retransplantation.

Bedside care and rehabilitation with mechanical circulatory support and thoracic transplantation

Introduction

Myopathy and polyneuropathy of critical illness is a well-recognized major complication in ICU patients. Hence, there is a move towards early mobilization and physical therapy (PT) to optimize postoperative recovery and to reduce the rate of physical and psychological deconditioning.

In this chapter, we present strategies for ambulation and rehabilitation in patients with long-term IABP, MCS, and those who have undergone cardiopulmonary transplantation.

Rehabilitation of patients with IABP and MCS

There is ample evidence that early mobilization after implantation of IABP and MCS confers great benefits to patients both physically and psychologically while they await organ transplantation. However, there are some inherent risks with ambulation, which should be weighed against its benefits. Furthermore, ambulation of HF patients on IABP or MCS is very time and resource consuming. There are a few barriers to ambulation, some of which include haemodynamic instability, presence of multiple lines and cannulas, muscle weakness, altered mental status, and shortage of staff or equipment required to ambulate the patient safely.

MCS patients may have up to four additional cannulas in the case of extracorporeal biventricular support as compared to the routine adult cardiac surgery patients. On transport, ECG, pulse oximetry, and PA and arterial lines pressures should be monitored closely. However, interpretation of haemodynamic parameters for MCS patients may be more difficult. The pump speed and flow parameters should also be taken into consideration prior to ambulation.

Prior to ambulation of the IABP or MCS patient, anticoagulation status should be noted; suboptimal anticoagulation and presence of thrombus in the oxygenator/external tubing may preclude ambulation due to risk of embolization. Overzealous anticoagulation predisposes patients to bleeding (trauma from falls, stress on cannulation sites and wounds).

IABP ambulation strategy

IABPs are traditionally inserted via the femoral artery, which limits the patient in terms of PT, as ambulation is often institutionally prohibited with the device in the femoral artery position. Not only is insertion site bleeding a possibility, but the IABP may become kinked with hip flexion leading to malfunction or rupture during ambulation. Patients with femoral IABPs should be turned at least 30° from side to side every 2 hours, have active and passive range of motion, and have the bed placed in reverse Trendelenburg position.

Alternative sites which would allow for more liberal ambulation are where IABP catheters are sited in the axillary or subclavian positions (see Chapter 9). These alternative positions would allow for mobilization out of bed, sitting on the chair or the commode, and walking. However, axillary or subclavian positions preclude arm raising above the head level on the side of the IABP to avoid the risk of catheter displacement. An elbow immobilizer may be used.

Ambulation should be performed in stages to avoid orthostatic hypotension. The patient and the medical team should be mindful of the increased risk of catheter migration with ambulation, which may require IABP repositioning. Patients with an axillary IABP should have the radial pulse on the ipsilateral side verified and the function and sensation of the upper extremity assessed before and after ambulation. If there is a suspicion of IABP displacement, a plain CXR would be indicated and repositioning can be undertaken at the bedside using fluoroscopy.

MCS ambulation strategy

ECMO and LVAD may be instituted centrally or peripherally. Common peripheral sites include the IJ veins, subclavian veins, the subclavian or axillary arteries, and femoral arteries and veins. Ambulation with an open sternum is contraindicated. Femoral cannulation may prove ambulation more challenging but is not a contraindication. While all cannulas are affixed securely at the time of cannulation, these should be examined before and after ambulation regimentally as there remains an inherent risk of cannula displacement leading to flow interruptions, limb ischaemia, and vascular injury.

The procedure for mobilizing patients with all forms of MCS is similar, although patients requiring ECMO are typically more acutely ill and require more support.

The following checklist should be completed prior to ambulation of MCS patients:

- All team members have discussed pertinent information and safety concerns.
- The patient can follow verbal directions and communicate answers to questions.
- For patients unable to verbalize, 'yes' and 'no' signals are clearly demonstrated.
- Body strength assessment is adequate.
- The patient is doing well (no significant bleeding, excessive fluid volume requirements, or electrolyte abnormalities).
- The patient has maintained adequate baseline oxygenation and haemodynamic stability in the sitting and standing positions.

If the patient does not meet all of these criteria or if adequate resources are not available to ambulate the patient safely, ambulation session should be postponed. Ideally, the patient should receive daily ambulation with PT which should be detailed in their occupational therapy plan of care.

Recommended ambulation procedure checklist

- Prior to each ambulation session, the aforementioned checklist is validated.
- Roles are clearly assigned and defined among the ambulating team.
- The route along the ward is created and decluttered.
- Two personnel jointly assess that the cannula sites are secure for ambulation (e.g. an arm sling for upper chest cannulation immobilizes that arm). A headband with self-adhering wrap or indwelling catheter securing devices secures neck cannulas to the head. Binders are worn for tunnelled cannulas.

- The MCS device console battery is checked prior to each ambulation and the gas tanks are verified to be adequately filled. Emergency back-up equipment or hand cranks are available as are tubing clamps and hospital standard MCS emergency supplies.
- The patient should stand only with the assistance of a fully trained physical therapist.
- Prior to each ambulation, the patient will perform weight shifting and marching on the spot. If stable with these, the patient will then take a few test steps prior to leaving the room. If a concern is raised by the patient or any member of the team regarding ambulation at this time, the effort will be paused, and issues rectified.
- The primary nurse will watch the monitor at all times and alert the team of any changes.
- A staff member will be in direct physical contact with the patient at all times.
- One clinical provider should carry a chair behind the patient. Should ambulation need to stop prior to returning to the room, the patient will sit on a chair and be wheeled back.
- Upon returning to the room, the care providers should reinstitute monitoring in the patient's room as per routine, remove stabilization equipment, and secure cannulation sites.
- Two staff members will re-examine cannulation sites.

Durable LVAD ambulation strategy

Durable (long-term) LVAD patients should be educated on how to incorporate the controller and batteries into their day-to-day activities, and physically adjust to the additional weight of the batteries and controller. The changes in gait, posture, and balance from the additional weight of the device and its batteries may result in early fatigue and can lead to falls.

PT in durable LVAD patients should be commenced in the immediate post-LVAD implantation period in the ICU, once the chest is closed, the patient is extubated, and is haemodynamically stable. A physiotherapist familiar with LVADs should evaluate the patient, set goals, and create a treatment plan. PT usually starts with lower extremity exercises in bed, followed by sitting on the edge of the bed, standing, and then gait training with a walker. Adverse effects of PT with durable LVAD patients are few and decreased pump flows are common. Keeping LVAD flows at >3 L/min during PT is recommended.

The driveline should be well secured to the skin and immobilized with a binder since excessive movement and jarring can result in driveline infections. Movements should be slow and steady, as rapid standing can cause orthostatic hypotension. Kinking or twisting of the driveline should be avoided. The PT session should be discontinued if there are significant fluctuations in LVAD flows, hypotension, chest pains, extreme fatigue, or by patient request.

Outpatient cardiac rehabilitation in durable VAD recipients has been associated with lower re-hospitalization rates and mortality risk.

Nutrition

Commencing feeds within 24 hours is recommended in the LVAD patient to prevent weight loss and ileus; feeding in VA ECMO patients within 2 days of its initiation has been associated with decreased mortality.

In many cases, enteric feeding tubes are placed as soon as the patient is haemodynamically stable and coagulation screen is appropriate. If the nasoenteric feeding tube can be placed before systemic anticoagulation is started, the risk of epistaxis is lower; epistaxis can be severe in the anticoagulated patient and can lead to aspiration.

Lung transplant patients with gastro-oesophageal reflux disease have a higher incidence of PGD, and should ideally be fed via a post-pyloric enteric tube (initiated at 10–15 cc/hour, then advanced to meet caloric goals). Swallowing assessment should be performed prior to commencing oral nutrition to avoid aspiration.

The ICU cardiopulmonary transplant and MCS patients are routinely suboptimally fed, for example, due to haemodynamic instability, GI intolerance, or if they are fasted pending further procedures or operations. Signs such as abdominal distention/pain, vomiting, residual gastric volumes >200 mL (if feeding in the stomach), and diarrhoea can indicate intolerance of enteral nutrition, which may be helped by prokinetic agents. Use of muscle relaxants, sedation, or prone positioning are not contraindications to nasoenteric feeding.

Daily protein requirements for patients on ECMO have been recommended at 1.2 g/kg ideal body weight, with energy requirements determined by using the Schofield equation and multiplying by 1.1–1.2; sodium administration should be kept to <2000 mg/day. If the patient is obese (BMI >30 kg/m^2), consider using the patient's ideal body weight to determine protein and caloric needs.

Rehabilitation post heart/ lung transplantation

Following heart/lung transplantation, close observation and monitoring is of paramount importance. Some of these observations are as follows:
- Respiration rate, oxygen saturations, oxygen therapy, and arterial blood gases.
- Blood pressure, heart rate, and temperature.
- CVP.
- Temporary pacing.
- Telemetry.
- Chest drain output.
- Fluid balance (avoid fluid overload).
- Daily weight (echocardiogram and diuretics if weight increasing).
- Blood tests (complete blood count, renal function, and coagulation screen).
- CXR (looking for fluid overload, effusion, pneumothorax, etc.).
- Immunosuppressant level assay.
- Nutritional assessment.
- Serum glucose measurement.
- Evidence of infection (wounds, respiratory, lines).

Pain management

Optimal pain management is key to patient comfort, and speedy recovery in the postoperative period. Effective pain management improves the ability to take deep breaths, cough and expectorate, sleep, mobilize, and perform self-care. The World Health Organization (WHO) pain ladder should be adhered to. In cases of inadequate pain control, consultation with the 'chronic pain team' would ensure sufficient follow-up and continuity of care regarding pain management.

Wound management

Sternotomy, thoracotomy, and clamshell wounds can take up to 4 months to fully heal in routine heart–lung surgery. However, the impact of major surgery, combined with long-term chronic illness, deconditioned state, comorbidities, and immunosuppressive drug regimen, means that the transplant recipients often experience a longer period of wound healing and carry a higher risk of wound complications such as superficial (involving skin/subcutaneous tissue) or deep wound infections (involving the mediastinum/sternum).

Psychological rehabilitation

Emotional health affects physical health. The most common presentations, following the acute physiological impact of cardiopulmonary transplantation include anxiety, depression, post-traumatic stress, and 'survival guilt'. Occasionally, recipients may develop steroid psychosis, delirium, delusions, or hallucinations. It is important, therefore, to consider the role of medications in any psychological presentation. Patient concerns regarding physical challenges of lifestyle modification following cardiopulmonary transplantation, fear of life- or limb-threatening complications, and mortality, as well as non-physical challenges (e.g. financial and social), lead to psychological burden which would require support and intervention. Psychological/psychiatric support should be sought readily in such patients. The use of antidepressants, antipsychotics, or anxiolytics can be helpful in overcoming some of the sequalae of acute psychiatric decompensation. However, the medical and social services team should, whenever possible, strive to resolve the underlying aetiology of the stressors, for example, by providing social support or fund raising for financial support to ensure the best possible prognosis.

Physical rehabilitation

Rehabilitation is influenced by the length of time in ICU. Skeletal muscle mass loss can be as much as 5–20% after 7–10 days in the ICU.

A programme of physical exercise post transplantation would aim to improve muscle strength and exercise tolerance. It is also beneficial in reducing risks of hypertension, obesity, and osteoporosis and psychological dysfunction.

A combination of aerobic, resistance, and endurance exercise and physical rehabilitation is beneficial to both heart and lung recipients. Physiotherapy is implemented immediately post transplantation to optimize recovery and continues to be expanded throughout the rehabilitation programme.

A programme is determined by the multidisciplinary team of clinicians, physiotherapists, and occupational therapists and depends on various factors including:

- Degree of frailty prior to transplantation.
- Organ implanted (heart or lung).
- Physiological alterations post transplantation.
- Complications post surgery.
- Comorbidities.

Physiological alterations post cardiac transplantation which influence exercise capacity may include surgical denervation of the transplanted heart, decrease in chronotropic competence, cardiac function, vascular endothelium, and pulmonary diffusion.

In the absence of clear evidence to support a 'one-size-fits-all' exercise programme, an individually tailored plan is required. Currently, there is no evidence to categorically indicate a recommendation for one rehabilitation programme over another. Exercise regimens are currently based on developing the frequency, intensity, timing, and type of exercise and adopting an integrative approach to building individual programmes, which incorporate both cardiac and respiratory rehabilitation.

Patient education programme

Successful transplantation requires the recipient's full cooperation as well as adequate social support. It is imperative that the organ recipients are made aware of the risks and what is required of them.

Patient education before transplantation provides the opportunity for recipients to gain information on the following topics:

- Transplant-specific information.
- Surgical procedure and complications.
- In-hospital course.
- PGD and rejection.
- Importance of compliance with treatment.
- Implications for employment.
- Outcomes.

Leaflets and patient information sheets should be provided in the pre-transplantation interval to the patient and family members.

Self-medication programme

The success of the transplant patient is dependent on adherence to the self-medication programme. This is a lifetime commitment. Recipients are educated in the importance of adherence to a strict regimen. They should be educated in the role of each medication, the time and method of administration of each, maintaining a meticulous medication diary, as well as any changes in their weight and temperature. Such information may prove invaluable for the transplant team in subsequent clinic visits.

Infection

Transplant recipients are prone to opportunistic infections which could be bacterial, viral, or fungal, due to the high levels of immunosuppressive medications (see Chapters 21 and 30).

Rejection

Rejection is unpredictable in its frequency and severity. The recipient is educated in the signs of rejection (see Chapters 20 and 28).

Follow-up clinic

In the first 6 months, frequent visits are scheduled and the intervals are variable depending on unit protocols. In the interval period between clinic visits, the organ recipient will have an assigned contact in the transplant unit whom they can get in touch with for any queries or concerns. Education continues in follow-up clinics and recipients are made aware of the importance of continued dose monitoring, identification of complications, infection, rejection, and prompt intervention.

Management of rejection following cardiac transplantation

Induction of immunosuppression

Acute rejection and graft failure continue to be common causes of death in the first 30 days after cardiac transplantation. Induction immunosuppression regimens are therefore administered immediately after cardiac transplantation to decrease the risk of acute rejection while maintenance immunosuppressive regimens are initiated and titrated. The potential benefits of induction therapy include (1) decreased early rejection, (2) the ability to delay initiation of nephrotoxic maintenance CNIs, and (3) the opportunity to decrease corticosteroid dosing. There are potential risks including early infections and increased risk of malignancy hence the decision to utilize induction immunosuppression is often individualized, taking into account individual recipient factors (e.g. baseline renal function, pre-sensitization, younger age, female sex, and African American race) that may confer higher rejection risks.

Induction immunosuppression regimens typically include one of the following: interleukin-2 receptor antagonist (IL2RA; basiliximab), polyclonal anti-thymocyte antibodies (ATG), or historically and least commonly a murine monoclonal antibody that binds to the T-cell receptor–CD3 complex (OKT3) (Table 20.1). These agents, when given, are administered along with high-dose corticosteroids.

International Heart and Lung Transplant Registry data suggest more than half of transplant recipients receive some form of induction immunosuppression with approximately 30% of recipients receiving IL2RA and approximately 20% receiving polyclonal ATG. However, the recommendation for induction therapy is based on limited prospective randomized controlled clinical trial data. Data from recent meta-analyses do not suggest any difference in all-cause mortality, infection, or malignancy with the use of induction immunosuppression with either IL2RA or ATG. The data are mixed in terms of impact on rejection, with some analyses suggesting a reduction in acute rejection with induction therapy with either IL2RA or ATG compared to no induction, and others reporting no difference in moderate or severe rejection with induction therapy. In non-randomized studies, there are also data to suggest that ATG-based induction therapy may be associated with less acute rejection compared with IL2RA.

Anti-thymocyte globulin

ATGs are polyclonal immunoglobulin (Ig)-G antibodies derived from immunization of rabbits (rATG) or horses (eATG) with human thymocytes. As a result, ATG is comprised of cytotoxic antibodies directed against a wide array of epitopes found on antigens expressed by human T lymphocytes. The antibody–antigen interactions have been found to affect a spectrum of immune processes both in the peripheral blood and lymphoid tissue. Antibody binding has been implicated in the following: (1) depletion of T and B cells by both cytolysis and apoptosis, (2) modulation of cell adhesion, (3) interruption of cell signalling necessary for immune activation, (4) depletion of both immature and mature dendritic cells responsible for tolerance and T-cell activation, and (5) expansion of regulatory T cells necessary for immune tolerance.

ATG is highly immunosuppressive in the timespan of weeks to months after administration and causes a dose-dependent depletion of T cells.

Table 20.1 Induction immunosuppression

Agent	Mechanism of action	Typical dosage	Considerations
Basiliximab	IL2RA	2D mg IV post operative day 0 and 4	Common indications: abnormal baseline renal function, diabetes, elevated panel-reactive antibodies (PRAs), transplant from LVAD, young female recipients
ATG	Polyclonal, cytotoxic anti-thymocyte antibodies	1.5 mg/ kg/day for 3–5 days	Prophylaxis against infusion reactions is common. Monitor for leucopenia and thrombocytopenia
Alemtuzumab	Monoclonal antibody against CD52 receptor	3D mg IV once intra operatively	Can cause serious infusion reaction, bone marrow suppression, and lymphopenia
Muromonab	Monoclonal antibody against T-cell receptor–CD3 complex	5 mg/day	Can cause fatal cytokine release syndrome usually between the first and second doses

Given that these antibodies are rabbit or horse derived, they are contra-indicated in individuals who have allergy or anaphylaxis to rabbit or horse proteins. Prophylaxis against infusion reactions is commonly administered including diphenhydramine, acetaminophen, and corticosteroids (which are given in high doses during induction). The most common adverse effects include leucopenia and thrombocytopenia which may require dose reduction by 50% for white blood cell count of $2-3 \times 10^9$/L or platelets $50-75 \times 10^9$/l or discontinuation if white blood cell count $<2 \times 10^9$/L or platelets $<50 \times 10^9$/L. Prophylaxis against CMV is necessary in moderate to higher risk recipients during treatment with IV ganciclovir with a transition to oral valganciclovir after treatment.

Basiliximab

Basiliximab is a chimeric mouse–human monoclonal antibody with specificity to CD25, the alpha chain of the interleukin-2 receptor (IL2R) on T cells. Antibody–antigen binding disrupts the subsequent clonal proliferation of activated T cells. Basiliximab is administered on postoperative day 0 and postoperative day 4 for induction therapy and saturates the IL2R for 4–6 weeks. Basiliximab has not been associated with a cytokine release syndrome.

Alemtuzumab

Alemtuzumab is a humanized rat monoclonal antibody with specificity to the CD52 receptor present on not only B and T cells but also other immune cells including neutrophils, natural killer cells, and eosinophils. Binding of alemtuzumab leads to initial activation but subsequent complement and antibody-mediated cytolysis of B and T cells. It is used less frequently in cardiac transplantation and is associated with infusion reactions and bone marrow suppression.

Muromonab

Muromonab (OKT3) is a murine-derived monoclonal antibody with specificity for the CD3 coreceptor on T cells. Antibody–antigen binding to the CD3–T-cell receptor complex leads to initial activation but subsequent rapid depletion in CD3+ T cells via apoptosis. The initial activation leads to a cytokine release syndrome with release of interferon gamma and tumour necrosis factor which can be life-threatening. Given the adverse effect profile, OKT3 is rarely used. Similar to ATG, premedication with diphenhydramine and acetaminophen is necessary.

Maintenance immunosuppression

The basis of maintenance immunosuppression regimens consists of three pharmacological classes of medications including CNIs such as tacrolimus or ciclosporin, antiproliferative agents such as MMF or azathioprine, and corticosteroids such as prednisone. In addition, inhibitors of the mTOR can be used in lieu of or in addition to CNIs when CAV is detected or instead of CNIs when there is intolerance or toxicity (i.e. renal toxicity).

The goal of triple drug therapy is to target separate biochemical pathways for immune-modulation while minimizing dose-dependent drug toxicities and oversuppression of the immune system that can increase infectious and malignancy risks. Since the risk of acute rejection is highest in the first year after transplantation, maintenance regimens are designed to begin with higher levels of drug therapy that tapers during the first year with more frequent surveillance until a low-dose two- or three-drug regimen can be achieved without significant graft rejection.

Calcineurin inhibitors

The CNIs ciclosporin and tacrolimus form the foundation of immunosuppressive regimens in cardiac transplant. Both drugs ultimately inhibit the transcription of IL-2 among several other proinflammatory cytokines but do so with slightly different mechanisms.

Ciclosporin is a cyclic peptide consisting of 11 amino acids derived from fungus and binds to cyclophilin in the cell cytoplasm; this complex inhibits calcineurin. Under normal conditions, calcineurin is a phosphatase which dephosphorylates the transcription factor NF-AT which allows for transcription of IL-2 and other related cytokines such as tumour necrosis factor alpha, granulocyte colony-stimulating factor, interferon gamma, IL-4, and CD40L. Calcineurin inhibition impairs the transcription of these cytokines, particularly in helper T cells and decreases effector T-cell activation and proliferation.

Tacrolimus is a macrolide also derived from fungus which inhibits calcineurin by binding to a different cytoplasmic protein called FKBP with similar downstream reduction in transcription of IL-2 and related cytokines.

There are several important toxicities to CNIs that require careful monitoring and these include hypertension, dyslipidaemia, new-onset diabetes, renal insufficiency, hypomagnesaemia, and hyperkalaemia for tacrolimus versus hypokalaemia for ciclosporin, and neurological side effect such as seizures, headache, tremors, and posterior reversible encephalopathy syndrome (i.e. PRES). Ciclosporin has a few unique adverse effects including hirsutism and gingival hyperplasia.

Several randomized controlled trials compared tacrolimus to ciclosporin-based regimens and, overall, the survival is similar but tacrolimus has a better side effect profile and lower rejection rates. Given the variable toxicities and risk for both infection and malignancy with CNIs, serum drug level monitoring is imperative. While target trough concentrations are individualized based on balancing history of rejection, infection, and other toxicities, general guidelines are tabulated for reference (Fig. 20.1 and Table 20.2).

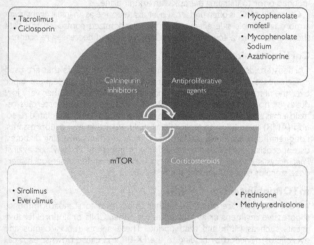

Fig. 20.1 Maintenance Immunosuppression

Antiproliferative agents

Antiproliferative agents include MMF and azathioprine and are used as adjuncts to CNIs and corticosteroids. Both drugs impair nucleic acid synthesis and thus inhibit proliferation of both B and T cells.

Azathioprine is a prodrug that is hydrolysed within tissues to 6-mercaptopurine (6-MP) and undergoes a series of further biochemical modifications to become a purine analogue that is incorporated into DNA and interrupts cell replication. The purine analogue also impairs purine biosynthesis in actively replicating B and T cells.

MMF is a newer class of antiproliferative agent that is also a prodrug which is hydrolysed to mycophenolic acid which inhibits the enzyme inosine monophosphate dehydrogenase involved in the *de novo* pathway of guanine nucleotide synthesis. B and T cells rely on the *de novo* pathway for purine synthesis and thus are selectively inhibited.

Important toxicities for antiproliferative agents include myelosuppression and notably leucopenia, and increased risk for both bacterial and viral infections such as CMV which requires surveillance. MMF can also cause notable GI side effects with nausea, vomiting, and diarrhoea which often require either dose adjustment or substitution with mycophenolate sodium which is an enterically coated delayed-release formulation.

Azathioprine is associated with more myelosuppression than MMF but less diarrhoea and can cause pancreatitis and hepatic dysfunction. Importantly, patients with impaired function or expression of a particular enzyme, thiopurine methyltransferase (TPMT), are at increased risk for myelosuppression with azathioprine and testing for TPMT activity is recommended prior to initiating therapy with azathioprine.

Currently, MMF is often preferred over azathioprine as an initial agent given a more favourable side effect profile with randomized controlled trial data showing some signal towards decreased mortality and decreased rejection.

Corticosteroids

Corticosteroids are non-specific immunosuppressive agents that are used in high doses early after cardiac transplantation with a subsequent taper over the first year with the goal of maintaining patients on either very low doses or no corticosteroids at all after the first year. Corticosteroids remain a mainstay of treatment of acute cellular and antibody-mediated rejection (AMR) in addition to their role as maintenance immunosuppressants. Long-term corticosteroid use has many adverse effects including diabetes, osteoporosis, gastritis, and increased risk of infection. Prophylaxis against *Pneumocystis jirovecii* and GI candidiasis is recommended when on higher-dose steroids especially during the first year.

mTOR inhibitors

mTOR inhibitors are often used either as adjuncts to standard immunosuppressive regimens or as substitutes for either CNIs or antiproliferative agents such as MMF and azathioprine. These agents (i.e. sirolimus and everolimus) function by binding to the FK-BP and cause downstream cell cycle arrest, leading to decreased T and B cell proliferation. Although mTOR inhibitors bind to the same cytoplasmic protein as tacrolimus, their mechanism of action signalling is independent of the calcineurin pathway. The benefits of these agents are severalfold: (1) allow for reduction in dose or substitution of CNIs when there is concern for nephrotoxicity, (2) reduce the progression of CAV, and (3) reduce malignancy risk associated with CNIs and antiproliferative agents. The toxicities of mTOR inhibitors include hyperlipidaemia, myelosuppression, oral ulcers, and proteinuria. Delayed wound healing is an important adverse effect and thus mTOR inhibitors are not used immediately after transplantation and careful consideration must be made prior to other surgical procedures. There are no official guideline recommendations for therapeutic drug troughs for these agents but often CNI dosing is reduced when used as an adjunct. Drug levels depend on each clinical scenario and are usually programme and assay dependent. Typical drug trough levels for sirolimus and everolimus are listed in Table 20.2.

Table 20.2 Maintenance immunosuppression

Pharmacological class	Agent	Dose	Therapeutic trough levels[a]
CNI	Ciclosporin	4–8 mg/kg/day at twice a day dosing	275–375 ng/mL; 0–6 weeks
			200–350 ng/mL; 6–12 weeks
			150–300 ng/mL; 3–6 months
			150–250 ng/mL; 6–12 months
			~200 ng/mL; 12–24 months
			~150 ng/mL; >24 months
	Tacrolimus	0.075 mg/kg/day at twice a day dosing	10–15 ng/mL; 0–6 months
			8–12 ng/mL; 6–12 months
			5–10 ng/mL; >12 months
Anti proliferative agent	MMF	2000–3000 mg/day at twice a day dosing; maintain white blood cell count >3.5 × 10⁹/L	Myrophenolic acid 2–5 mcg/mL
	Azathioprine	2 mg/kg/day; maintain white blood cell count >3.5 × 10⁹/L	—
	Mycophenolate sodium	720–2160 mg/day at twice a day dosing	—
mTOR inhibitor	Sirolimus	1–5 mg/day	4–12 ng/mL
	Everolimus	1.5 mg/day at twice a day dosing	3–8 ng/mL

continued

Table 20.2 Continued

Pharmacological class	Agent	Dose	Therapeutic trough levels[a]
Corticosteroid	Methyl prednisolone	1000 mg IV on day 1 125 mg IV every 8 hours on day 2	—
	Prednisone	0.5mg/kg twice daily and decrease by 5 mg twice daily every 2 days until 10 mg twice daily 15mg PO four times daily; month 1–2 12.5mg PO four times daily; month 2–3 10mg PO four times daily; month 3–4 7.5mg PO four times daily; month 4–5 5mg PO four times daily; month 5–6 2.5mg PO four times daily; month 6–8	—

[a] Dosing and therapeutic trough levels intended to be representative and general guidelines; each immunosuppressive regimen must be tailored based on balancing rejection history with adverse effects

Rejection surveillance

Down-titration of triple drug immunosuppression during the first year of transplantation necessitates frequent monitoring and surveillance for cellular mediated rejection and AMR as acute rejection is inversely related to time from cardiac transplantation. The most recent International Heart and Lung Transplant Registry data suggest a 12.6% incidence of treated rejection within the first year of transplant. Endomyocardial biopsies are the standard of care with frequent biopsies in the first 6 months following transplantation. While the exact schedule for biopsies is dependent on individual patient level factors such as previous history of rejection, baseline immunological response of the recipient, clinical signs and symptoms of rejection, concurrent infection, or rapid changes in immunosuppression regimens, biopsies at our institutions are performed on the following schedule: a weekly basis during the first month; every 2 weeks through post-transplant month 2; monthly through post-transplant month 6; and finally every other month until post-transplant month 12 (Table 20.3).

After the first postoperative year, surveillance with endomyocardial biopsies can be further spaced out to every 4–6 months in higher-risk recipients and often is not utilized in those who have not had any significant rejection history and are otherwise clinically stable. Under these circumstances non-invasive testing with echocardiograms or gene expression profiling assays (AlloMap (CareDx, Brisbane, CA, USA)) can be utilized as a surrogate. AlloMap testing may be a useful alternative in patients who have reached the nadir of their immunosuppression regimen and can help reduce the number of endomyocardial biopsies. For example, for low-risk transplant recipients who are >6 months from transplantation, if AlloMap scores are ≤34 then surveillance with this method can be continued. If there is an abnormal AlloMap score >34 then further characterization with an endomyocardial biopsy may be warranted for a pathological diagnosis. Among these lower-risk individuals without significant prior rejection or graft dysfunction, AlloMap profiling has been associated with a high negative predictive value for acute cellular rejection (ACR) surveillance. Additionally, low serial test variability which is measured as the standard deviation of 4 AlloMap scores (≤0.6) has also been shown to have prognostic value related to a high negative predictive value. These strategies are intended for surveillance and if there is any concern for rejection by history, physical examination, or laboratory findings then non-invasive modalities should not supplant histopathological determination with biopsy.

CAV manifests as a chronic pan-arterial concentric intimal hyperplasia in the epicardial arteries and concentric hyperplasia of the media of the microvasculature of the cardiac allograft. Factors associated with CAV include immunological factors such as prior cellular mediated rejection and AMR, presence of donor-specific anti-HLA antibodies, and non-immunological factors such as CMV infection, diabetes, hypertension, obesity, smoking, and hypercholesterolaemia. Progression of CAV can lead to allograft dysfunction from myocardial ischaemia leading to symptoms of dyspnoea on exertion and chest pain, progressive conduction disease leading to symptoms of palpitations, presyncope, or syncope. Monitoring and surveillance of CAV with angiography with or without intravascular imaging such as intravascular ultrasound or stress imaging are important as changes in immunosuppression, namely introduction of mTOR inhibitors, can curb progression. CT coronary angiography can be used as well when technically feasible. Statin therapy has also been shown to reduce CAV independent of lipid levels. PCI with drug-eluting stents is recommended for angiographically amenable vessels. Retransplantation is required in severe cases.

Table 20.3 Rejection surveillance schedule

Months	Example biopsy schedule	Example CAV screening	Gene expression profiling assays (AlloMap)
0–1	Every week	—	
1–2	Every 2 weeks	Baseline angiogram ± intravascular ultrasound	
2–6	Every 4 weeks	—	
6–12	Every 8 weeks	Repeat angiogram at ~1 year ± intravascular ultrasound	Begin AlloMap at 6–10 months
12–24	Every 4–6 months in higher-risk individuals	Stress imaging alternating with angiogram pending renal function	Annually
>24	As needed		

Cellular rejection

ACR is diagnosed with endomyocardial biopsy. Histological examination demonstrates inflammatory infiltrate comprising lymphocytes, macrophages, and less commonly eosinophils. Neutrophils are not characteristic of cellular rejection and suggestive of alternative processes such as healing ischaemic injury, AMR, or infection. The presence of plasma cells may suggest an alternative process such as healing ischaemic injury, nodular endocardial infiltrates (i.e. Quilty effect), or lymphoproliferative disorders. In addition to inflammatory infiltrate, myocyte damage is an additional feature used to grade severity of rejection. Myocyte damage is histologically characterized by myocytolysis with encroachment of mononuclear cells at the periphery of the myocytes resulting in scalloped myocyte borders and distortion of cellular architecture.

The incidence of ACR has decreased with the development of more robust immunosuppressive drugs. The risk is inversely proportional to time, with a higher risk immediately after transplant. The ISHLT revised its grading system in 2004 to address inconsistencies in classification among pathologists and variability in treatment related to the previous classification scheme.

Treatment options for ACR consist of oral or IV corticosteroids with the option to add ATG or less commonly OKT3. The intensity of immunosuppressive treatment depends on histological severity of the rejection episode in combination with the degree of haemodynamic compromise. Graft dysfunction from rejection can be ascertained by invasive haemodynamic study with a right heart catheterization well as by echocardiography where wall thickening from myogenic oedema and systolic dysfunction are characteristic.

Grade 1R typically does not require treatment unless there is haemodynamic compromise, in which case a short pulse of oral or IV steroids is administered. If there is severe graft dysfunction, cytolytic therapy can be given but this is rare. Grade 2R rejection without haemodynamic compromise is often treated with oral or IV steroids with resumption of the original steroid taper. Background immunosuppression therapy is adjusted if serum levels are subtherapeutic. Grade 2R with haemodynamic compromise or grade 3R rejection or recurrent lower grade rejection refractory to steroid treatment is treated with cytolytic therapy, most commonly ATG on the background of pulse IV steroids. Addition of ATG in severe ACR requires premedication with steroids, antipyretics, and antihistamine to reduce the risk of infusion-related reactions. Antiproliferative agents such as MMF or azathioprine can be held to reduce the effect of leucopenia. Antiviral prophylaxis can be escalated with IV ganciclovir during treatment and then transitioned to oral valganciclovir among patients who are medium to high risk for CMV. Histological evaluation of response to treatment should be performed with an endomyocardial biopsy within 1–2 weeks of treatment for severe symptomatic rejection and can be within 2–4 weeks for mild to moderate asymptomatic rejection. Serial echocardiograms are recommended to assess functional improvement after treatment.

Importantly, severe ACR with haemodynamic compromise is a global biventricular inflammatory process and, as such, circulatory support with inotropic or vasopressor therapy is frequently needed while anti-rejection

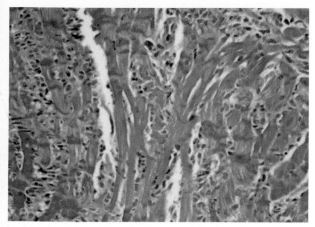

Fig. 2.1: haematoxylin–eosin staining of an endomyocardial biopsy sample showing an inflammatory infiltrate with associated cellular necrosis consistent with acute myocarditis.

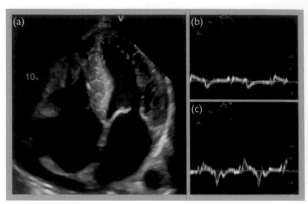

Fig. 3.1: Still image of infiltrative RCM highlighting normal LV size, thickened ventricular walls, enlarged RV, and biatrial enlargement indicative of late-stage disease (a). Figure on right reveals low tissue Doppler velocities at medial (b) and lateral (c) mitral annulus.

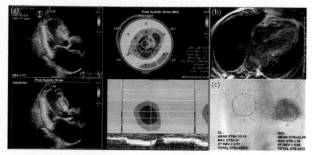

Fig. 3.2: Characteristic imaging findings of cardiac amyloidosis. (a) Typical findings of longitudinal strain imaging with characteristic 'bullseye' pattern. (b) MRI with diffuse subendocardial late gadolinium enhancement. (c) Pyrophosphate (PYP) scan with heart/ contralateral (H/ Cl) ratio >1.5.

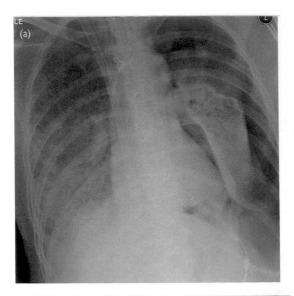

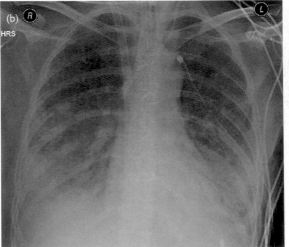

Fig. 18.1: Anteroposterior CXRs demonstrating Pneumocystis jirovecii infection. Sternotomy wires from cardiac transplantation, VV ECMO cannula in situ (a), and left intercostal chest drain for associated left- sided pneumothorax (b) are also seen.

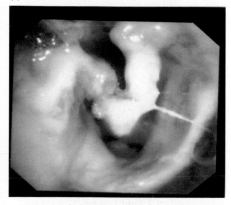

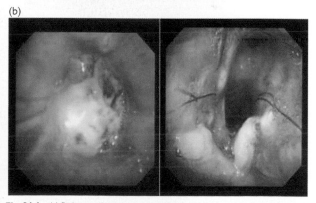

Fig. 31.1: (a) Right main bronchus with severe peri-anastomotic ischaemic necrosis of the airway. (b) Complete occlusion of right main bronchus with granulation tissue, successfully removed by cryotherapy.

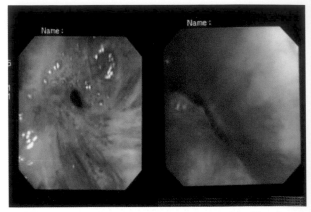

Fig. 31.2: Ischaemic stricture with severe airway narrowing of the right main bronchus. total dynamic obstruction of right main bronchus secondary to bronchomalacia

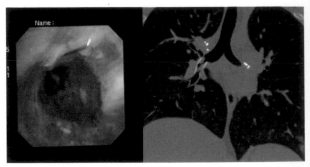

Fig. 31.3: Right main bronchus stent with in-stent bronchial granulation tissue. CT demonstrating in-stent stenosis

(a)

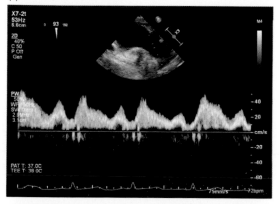

(b)

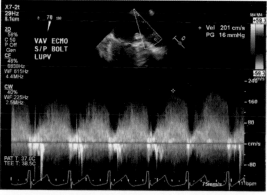

Fig. 37.1: (a) pulsed wave Doppler of the left superior pulmonary vein in the mid-oesophageal, two-chamber view. Systolic dominance of a normal pulmonary vein tracing, with velocities <100 cm/s and without turbulence is noted (colour flow Doppler not shown). (b) abnormal continuous-wave Doppler of the left superior pulmonary vein in the mid-oesophageal, two-chamber view. here velocities throughout systole and diastole exceed 200 cm/s, and pulsed wave Doppler is not possible because the velocities are too high.

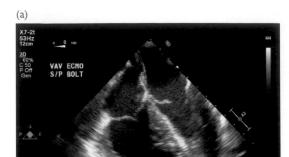

(a)

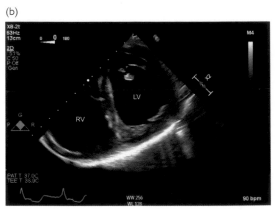

(b)

Fig. 37.2: (a) TOE demonstrating RV dilation and dysfunction in the mid-oesophageal, four- chamber view. This patient required VAV ECMO for support during lung transplantation. (b) TOE demonstrating RV dilation, hypertrophy, and dysfunction in the transgastric, short- axis view of the RV. This patient has the classically described 'D-shaped left ventricle' suggestive of both pressure and volume overload, and required VAV ECMO for support during lung transplantation.

treatment is administered to protect end-organ function. In the most severe cases, MCS may need to be implemented spanning from percutaneous mechanical circulatory support (e.g. IABP) to full biventricular mechanical circulatory assistance (e.g. VA-ECMO) (Table 20.4).

Table 20.4 Endomyocardial biopsy grading criteria

Grade	Histological features	Treatment considerations	Dosage range
ISHLT standardized cardiac biopsy grading: ACR (revised 2004)			
0	No rejection	No treatment	—
1R (mild)	Interstitial and/or perivascular infiltrate with up to 1 focus of myocyte damage	Treat with steroids if haemodynamic compromise	Prednisone 1–3 mg/kg/day (3–5 days) Methylprednisolone 250–1000 mg/day (3 days)
2R (moderate)	Two or more foci of infiltrate with associated myocyte damage	Treat with steroid pulse if no haemodynamic compromise. With haemodynamic compromise add cytolytic therapy with ATG	Methylprednisolone 1000 mg/day (3 days) Thymoglobulin 0.75–1.5 mg/kg/day for 5–14 days Atgam 10 mg/kg/day for 5–14 days ATG-Fresenius 3 mg/kg/day for 5–14 days
3R (severe)	Diffuse infiltrate with multifocal myocyte damage ± oedema ± haemorrhage ± vasculitis	High-dose IV steroids with cytolytic therapy	Methylprednisolone 1000 mg/day for 3 days ATG (as above)

Antibody-mediated rejection

AMR is thought to occur when recipient antibodies interact with specific HLA antigens on the endothelial cells of the cardiac allograft leading to complement activation and tissue injury. The diagnosis is made with endomyocardial biopsy. Histologically, AMR is characterized by myocardial capillary injury with endothelial cell swelling, intravascular accumulation of macrophages, cytokine-mediated inflammatory changes, and microvascular thrombosis. Risk factors for AMR include pre-sensitized recipients such as those with a history of prior transplantation, multiple blood product transfusions, female sex, pregnancy, CMV seropositivity, or LVAD implantation. Importantly, pre-existing and *de novo* anti-HLA antibodies have been associated with cellular rejection, the development of CAV, and decreased survival.

In addition to standard histological evaluation, immunohistochemical and immunofluorescent assays intended to detect complement deposition are utilized to make the diagnosis of AMR. C4d, which covalently binds to the endothelium and thus has a longer half-life than other complement cascade intermediates, can be detected in the capillaries by immunohistochemistry and immunofluorescence. The presence of C4d along with histological features is suggestive of AMR. Detection of C3d in capillaries, which is another complement split product, is also useful in conjunction with C4d staining and the combination of C4d and C3d increases the likelihood of AMR. HLA-DR staining can also be utilized to assess the integrity of the capillary endothelium which can be disrupted with AMR-mediated endothelial damage. Since AMR can be concurrent with cellular rejection, delineation of the two processes can be aided by macrophage-specific staining such as CD68 which is more specific for AMR. In addition, CD34 and CD31 which are endothelial cell markers can be stained to understand intravascular localization of macrophages which occurs in AMR.

Other diagnostic information that can aid in the diagnosis is detection of circulating donor-specific antibodies (DSAs) along with clinical allograft dysfunction. In addition to anti-HLA antibodies, non-HLA antibodies may also contribute to endothelial cell injury via apoptosis and can be implicated in AMR when there is pathological evidence of AMR in the absence of detectable circulating DSAs. These non-HLA antibodies bind to autoantigens such as endothelial cytoskeletal proteins, polymorphic minor antigens, and polymorphic non-HLA antigens such as major histocompatibility complex class I chain-related antigens A and B (MICA, MICB).

Similar to cellular rejection, AMR (Table 20.5) can be subclinical and asymptomatic but can also lead to allograft dysfunction and HF symptoms and in severe cases can lead to cardiogenic shock. Treatment guidelines for AMR are based on expert consensus and typically involve a combination of high-dose IV corticosteroids, removal of circulating antibodies with plasmapheresis, inhibition of circulating antibodies with IVIGs, anti-lymphocyte antibodies (ATG), B-cell depleting therapy (rituximab), plasma cell depleting therapy (bortezomib), complement inhibition (eculizumab), and B- and T-cell depletion (alemtuzumab).

Table 20.5 AMR classification

Category	Histological and immunopathological features
pAMR 0	Negative for pathological AMR
pAMR 1 (H+)	Histological findings present and immunopathological findings negative
pAMR 1 (I+)	Histological findings negative and immunopathological findings positive
pAMR 2	Both histological and immunopathological findings present
pAMR 3	Severe AMR with histological findings of interstitial haemorrhage, capillary fragmentation, mixed inflammatory infiltrates, oedema, endothelial cell pyknosis, and/or karyorrhexis

Management of sensitized patients

Sensitization occurs when the transplant recipient has pre-existing anti-HLA antibodies which are associated with increased risk of rejection and CAV. Moreover, pre-sensitization has been associated with longer wait times to transplantation and impacts post-transplant survival. HLA cell surface proteins are encoded by genes within the major histocompatibility complex and there are two subgroups of HLA antibodies; namely, class I (A, B, C) and class II (DR, DQ, DP).

Risk factors for sensitization include prior exposure to foreign HLA antigens through blood transfusion, prior transplantation, pregnancy, and implanted tissue allografts. Other risk factors include African American race, prior viral infection, MCS, and LVAD implantation.

The degree of sensitization is determined by detection of circulating antibodies using PRA testing. Contemporary methods utilize solid phase immunoassays where purified or recombinant HLAs are attached to polystyrene beads that can be distinguished by differences in internal fluorescence when interrogated by flow cytometry or a commercial Luminex fluoroanalyser. The polystyrene beads contain distinct concentrations of two fluorescent dyes and can be segregated into 100 different bead populations with each population conjugated to either a known pool of HLA antigens or single HLA antigen. Recipient serum is introduced to these beads and recipient antibody and bead antigen binding is detected with a reporter dye that binds to the recipient antibodies. The combination of the individual bead fluorescent signal along with the reporter signal indicates specific binding which is reported as a mean fluorescent intensity (MFI). Importantly, MFI is a marker of binding or bead saturation and not of actual antibody titre. Serum dilution is performed instead to quantitate the highest dilution at which antibody–antigen binding is detected. Often antibody–antigen binding can become undetectable at low serial dilutions and suggest lower antibody concentrations independent of the MFI.

The bead composition ranges in terms of specificity. For example, basic screening for sensitization can be determined with a pooled antigen panel where beads are coated with either class I or class II proteins. This method is mostly qualitative and indicates whether there is positive or negative signal. Phenotype panels include bead populations that have either class I or class II proteins from 98 individuals and offer more specificity in tracking changes in the level of class I or class II antibody binding. The most specific assays utilize single antigen beads where each bead population is coated with a unique HLA antigen and thus individual antibody–antigen interactions can be identified. The percentage of positive reactions is quantified as a percentage PRA and a percentage PRA>10% indicates significant allosensitization. Determination of unacceptable antigens is determined using these assays for donor–recipient matching.

A separate entity known as a calculated PRA (cPRA) is also routinely determined. A cPRA represents the percentage of actual organ donors from an ethnically weighted database who express more than one of the unacceptable HLAs. That is, a high cPRA would correspond to more sensitization and less compatibility. A cPRA >50–80% has been cited as significant sensitization warranting consideration for desensitization therapies.

When sensitization is quantified and significant, desensitization strategies can be used to clear circulating antibodies and thus increase donor compatibility and improve post-transplant outcomes associated with pre-sensitization. There are limited data evaluating and comparing various desensitization protocols and thus treatment choices are often based on programmatic experience. In general, treatment strategies often involve some combination of mechanical removal of antibodies with either plasmapheresis or immunoadsorption, addition of immunosuppressive medications to reduce antibody production with rituximab, bortezomib, alemtuzumab, eculizumab, ATG, cyclophosphamide, and treatment with IVIG. The optimal regimen, treatment goal, and timing of desensitization is variable and programme specific.

Cross-matching is performed to determine recipient antibody to donor antigen interaction and can be done directly with donor cells in a prospective fashion; this is frequently done when feasible geographically and when there is concern for recent sensitization in the recipient. Alternatively, virtual cross-matching is performed which compares recipient HLA antibodies detected with single antigen bead assays with donor HLA antigens using prespecified thresholds based on either MFI or serial dilution to determine which antigens are unacceptable. Physical cross-match is performed regardless immediately after transplant. Transplanting across a positive cross-match can be done with added risk of rejection and graft dysfunction but can be considered on a case-by-case basis with addition of desensitization therapies. A positive physical cross-match is generally treated with induction therapy, plasmapheresis, and IVIG. Addition of more long-lasting immunosuppression outside of conventional maintenance therapy including rituximab, cyclophosphamide, alemtuzumab, and bortezomib can be considered if there is ongoing rejection, graft dysfunction, or presence of DSAs.

The detection of DSAs and particularly de novo DSAs is associated with AMR, decreased graft survival, and CAV. While the presence of DSAs is not synonymous with AMR, it can be an important clue to the immune environment of the cardiac allograft. Monitoring of DSAs is recommended at months 1, 3, 6, and 12 post transplantation and more frequently among sensitized recipients. Furthermore, DSAs are often checked when there are concerns for graft dysfunction, CAV, or signs of RCM. Whether to treat detected DSAs is a multifactorial decision with several factors that need to be considered case by case including whether background immunosuppression is at optimal levels, associated biopsy pathology, and whether there is clinical or haemodynamic evidence of graft dysfunction.

Conclusion

Advancements in immunomodulatory agents have been critical in improving survival among heart transplant recipients. However, there are still formidable challenges with the longer-term adverse effects of immunosuppression. As such, there is a strong need to have an improved mechanistic understanding of the alloimmune response that will inform newer therapeutics and prolong the longevity of donor organs. With newer biological-based therapies and a deeper understanding of allograft tolerance, there is a compelling opportunity for a more personalized approach towards immunosuppression.

Antimicrobial prophylaxis and treatment of infection after cardiac transplantation

Pre-transplant evaluation

Prior to listing for transplantation, recipients need to undergo a thorough infectious diseases evaluation. The aim of this is to:

* Identify any latent or active infections that need to be addressed.
* Determine the patient's immune status against vaccine-preventable infections and other potential donor-derived infections.
* Identify colonization with multidrug-resistant organisms that require modification of standard post-transplant antimicrobial prophylaxis or infection control procedures or that could preclude transplantation.

As part of the evaluation, a comprehensive lifelong infection history should be obtained, including review of specific pertinent microbiological records. Important areas to review include:

* Social history; examples of key risk factors to address are listed in Table 21.1.
* Current medications including use of immunosuppressive agents that could predispose to atypical infections earlier than otherwise expected in the post-transplant course.
* Complete immunization record.
* Drug allergies including exact reactions and severity.

Table 21.1 Risk factors associated with specific infections

Risk factor	Examples of associated infections
Travel or residence in areas with known endemic infections	*Mycobacterium tuberculosis*, *Trypanosoma* spp., *Histoplasma*, *Coccidioides*, *Strongyloides*, etc.
Travel to areas with recent outbreaks	Zika virus, Ebola virus, West Nile virus, *Candida auris*, etc.
Close contact with certain animals	Cats (*Toxoplasma*), birds (*Cryptococcus*), horses (*Rhodococcus*), bats (rabies), etc.
Occupational exposures	Soil (*Nocardia* and moulds), water (non-tuberculous *Mycobacteria*, *Legionella*), etc.
Unpasteurized dairy products	*Listeria monocytogenes*, *Brucella* spp.
Well water	*Cryptosporidium*
Time spent in homeless shelter or prison	*Mycobacterium tuberculosis*
IV drug use	HIV, hepatitis B, hepatitis C

Routine testing is performed for certain pathogens pre transplantation (see Box 21.1); however, unique epidemiological exposures may require additional testing in some cases (e.g. need for *Strongyloides* or *Coccidioides* antibody screening in patients who have spent time in endemic regions).

Box 21.1 Recommended pre-transplant testing

Serologies

Cytomegalovirus (CMV) antibody
Epstein–Barr virus (EBV) antibody
Varicella zoster virus (VZV) antibody
Herpes simplex virus (HSV) antibody
Hepatitis B (HB) virus: HB surface antigen and antibody, HB core antibody
Hepatitis C virus (HCV) antibody
HIV antibody/antigen
Mumps, measles, rubella antibodies
Toxoplasma gondii antibody
Treponema pallidum screening (rapid plasma regain (RPR) or fluorescent treponema antibody absorption (FTA-ABS))

Other tests

Tuberculin skin test (purified protein derivative (PPD)) or interferon gamma release assay for *Mycobacterium tuberculosis*
Tests individualized per patient's unique exposures (e.g. *Coccidioides* antibody, *Strongyloides* antibody, etc.)

Prophylaxis of infections

Various strategies have been implemented to aid in prevention of infection after transplantation. Based on timing relative to the transplant procedure, these include:

- Pre transplantation: update vaccines (see Table 21.5, p. 262).
- Peri transplantation: administer antimicrobials at the time of surgery to prevent nosocomial infections (see following discussion on peri-transplant prophylaxis).
- Post transplantation:
  - Prescribe 'universal prophylaxis'—administer an antimicrobial agent to all recipients for a defined period of time post transplantation to prevent infection.
  - 'Pre-emptively monitor' for infection—serially screen the recipient with specific tests at defined intervals to monitor for early reactivation or acquisition of an infection.

Table 21.2 provides some commonly used preventative regimens in heart transplant recipients.

Peri-transplant antimicrobial prophylaxis

Surgical site infections, which occur in 4–19% of heart transplant recipients, are associated with significant morbidity and mortality. Risk factors for surgical site infections include a BMI >30 kg/m², prior cardiac surgery, LVAD as a BTT, prolonged mechanical ventilation, and use of sirolimus in the immunosuppressive regimen. Bacterial infections tend to be the most common, though *Candida* species and other fungi can be encountered as well. Antimicrobial prophylaxis is recommended at the time of surgery to decrease the frequency of surgical site infections. Because there are no formal guidelines on choice of drug or duration, transplant centres formulate their own protocols. Antibiotic regimens should have good anti-staphylococcal activity and be individualized based on patient-specific factors such as colonization with multidrug resistant organisms (e.g. methicillin-resistant *Staphylococcus aureus* (MRSA)). Additionally, if the patient has a history of an infected LVAD or other cardiac hardware, susceptibility data from those infections should be used to guide antibiotic selection. Modification to the antibiotic regimen may also be required based on positive donor cultures. Routine antifungal prophylaxis in the heart transplant population is controversial and not routinely recommended unless the recipient has multiple and specific risks for invasive candidiasis (e.g. acute kidney injury, prolonged central venous catheter, etc.) or there is an outbreak of mould infections within the institution.

Table 21.2 Post-transplant prophylactic regimens

Pathogen	Prophylactic regimen
Pneumocystis jirovecii	TMP–SMX SS daily or TMP–SMX DS 3× weekly or daily for 6–12 months[a]
Toxoplasmosis gondii	TMP–SMX DS 3× weekly for 6–12 months
CMV D+/R– serostatus (high risk) *or* CMV R + and anti-lymphocyte antibody therapy	Valganciclovir or IV ganciclovir for 3–6 months
CMV R+ serostatus (intermediate risk)	Valganciclovir or pre-emptive monitoring for 3–6 months
CMV D–/R– serostatus (low risk)	Valaciclovir or aciclovir for 3 months (for prevention of HSV/VZV)
EBV	Pre-emptive monitoring and reduction of immunosuppression if detected (antivirals not effective)[b]

D, donor; DS, double strength; R, recipient; SS, single strength; TMP–SMX, trimethoprim–sulfamethoxazole.

[a] Second-line agents include dapsone, atovaquone, and aerosolized pentamidine.

[b] Reduction in immunosuppression needs to be weighed against risk of rejection. There is no consensus as to monitoring algorithms or viral load threshold for intervention. There is variability between quantitative NAATs and controversy regarding best sample type (whole blood vs plasma) for testing; the same NAAT and sample type should be used for the individual patient.

Infection diagnosis and management

A single-centre study of 600 OHT recipients over a 16-year time period reported infectious episodes as 44% bacterial, 42% viral, 10% fungal excluding *Pneumocystis jirovecii*, 4% *P. jirovecii*, and 0.6% parasitic. The timing and type of infection after transplantation is influenced by prophylactic regimens, enhanced immunosuppression, and environmental exposures. Because of their immunosuppressed status and altered anatomy, transplant recipients may not mount a robust inflammatory response and may have minimal or atypical signs and symptoms of infection. Accordingly, a high index of suspicion for infection has to be maintained. Concurrently, non-infectious syndromes such as rejection and drug reactions (e.g. sirolimus-induced pneumonitis, dapsone-induced methemoglobinemia/hypoxia, etc.) need to be kept in mind in the heart transplant recipient presenting with signs and symptoms concerning for infection. The diagnostic work-up for infection has to be individualized in accordance with the patient's presentation and history. Cultures relative to the infected body site should be obtained to aid in reaching a specific diagnosis. Conventional radiographs frequently lack sensitivity and the patient may need a CT scan or an MRI scan to delineate the presence and characteristics of specific radiological findings.

Donor-derived infections

Donor-derived infections are characterized by UNOS as *expected* or *unexpected*. Expected transmissions are those in which the donor was known to be infected with the pathogen prior to donation and for which routine prophylaxis or monitoring is employed in the recipient post transplantation (e.g. CMV, EBV, etc.). Unexpected transmissions are those wherein a donor was not known to harbour a pathogen but transmitted it to a recipient. Unexpected donor-derived infections, while rare, are often associated with high mortality as their diagnosis is frequently delayed in the recipient and treatment options may be limited. Clearly, maintaining a high index of suspicion for donor-derived infections is necessary. Most donor-derived infections present in the recipient within the first 3 months after transplant. Thus, if a recipient presents with unusual or unexplained symptoms within the first 3 months of transplant, a donor-derived infection should be considered and epidemiological clues for potential donor exposures should be investigated. In the US, when donor-derived infection is suspected, the Potential Donor-Derived Disease Transmission Event (PDTE) should be reported using the Secure Enterprise UNOS Improving Patient Safety portal (instructions available at: https://unos.org/wp-content/uploads/unos/Guidance_DTAC_PDDTE_06-2011.pdf).

HBV/ HCV/HIV

US Public Health Service (PHS) guidelines outline criteria that could indicate if a recipient would be at risk for acquiring HBV, HCV, and HIV. As part of donor screening, hepatitis B (HB) surface antigen, HB core antibody, HIV antigen and antibody, HCV antibody, and NAAT testing for HBV, HCV and HIV are performed. NAAT testing supplements antibody tests which can be falsely negative as a consequence of haemodilution/large volume resuscitation of the donor and during the 'window' period after acute infection if adequate viral replication has not taken place by the time the test is performed. While the window periods of new-generation NAAT testing are very small (<5 days for HIV and HCV, ~20 days for HBV), it is still possible for disease transmission to occur. Therefore, repeat testing in all recipients is recommended within 4-8 weeks of transplantation.

The advent of safe and effective HCV therapy in recent years has allowed for use of HCV-positive organs in HCV-negative recipients. Preliminary data on heart transplantation from HCV viraemic donors look promising though long-term outcomes are not yet available. These recipients are typically treated with direct-acting HCV therapy post transplantation and require close monitoring of therapy by either a hepatologist or infectious disease physician.

Unlike HCV, current therapeutic options for HBV only suppress the virus and are not curative. HBV serologies have to be carefully interpreted to determine patient status (Table 21.3). In the US, organs from donors who are HBV surface antigen positive (i.e. have active infection) are not considered for transplantation apart from urgent circumstances. However, in countries where HBV is highly endemic, organs from donors with active infection may also be accepted for transplantation, with plans for treatment with HB immunoglobulin and antivirals post transplantation. HB core antibody positive donors can be accepted for transplantation as cases of transmission have been rare and outcomes have been similar to recipients who received a HBV-negative organ. Based on individual recipient factors, some patients may require revaccination and antiviral therapy as prophylaxis, therefore it is important to involve your local infectious diseases physician or hepatologist in the management of these patients.

Other donor-derived pathogens

Table 21.3 Interpretation of hepatitis B serology

Interpretation	HBV surface antigen	HBV surface antibody	HBV core antibody
Active infection	+	–	+
Immunity due to natural infection	–	+	+
Immunity due to vaccination	–	+	–
Possible interpretations: chronic infection, false-positive test, resolving acute infection	–	–	+

There is a wide range of other pathogens which can be transmitted via donor organs. For example, rabies, lymphocytic choriomeningitis virus, West Nile virus, *Mycobacterium tuberculosis, Cryptococcus, Coccidioides immitis, Aspergillus,* and free-living amoebae (*Balamuthia, Acanthamoeba*) have all been transmitted from donors with meningitis or encephalitis of unknown cause. Numerous cases of unexpected tuberculosis transmission from donors to recipients have been reported including via heart, liver, kidney, and lung allografts. Table 21.4 provides a partial list of some of the more common 'unexpected' potential donor-derived pathogens and the most common clinical presentation in the recipient. Bottom line, if donor-derived infection is a concern, infectious diseases should be immediately consulted to aid in the diagnostic work-up and management of the recipient.

Table 21.4 Possible donor-derived infections

Pathogen	Donor exposure risks	Recipient presentation
Lymphocytic choriomeningitis virus	Rodent exposure, including pets (hamsters, etc.)	Encephalitis
Rabies	Unreported bat bites	Encephalitis
Toxoplasmosis	Travel to endemic area (Latin America, parts of Europe); ingestion of cat faeces or undercooked meat	Diffuse pneumonia myocarditis Retinitis Encephalitis
West Nile virus	Mosquito exposure	Meningitis Encephalitis Poliomyelitis-like flaccid paralysis
Chagas' disease (*Trypanosoma cruzi*)	Travel to endemic area (Latin America)	Fever Myocarditis
Acanthamoeba	Warm, fresh water exposure (drowning/near drowning in a lake/pond, tap water nasal irrigation)	Skin lesion Encephalitis
Strongyloides	Travel to endemic area (Southeast Asia, Central and South America, Africa)	GI complaints; hyperinfection syndrome (polymicrobial bloodstream infection, pneumonitis, meningitis)
Malaria	Travel to endemic area (Southeast Asia, Central and South America, Africa)	Fever

Sepsis

Transplant recipients are at a higher risk for developing sepsis than the general population and are more likely to have an atypical pathogen. Specific studies looking at sepsis mortality in heart transplant recipients are limited; one retrospective review of a national US database showed the mortality rate to be 15.7%. Empiric broad-spectrum antibiotics should be started promptly, as delay in initiation is associated with increased mortality. The antibiotic regimen should be tailored according to the suspected site of infection, susceptibility of prior infections, and local antimicrobial resistance patterns. It should typically include an antibiotic with MRSA coverage such as vancomycin or linezolid and a Gram-negative agent with anti-pseudomonal activity such as piperacillin–tazobactam or a carbapenem. An echinocandin for *Candida* coverage may be considered, depending on the risk. In cases where there is concern for a mould infection such as *Aspergillus*, therapy with a mould active azole may be required. We recommend prompt consultation with your local infectious diseases physician to help in the management of these complex cases.

Other specific pathogens

Listeria

L. monocytogenes is a Gram-positive rod usually acquired by eating food contaminated with the bacterium, most commonly unpasteurized dairy products, deli meats, smoked salmon, and produce (recent outbreaks have been traced to celery, sprouts, and cantaloupe). Solid organ transplant (SOT) recipients, owing to their suppressed cell-mediated immunity, can present with febrile gastroenteritis associated with sepsis and meningoencephalitis. In one case–control study, the median duration of symptoms prior to hospitalization in 30 SOT recipients with listeriosis was 3 days; at presentation, 87% of patients had bacteraemia, 33% had meningoencephalitis, and 23% had septic shock. Mortality at 30 days was high (27%). Blood and cerebrospinal fluid (CSF) should be submitted for culture; stool can also be cultured but requires special media for recovery. Thus, communication directly with the microbiology laboratory is recommended before sending stool for culture. *Listeria* should be considered when 'diphtheroids' are reported to be growing from blood or CSF cultures.

High-dose ampicillin (2 g IV every 4 hours renally adjusted for adults) is the drug of choice for listeriosis; trimethoprim–sulfamethoxazole (TMP–SMX) may be used for patients allergic to penicillin. Duration of therapy depends on site of infection, but typically 3–6 weeks in SOT recipients with bacteraemia and longer in those with CNS disease. Of particular note, *Listeria* is intrinsically resistant to cephalosporins and these agents should *not* be used for empiric treatment for *Listeria*. TMP–SMX used as prophylaxis after SOT has protective activity against *Listeria*.

Nocardia

At least 33 *Nocardia* species can cause disease in humans. Nocardiosis is most often acquired via inhalation of spores, and classically presents as a respiratory infection characterized by pulmonary nodules often mistaken radiographically for invasive pulmonary aspergillosis. It also frequently disseminates and based on its neurotropism, recovery of *Nocardia* from any body site should prompt imaging of the CNS to rule out an asymptomatic brain abscess. In one retrospective review, the median time to diagnosis among 37 SOT recipients was 370 days post transplantation. Blood, CSF, and tissue biopsies may be submitted for routine bacterial and fungal culture; *Nocardia* is frequently recovered from fungal culture as the media used supports its growth and fungal cultures are typically held longer than bacterial cultures. Because it grows more slowly than other bacteria, the microbiology laboratory should be notified when this pathogen is suspected. *Nocardia* appear as delicate, filamentous, branching Gram-positive rods that can be confirmed as *Nocardia* based on partial acid fastness on modified acid-fast stains.

High-dose TMP–SMX is considered the drug of choice for *Nocardia*; in cases of intolerance, treatment should be based on susceptibility results and site of infection. The duration of therapy ranges from 3 months up to 1 year or longer depending on disease severity, location, and response. Of note, while TMP–SMX is the treatment of choice for *Nocardia*, doses used for *Pneumocystis* prophylaxis are not protective against *Nocardia*.

Clostridium difficile-associated diarrhoea (CDAD)

C. difficile is an anaerobic Gram-positive rod that can be part of the normal stool flora in up to 5% of healthy adults and up to 30% of healthy neonates. Colonization with *C. difficile* alone does not result in CDAD. Only strains that are able to produce *C. difficile* enterotoxin (TcdA) and/or cytotoxin (TcdB) are capable of causing CDAD. In addition to being colonized with a TcdA/TcdB-producing *C. difficile* strain, other risks (e.g. antibiotic exposure, proton pump inhibitor use, etc.) combine to influence toxin production resulting in CDAD. *C. difficile* is highly transmissible via the faecal–oral route which is facilitated by the production of spores that can persist on environmental surfaces for months and which are resistant to commonly used cleaning agents and alcohol-based hand gels (hence the need for washing hands with soap and water after contact with infected patients). Diagnosis of CDAD should be pursued only in patients with acute diarrhoea (≥ 3 loose stools in 24 hours) and with no other obvious explanation for the diarrhoea. Diagnosis typically includes testing a liquid stool sample with an enzyme immunoassay (EIA) for *C. difficile* toxins A and B. Use of the newer NAAT, which only detects the presence of toxin-producing *C. difficile* but not the actual toxin itself, has been associated with false-positive tests.

Heart transplant recipients have a CDAD incidence ranging from 1% to 8%. Patients with CDAD should be assessed for disease severity. Criteria proposed for severe CDAD include white blood cell count >15,000 cells/ mL or serum creatinine >1.5 mg/dL. Complications may include pseudomembranous colitis, toxic megacolon, perforation of the colon, and sepsis. Oral vancomycin or oral fidaxomicin are typically first-line therapy for CDAD. Fidaxomicin is more expensive than vancomycin but is associated with a lower recurrence rate. Alternatively, oral metronidazole, may be used for non-severe CDAD. Treatment duration is typically 10 days. Test of cure is not indicated as tests may remain positive during or after clinical recovery.

CMV

The most common presentation of CMV is CMV viral syndrome, a mononucleosis-like syndrome which consists of the presence of CMV in blood and fever and one or more of the following: malaise, leucopenia, atypical lymphocytes, thrombocytopenia, or elevated hepatic enzymes. CMV may also cause tissue-invasive disease with end-organ damage, with predilection to involve the allograft and presenting as myocarditis in heart transplant recipients. As CMV is a known immunomodulatory virus, it also plays an indirect role in driving other post-transplant infections, such as invasive fungal infections, *P. jirovecii* pneumonia, EBV-related PTLD, as well as allograft rejection. The risk for CMV disease is based on the SOT recipient's immune status prior to transplantation and the type of organ transplanted. Heart is considered an intermediate-risk organ. Quantitative NAAT is the method of choice for rapid diagnosis of CMV in blood.

IV ganciclovir is recommended for severe or life-threatening disease. Antiviral treatment should be administered for 2–3 weeks, and continued until viremia clears or reaches a negative threshold, *and* there is resolution of clinical symptoms. Oral valganciclovir may be used in mild to moderate disease. Drug resistance should be suspected if there is prolonged ganciclovir exposure (>6 weeks) and no reduction in viral load or lack of clinical improvement after 14 days of treatment in which case genotypic testing for specific resistance mutations (UL97 and UL54) should be performed. Based on the specific mutation present, therapeutic options include high-dose IV ganciclovir, foscarnet, maribavir or cidofovir.

EBV

EBV, the aetiological agent of mononucleosis, is also involved in the uncontrolled proliferation of EBV-infected lymphocytes resulting in PTLD. Clinical manifestations vary from a non-specific febrile mononucleosis-like illness with lymphadenopathy to solid tumours. Being an EBV seronegative recipient is a well-known risk for PTLD which is a significant complication after paediatric heart transplantation in particular. In a retrospective cohort, 80% of heart transplant recipients presented with late-onset PTLD (>1 year post transplantation) and the GI tract, with its high content of lymphoid tissue was the site most frequently involved, followed by hilar lymph nodes, then lung, cervical, axillary, para-aortic, and inguinal lymph nodes, and finally skin. Involvement of the GI tract may present as abdominal discomfort, nausea, or diarrhoea and requires a high index of suspicion. Overall 5-year mortality was 29%, mainly related to disease progression or treatment-related mortality. Tissue biopsy and histopathology is the gold standard for the diagnosis of PTLD.

The mainstay of management is reduction in immunosuppression. Treatment regimens that include rituximab, an anti-CD20 monoclonal antibody, are also used. Though antivirals have been used in this setting, they lack activity on latently infected lymphocytes. Factors which may affect overall survival after PTLD include bone marrow involvement and hypoalbuminemia, both poor prognostic factors which suggest advanced disease at presentation. Complete response to therapy is associated with improved survival.

VZV

VZV is the aetiological agent for varicella, or chicken pox, and for herpes zoster (HZ). Most primary infections occur in childhood, though immunity may also be acquired by vaccination with a live attenuated VZV vaccine. After infection, VZV establishes lifelong latency. Primary varicella infection in SOT may present with fever, constitutional symptoms, and a vesicular disseminated rash. SOT patients are at increased risk for complications, such as pneumonia. The incidence of HZ reactivation, or shingles, in heart transplant recipient ranges from 5.5% to 16.8%. While most cases of HZ occur in the first year post transplantation, in a multicentre cohort of mixed SOTs, HZ occurred a median of 2.6 years after transplantation. Complications such as post-herpetic neuralgia was reported in 26–45% of patients and HZ ophthalmicus in 14%. Risk factors for HZ include MMF use, being African American, and older age at time of transplant. Severe, disseminated or CNS infection with VZV may require additional testing. Laboratory tests include VZV NAATs, direct fluorescent antibody assay, and viral culture, though the latter is used principally for epidemiological purposes.

SOT patients who develop primary varicella should be treated with IV aciclovir. For limited dermatomal HZ, oral agents such as aciclovir, valaciclovir, or famciclovir, may be used. Severe HZ necessitates IV aciclovir, and, for HZ ophthalmicus, an ophthalmology consult.

Influenza

Influenza virus usually causes a self-limited illness characterized by fever, rhinorrhoea, and cough. In SOT recipients, however, fever may be absent, though upper respiratory symptoms, with or without myalgia, headache, and dyspnoea during influenza season are highly suspicious. In this patient population, approximately 22% of patients present with pneumonia, and may have co-infection with other viruses or bacteria. Influenza infection may occur at any time post transplantation and early infections, <3 months post transplantation, may be associated with severe illness. Risk factors for severe influenza in SOT recipients include age, use of MMF, and early infection (<3 months) after transplantation. NAAT is the preferred diagnostic method. Since it is not possible to clinically differentiate disease caused by respiratory viruses, multiplex PCR assays that test for influenza and other respiratory viruses are recommended. Preferred clinical specimens in early illness include nasopharyngeal swab, wash, or aspirate. If negative or if diagnostic uncertainty, or if symptoms and signs of lower tract disease are present, a lower respiratory tract specimen obtained via bronchoalveolar lavage (BAL) may have higher diagnostic yield.

Neuraminidase inhibitors, oseltamivir and zanamivir, are associated with improved outcomes in SOT. Early initiation of antiviral therapy is associated with lower risk of progression to pneumonia, as is influenza vaccination in the same season.

Other respiratory viruses

Other respiratory viral pathogens causing infection in SOT recipients include parainfluenza (PIV), respiratory syncytial virus (RSV), human metapneumovirus (hMPV), rhinovirus (hRV), severe acute respiratory syndrome coronavirus 2 (SARS-CoV-2) and adenovirus (ADV). Most are community acquired and cause upper respiratory tract infections. In SOT, however, these may be nosocomially acquired and have increased risk of progression to lower respiratory tract infections (pneumonia) as well as prolonged duration of illness and viral shedding. Some viruses have year-round prevalence while others circulate with a seasonal pattern. Transmission of the different respiratory viruses may be via direct or indirect contact through droplet or aerosol. For ADV, there is also the faecal–oral route. In hospital settings, appropriate infection control measures including consistent hand washing, standard and contact precautions, droplet precautions, and, depending on the virus, airborne precautions should be instituted. Molecular diagnostic tools, such as multiplex PCR is the diagnostic method of choice. In cases with tissue invasive disease, histopathology with immunohistochemistry is used to evaluate for select viruses and to distinguish between infection and rejection.

Supportive treatment is the mainstay of therapy, with reduction in immunosuppression when possible. Antiviral agents with effect against some of these viruses include ribavirin, cidofovir, remdesivir and possibly palivizumab. IVIG in conjunction with antiviral therapy is occasionally used in select patients. Management should be individualized with consultation by an infectious disease specialist.

Pneumocystis jirovecii

P. jirovecii is an opportunistic fungal pathogen that causes pneumonia in SOT not receiving effective prophylaxis. Primary infection is acquired via the respiratory route usually in childhood, which then may enter a latent phase. Reactivation or *de novo* exposure can lead to *P. jirovecii* pneumonia (PJP), presenting with fever, non-productive cough, and dyspnoea with hypoxaemia. Increased risk for PJP is seen with lack of effective prophylaxis, increased immunosuppression (corticosteroids or antilymphocyte therapy), CMV reactivation, allograft rejection, older age, and low absolute lymphocyte count post transplantation. Nosocomial infections via interhuman transmission in outbreak situations have been reported in heart transplant recipients. Without prophylaxis, the risk of PJP is high in the first 6 months following SOT and during periods of increased immunosuppression. The use of prophylaxis may lead to delayed-onset PJP. Diagnosis of PJP is made through a combination of clinical, radiological, and laboratory features. The preferred specimens for diagnosis include induced sputum, BAL, or biopsy. Immunofluorescence testing of specimens, or validated NAATs will detect *P. jirovecii*. Calcofluor stains of respiratory specimens, and lung tissue histopathology stained with polychrome or silver, will also demonstrate the organisms. Serum testing of lactate dehydrogenase and $(1{\to}3)$ β-D-glucan may be useful adjuncts. Abnormal CXR is present in most patients, with patterns ranging from bilateral interstitial infiltrates to alveolar infiltrates, nodules, or consolidation.

TMP–SMX is the drug of choice for treatment of PJP. Clindamycin with primaquine is a second line regimen. IV pentamidine use is limited by numerous adverse effects. Atovaquone at higher doses has also been used. Adjunctive steroids are controversial but may have a role in severe hypoxaemia.

Aspergillus

Aspergillus is the most frequent cause of invasive mould infection following heart transplant and *A. fumigatus* is the most common species causing invasive aspergillosis (IA). Incidence of IA in heart transplant recipients ranges between 3.5% and 7.1%. Though the time of IA onset varies in heart transplant recipients, most occur in the first year post transplantation. Risk factors for IA in heart transplant recipients include *Aspergillus* colonization, reoperation, CMV disease, post-transplant haemodialysis, and an episode of IA in the heart transplant programme within 2 months prior to or post transplantation. Older age has been associated with late IA. Infection is acquired most commonly by the inhalation of *Aspergillus* spores and accordingly, the site most frequently involved is the lower respiratory tract, followed by dissemination, with or without CNS infection. Mediastinitis and surgical site infection have also been reported. Mortality due to IA in a Swiss cohort was 26.7% for heart transplant recipients and in a Spanish cohort, IA mortality ranged from 26% for early IA to 63% for late IA. Clinical signs and symptoms, together with laboratory results and radiographic findings on CXR or chest CT, are used to make the diagnosis of IA. Isolation of *A. fumigatus* from a respiratory site in a heart transplant recipient has a high positive predictive value and is highly suggestive of IA. BAL specimens should be sent for culture and a galactomannan test and tissue should be sent for histopathology and culture. Culture allows for identification of the *Aspergillus* species and susceptibility testing. Radiographic findings suggestive of IA include nodules or cavitation, though more than half may present with atypical finding such as ground-glass opacities or pleural effusion.

Voriconazole is the drug of choice for the treatment of IA. Isavuconazole or lipid amphotericin are considered alternative agents, and posaconazole has been used in refractory IA. Some centres add an echinocandin as part of salvage therapy.

Non-Aspergillus fungal infections

Infections due to infrequently encountered fungi have increasingly been reported in immunocompromised patients. Some invasive moulds include non-Aspergillus hyalohyphomycetes, phaeohyphomycetes, or dematiaceous (black) moulds, and Mucorales (also referred to as Zygomycetes). The most commonly reported moulds in each category are as follows:

- Hyalohyphomycetes: Scedosporium, Lomentospora, and Fusarium.
- Phaeohyphomycetes: Alternaria, Bipolaris, Exophiala, Verruconis, and Cladophialophora.
- Mucormycetes: Rhizopus, Mucor, and Cunninghamella.

Portals of entry include the skin or the respiratory tract. If infection ensues, clinical signs and symptoms may be indistinguishable from those caused by Aspergillus or Nocardia. Clinical manifestations include cutaneous or sub-cutaneous infection, pulmonary disease, and disseminated infection, with or without CNS involvement. Other specific locations may be associated with underlying medical conditions, secondary to focal trauma, or be seeded during dissemination. The diagnostic approach includes a comprehensive history (with exposure if known), clinical findings, specimens for culture and histopathology, and radiographic studies. Response to treatment is predicated not only on the type of fungal pathogen and the minimum inhibitory concentration to the antifungal agent being considered, but also site of infection, underlying host factors, degree of immunosuppression, therapeutic drugs levels, and need for adjunctive surgical excision or debridement. Expert consultation with infectious disease physicians should be obtained when managing these infections.

Cryptococcus

Cryptococcus is an encapsulated yeast and the third most common invasive fungal infection in SOT after invasive candidiasis and IA. Acquisition may occur through inhalation or through the skin. Cryptococcosis is usually a subacute, late occurring infection in SOT due to reactivation of latent or quiescent infection. Very early-onset cryptococcosis may be due to early reactivation, unrecognized cryptococcosis pre transplantation, or in some cases, donor derived. The most common clinical presentation is pulmonary disease, with cough, dyspnoea, and sputum production. Fever may or may not be present. Extrapulmonary disease may include CNS disease/meningitis, skin/soft tissue infection, or fungemia. Clinical manifestations of cryptococcal meningitis may be subtle and include headache, gait disorder, hearing loss, and altered mental status. Necrotizing fasciitis and infection of the prostate have been reported in heart transplant recipients. It is important to determine site and extent of infection. Blood, sputum or BAL, and tissues should be sent for culture and tissues for histopathology (Cryptococcus appears as round yeasts with narrow budding and the mucicarmine stain reveals the organism's capsule). Serum cryptococcal antigen should also be submitted. In patients with a positive serum cryptococcal antigen or diagnosed with pulmonary disease, a lumbar puncture should be performed to evaluate for cryptococcal meningitis (send CSF for fungal culture and cryptococcal antigen); documenting the opening pressure is critical as this guides therapeutic taps as outlined below. Radiographic findings include pulmonary nodules which may be solitary or multiple and indistinguishable from other infections. Occasionally, findings include diffuse interstitial infiltrates or effusion. Some centres also conduct CNS imaging with CT prior to lumbar puncture.

For CNS disease, disseminated disease, or moderate to severe pulmonary disease, the primary induction regimen consists of a lipid formulation of amphotericin B plus 5-fluocytosine for ≥14 days or until CNS culture sterilization, followed by long-term fluconazole therapy for the maintenance phase. If the patient has elevated intracranial pressure (CSF opening pressure >25 cm), CSF drainage by lumbar puncture to reduce opening pressure by 50% or to 20 cm of CSF is recommended. Patients may require serial lumbar punctures or placement of a lumbar percutaneous drain for pressure control. For individuals with mild to moderate disease limited to the lung, azole therapy may be used as the primary regimen.

Toxoplasma
Toxoplasma gondii is a protozoan with seroprevalence varying by geographic region. In the US, the most recent seroprevalence was 12.4% in those ≥6 years, and 9.1% in women of child-bearing age. Information regarding the frequency of toxoplasmosis in SOTs is scarce; one multicentre study reported the overall frequency of toxoplasmosis to be 0.14%, and highest in heart transplant recipients at 0.6%. SOT recipients may acquire primary toxoplasmosis from ingesting food or water contaminated with oocysts from faces of infected felines or by eating undercooked meat containing cysts. SOT recipients are also at risk for endogenous reactivation of latent disease, and for acquisition from a cyst-containing donor organ. SOTs who have negative serostatus prior to transplantation, especially if discordant to the donor status (D+/R−), are at highest risk for primary infection in the first 6 months post transplantation. Reactivation toxoplasmosis in R+ recipients may be asymptomatic. However, in those who were seronegative prior to transplant and acquire primary infection, clinical manifestation may be severe, including pulmonary toxoplasmosis, cerebral toxoplasmosis, and disseminated disease. Fever is present in approximately two-thirds of patients. Lung infections present with cough and dyspnoea, with diffuse infiltrates on imaging. Myocarditis can present as HF resembling allograft rejection. CNS infections, including chorioretinitis, meningitis, encephalitis, brain abscess, and disseminated infection may present with headache, confusion, focal neurological signs, and visual abnormalities. Since infection may be asymptomatic or initially present with non-specific signs and symptoms, diagnosis depends on laboratory tests. PCR is the method of choice, especially in patients with discordant serostatus and those unable to tolerate TMP–SMX prophylaxis. PCR can be performed on BAL, blood, CSF, and other body fluids. Histopathology may also reveal the pathogen.

Based on studies in HIV patients, the preferred regimen for induction therapy is pyrimethamine *plus* sulfadiazine *plus* leucovorin, for at least 6 weeks, followed by lifelong chronic suppressive therapy with the same agents at a reduced dose. Alternative regimens are available but should be managed by an infectious disease consultant.

Strongyloides

S. stercoralis is a soil-transmitted nematode found worldwide, with a prevalence up to 60%-≥ 71% in resource-poor countries. Prevalence of *S. stercoralis* in the US ranged between 0% and 3.8% in areas of Appalachia and the southern US. Infective filariform larvae in the soil directly penetrate human host skin, migrate to the small intestine, then reach the lung either directly or via the bloodstream. They are then coughed and ingested, reaching the small intestine where they mature to adult form. Reproduction within the human host results in endogenous autoinfection. In the immunocompetent host, uncomplicated intestinal infection may present with nonspecific GI symptoms, such as diarrhoea and abdominal pain, but is typically asymptomatic. However, in SOT recipients, hyperinfection syndrome and disseminated disease resulting from reactivation of chronic latent infection, or primary infection from an infected donor may occur. Hyperinfection syndrome is characterized by a massive production of larvae in the GI system and invasion of the lungs by the parasite, often combined with polymicrobial bloodstream infection. Disseminated disease involves larval migration to other organs. Meningitis by enteric Gram-negative rods may also occur. Heart transplant patients with *Strongyloides* hyperinfection syndrome may present with nausea, vomiting or diarrhoea, cough, dyspnoea or respiratory failure, fever, malaise, headache, altered mental status, and cutaneous rash.

A combination of diagnostic methods is often need for the diagnosis of *Strongyloides* in the SOT recipient. Stool should be collected for ova and parasite exam and PCR testing. For hyperinfection or disseminated disease, stool studies along with lower respiratory specimens (BAL) or other affected body fluid or tissue should be evaluated. Larvae can be seen in respiratory secretions, BAL, CSF, peritoneal fluid, urine, pleural effusion, blood, and in other tissue specimens. Blood and CSF cultures should also be collected to evaluate for Gram-negative rods. Imaging of the chest often demonstrates diffuse bilateral alveolar and interstitial pulmonary infiltrates, reflecting underlying diffuse alveolar haemorrhage or acute respiratory distress syndrome. Brain imaging may reveal areas of new infarcts.

The drug of choice for *Strongyloides* is ivermectin by mouth then repeated 2 weeks later. Albendazole is considered a second line agent. *Strongyloides* hyperinfection syndrome and disseminated disease require longer duration of treatment. Management also involves a combination of broad-spectrum antimicrobials for systemic bacterial sepsis and reduction of immunosuppression, if feasible.

Immunizations post transplantation

Whenever possible, the recommended series of vaccines should be administered before transplantation, allowing for completion at least 2 weeks prior to transplantation (Table 21.5). Live-attenuated vaccines should be administered at least 4 weeks prior to transplantation to ensure resolution of viral replication. Vaccines noted to be safe for administration after transplantation may not be sufficiently immunogenic post transplantation and should be delayed at least 3–6 months following transplant. Live vaccines are *not* recommended after SOT. For patients who are unvaccinated or incompletely vaccinated prior to transplant, infectious disease consultation should be obtained.

Table 21.5 Vaccinations in the post-transplant period

Vaccine	Inactivated (I)/live attenuated (LA)	Can be given after transplant	Comments
Anthrax	I	No	
BCG	LA	No	
Cholera	LA	No	Travel vaccine
Cholera and traveller's diarrhoea	I	Yes	Travel vaccine; oral inactivated vaccine against cholera and enterotoxigenic *Escherichia coli* provides short-term protection. (Not available in the US)
Haemophilus influenzae B	I	Yes	If residential college student, receiving eculizumab, asplenic or functional asplenia (e.g. sickle cell disease)
Hepatitis A	I	Yes	If hepatitis A antibody negative (and vaccination *not* previously administered)
Hepatitis B	I	Yes	Hepatitis B series should be offered prior to transplantation. If HB surface antibody and surface antigen are negative, may administer
Human papillomavirus	I	Yes	If age ≤26 years and *not* previously administered (patients up to age 45 can receive the vaccine at patient/ provider discretion)
Influenza, inactivated	I	Yes	High-dose or booster during same season has higher immunogenicity than single dose
Influenza, intranasal	LA	NO	
Japanese encephalitis	I	Yes	Travel vaccine
Measles/ mumps/ rubella	LA	No	
Neisseria meningitides ACYW and *N. meningitides* B	I	Yes	If residential college student, receiving eculizumab, asplenic or functional asplenia (e.g. sickle cell disease)
Pertussis (Tdap)	I	Yes	
Polio, inactivated	I	Yes	
Polio, oral	LA	No	

Vaccine	Inactivated (I)/live attenuated (LA)	Can be given after transplant	Comments
Rabies	I	Yes	Not routinely administered. Recommend for exposure or potential exposure due to occupation
Rotavirus	LA	No	Usually administered prior to transplantation in paediatric patients
Salmonella typhi, oral	LA	No	Travel vaccine
S. typhi, intramuscular	I	Yes	Travel vaccine
Streptococcus pneumoniae conjugate or poly saccharide	I	Yes	PCV20 conjugate, PPSV23 polysaccharide
Smallpox	LA	No	Transplant recipients with face-to-face contact with smallpox should be vaccinated. Vaccinia immune globulin may be administered concurrently if available. With less intimate contact, vaccine should not be administered
Tetanus	I	Yes	
Varicella, subunit	I	Yes	Varicella IgG *positive* and age ≥50 years (and *not* previously administered)
Varicella, live	LA	No	
Yellow fever	LA	No	Travel vaccine. Severely immunosuppressed travellers are encouraged to *avoid* travel to areas where there is risk for yellow fever

Heart failure in paediatric patients

Heart transplant
for paediatric patients

Selection criteria and evaluation for donor and recipient

Paediatric heart transplant listing criteria are not rigid. The scarcity of donor organs means that each patient needs to be carefully assessed in order to identify patients with the greatest need and most favourable outcome post transplantation.

Recipient selection criteria

The following are used as guidance criteria for listing in the UK.

Indications for listing
- End-stage HF despite maximal medical therapy.
- Complex congenital heart disease with no further medical or surgical options.
- Progressive PH secondary to systemic ventricular failure that would preclude transplantation at a later date.
- Failing Fontan circulation with no medical or surgical option.
- Refractory malignant arrhythmia causing haemodynamic compromise.
- Unresectable cardiac tumours causing haemodynamic consequences.
- Unacceptable poor quality of life secondary to advanced HF.

Contraindications
- Active malignancy or history of previous treatment with a high recurrence risk.
- Irreversible end-organ failure:
  - Decompensated liver cirrhosis is a contraindication to heart-only transplantation.
  - Severe renal abnormality/dysfunction not likely to be reversible and not suitable for continuing dialysis or renal transplantation at a later stage.
  - Progressive or refractory multisystem organ failure unlikely to be resolved by heart-only transplantation.
  - Other significant organ dysfunction (including neurodevelopmental delay) likely to lead to an inability to adhere to post-transplant treatment regimens or poor quality of life.
- Progressive systemic disease with early mortality (genetic, metabolic, syndromic, or neurological disease).
- Anatomical concerns regarding appropriate anastomosis (e.g. severely hypoplastic pulmonary arteries or veins).
- Severe, fixed elevation of PVR is a contraindication to heart-only transplantation.
- History of recurrent medical non-compliance despite an appropriate multidisciplinary and safeguarding team involvement.
- Psychological or psychiatric conditions not amenable to treatment leading to non-compliance with treatment regimens after transplantation in spite of appropriate multidisciplinary team involvement.
- A lack of appropriate social support to enable compliance with treatment regimens after transplantation.

Relative contraindications

- Malignancy in remission, patients should be assessed on an individual basis.
- Severe renal impairment not likely to be reversible.
- Active sepsis from bacterial, fungal, or severe viral infection.
- Prior sensitization with high levels of HLA antibody.
- Diabetes mellitus with evidence of severe end-organ damage.
- Morbid obesity.
- Limited venous access.

Indication for retransplantation

- Significant CAV.
- Graft dysfunction without evidence of acute graft rejection.

Criteria for urgent listing

- Short-term MCS for acute haemodynamic instability (e.g. ECMO, Berlin heart VAD).
- Need for more than one IV inotrope.
- Need for IV inotrope and mechanical ventilatory support.

Donor evaluation

Essential donor information at first call includes

- Blood group.
- Weight and height.
- Cause of death.
- Duration of CPR (if any).
- Amount of inotropes required to maintain haemodynamic stability.
- Echocardiography.

The paediatric heart has great potential for recovery after acute events. A short run of ECMO support following transplant is not an uncommon practice. This has made the use of grafts with borderline function more acceptable than in adult population with no difference in outcome.

Donor–recipient size matching

Donor weight is the most commonly used size-matching criteria. Donor–recipient size mismatch is common in paediatric transplants. Oversizing up to three times is usually feasible. Delayed sternal closure should be performed following diuresis and resolution of allograft myocardial oedema. The disadvantage of oversizing are hypertension and possible left bronchial compression.

Smaller donors with >20% mismatch are usually avoided as this is associated with poor outcome.

Procurement

- Harvesting team assessment is crucial. Visual assessment, TOE (if available), and Swan–Ganz readings (in older donors) can confirm the quality of the graft.
- Proper communication between the implant and the harvesting teams is essential. Extra donor tissue (e.g. the entire length of the SVC, the left innominate vein, the aortic arch, the branch PAs, and even the pericardium) may be required for complex reconstruction.

Technical aspects of heart transplantation for congenital conditions

Heart transplantation in congenital populations is more technically challenging than in cardiomyopathy patients. Challenges commonly faced are:
• Multiple previous sternotomies.
• Proximity of the cardiac structures to the sternum.
• Anomalous systemic or pulmonary venous connections.
• Previous reconstruction of the great vessels.
• Previous catheter intervention and placed stents/devices.
• Questionable patency of peripheral vessels.
• Significant collateral load in cyanotic patients.

Conduct of bypass

Preoperative preparation
• Cross-sectional imaging is vital to plan entry strategy, CPB cannulation, and need for any technical modifications.
• Imaging of peripheral arterial and venous access.
• Planning monitoring and invasive lines with anaesthetic team.
• Coordination between the implant and the harvesting teams is essential to avoid any unnecessary long cold ischaemia time, especially in patients with VAD support, those with anticipated dense adhesions, or those who need reconstruction of the arterial or the venous pathway.

Operative steps
• Bicaval OHT is currently the most used technique.
• Set up is similar to any open-heart surgery with stress on redo precautions.
• Groin or neck vessels included in the surgical field and exposed or cannulated as planned.
• Standard median sternotomy is performed.
• Aortic and bicaval cannulation performed as distal as possible with caval tapes placed.
• CPB flow adjustment for collateral run-off and extra suction lines for significant pulmonary return or bleeding.
• A LA vent is placed to reduce the distension of the donor heart.
• Any required reconstruction of the arterial or venous pathway is done.
• In HLA and ABO incompatibility, plasma exchange is undertaken prior to commencing CPB using a short period of circulatory arrest.

Recipient cardiectomy
Usually performed just before the donor heart arrives in theatre:
• The great vessels are cut just distal to their respective valve.
• The SVC is cut at the SVC–RA junction and IVC to be cut with a generous cuff of RA.
• Caution is required when cutting the LA to leave sufficient cuff around the pulmonary veins.
• Cardiectomy may be done earlier if there is a need for extensive reconstruction of arterial or venous pathway.
• Haemostasis is addressed before implanting the donor heart as it is usually difficult to reach afterwards.

Preparation of the donor heart
- The aorta and PA are separated.
- LA cuff is created by connecting incisions between four pulmonary veins (if the lungs were not used).
- The fossa ovalis is inspected (some units prefer to keep PFO patent or create a small hole in the floor of the fossa ovalis that helps decompression of the left side if ECMO is required in the postoperative period).
- The SVC is trimmed to have as wide an anastomosis as possible.

Bicaval anastomosis
Usually carried out in the following order:
- LA anastomosis starting adjacent to the site of LAA.
- A vent is left in place to avoid distension of the donor heart and help de-airing.
- PA anastomosis avoiding a long cuff that may produce kinking.
- Anastomosis of the aorta. A dose of corticosteroids is usually given at this point before release of the aortic cross-clamp.
- Some centres prefer to inject warm cardioplegia and/or warm shot before release of THE clamp.
- The anastomosis of the IVC and finally SVC are to be performed on beating heart.
- Attention is required for SVC anastomosis. Interrupted or semi-continuous running sutures are used to avoid A purse-string effect.

Preparation for weaning off CPB
Once anastomosis is done and patient temperature is acceptable, the following has to be in place before weaning off CPB:
- Temporary pacing wires (multisite pacing is favourable to achieve the best biventricular synchronization possible).
- LA line is placed through the LA vent site to monitor LA pressure.
- Appropriate inotropic support is in place.
- NO is routinely introduced to lower the PVR which is commonly high in those patients.
- Proper de-airing is confirmed on TOE or epicardial echocardiography.

After weaning off CPB, drains are inserted and the chest closed in the usual fashion. In case of significant bleeding or borderline graft function, the chest can be left open and sealed with membrane until chest closure is possible.

If the graft function is not good enough, ECMO is used to support the circulation for few days until the graft recovers. ECMO cannulation could be central (RA–aorta) using CPB cannulas or peripheral, which would facilitate chest closure and reduce the risk of infection.

Technical considerations

Bicaval versus biatrial
- Bicaval transplant is the commonly used technique nowadays:
  - Lower risk of tricuspid insufficiency.
  - Less arrhythmogenic.
  - Avoids need for complex intra-atrial adjustments (e.g. baffle redirection as in Senning or Mustard procedure).

- Biatrial can be helpful in rare situations as in left SVC with azygos continuation of the interrupted IVC. It avoids the risk of SVC anastomosis commonly seen with the bicaval technique. Also, it can be used in neonatal heart transplantation to avoid stenosis at the caval anastomosis site.

Dextrocardia

- The pericardial cavity is usually big enough to accommodate the donor heart.
- You might need to cut the left side of the pericardium and open the left pleura (avoid phrenic nerve).
- There is usually a dead pericardial space that was previously occupied by the cardiac apex. The pericardium needs to be plicated and attached to the chest wall to obliterate this space and avoid pericardial collection or rightward rotation of the apex, which may distort the tricuspid valve and the interventricular septum.

Venous pathway

Left SVC

- Presence of additional left superior caval vein with a bridging (innominate) vein; it can be ligated and divided.
- Presence of a single left SVC or additional left superior caval vein without a bridging vein:
  - Anastomose to donor innominate.
  - Use a prosthetic conduit and place in pre- or retro-aortic position (Fig. 22.1.1).

Anomalous pulmonary veins

- Those are usually dealt with in a previous stage. The principle is to have wide confluence and enough cuff of tissue around to anastomose to the donor heart.

Great vessels

Aorta

- Arch hypoplasia or coarctation are usually dealt with at early stage.
- In presence of distortion, re-coarctation, or calcified patches: repair is carried out before the donor heart is brought into the chest. That might require a period of circulatory arrest or selective cerebral perfusion.
- In patients with ventriculoatrial discordance (transposition of the great arteries), restoring the normal relation between the aorta and the PA may require:
  - Reversing LeCompte manoeuvre with or without shortening of the ascending aorta.
  - Repositioning of the pulmonary confluence to the proximal left PA (Fig. 22.1.2).

Pulmonary arteries

- Diminutive branch PA is usually a contraindication to heart-alone transplantation.
- Reconstruction of any focal narrowing of branch PA (preferable with donor tissue).
- Resection/division of previously inserted stents may be required.
- Intraoperative hybrid stenting of branch PA may be needed to avoid kinking or compression.

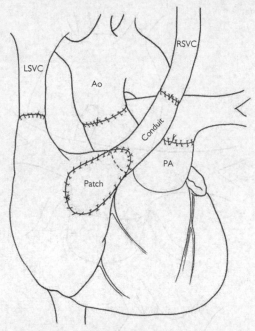

Fig. 22.1.1 In case of a single left SVC (LSVC), a conduit can be used to connect it to the RAA in a pre- or retro-aortic position. RSVC, right superior vena cava.

Transplantation in single-ventricle patients
- Usually shows higher complexity and combination of previously mentioned challenges.
- Patients are usually in poor general condition as result of Fontan failure (liver cirrhosis, PLE, chylothorax, plastic bronchitis, etc.).
- Higher collateral load (commonly assessed on MRI or aortic angiogram) requires higher CPB flows, avoidance of donor heart distension, and meticulous haemostasis.

Outcome

The outcome of transplantation in patients with congenital heart disease is relatively good and has improved over the years. However, considering all the previously mentioned challenges, early survival remains lower than in children with cardiomyopathy (3-year survival of 79% vs 88% respectively) this gap tends to get smaller with time (10-year survival 68% vs 70%). Although results have improved, patients with a single ventricle still have 10-year survival of 53%.

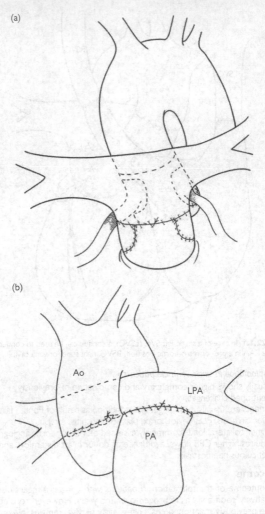

Fig. 22.1.2 (a) Typical aortopulmonary arrangement following LeCompte manoeuvre with the PA anterior to the aorta. (b) The donor main PA is anastomosed to the proximal left PA (LPA) while the distal cut end of the recipient's main PA (at previous confluence) is now closed.

Paediatric extracorporeal membrane oxygenation

Introduction

Extracorporeal membrane oxygenation (ECMO), also known as extracorporeal life support (ECLS), is well established as therapy for cardiorespiratory failure in the paediatric population.

The care of children on ECMO is a complex task, requiring the expertise of specialized intensivists, surgeons, haematologists, cardiologists, and respiratory physicians. ECMO is deployed in increasingly complex situations to provide the time required to tackle the underlying pathophysiology and allow intrinsic recovery of lungs and heart or bridging to decision.

Patient selection in paediatric ECMO

Patients who are potential ECMO candidates should be discussed at the earliest opportunity with the appropriate paediatric ICU/surgical team. Early initiation of ECLS can reduce end-organ malperfusion and failure.

The following inclusion and exclusion criteria are suggestive. Each case merits individual discussion with an ECMO centre.

Inclusion criteria

- >34 weeks of gestation.
- >2.5 kg body weight. Neonates with lower birth weight may be candidates in certain centres depending on assessment of vessel size for cannulation. Successful ECMO has been reported in preterm neonates of <32 weeks of gestation and <1.5 kg.

Exclusion criteria

- Major intracranial haemorrhage.
- Severe neurological injury.
- Lethal congenital malformation, chromosomal anomalies.

Indications

Cardiac

- Post cardiotomy:
  - Failure to wean from CPB.
  - Postoperative instability or cardiac arrest.
  - Post transplantation: donor heart dysfunction, RV failure secondary to PH.
- HF:
  - Cardiomyopathy (idiopathic, viral, nutritional), structural heart lesions (anomalous left coronary artery from the pulmonary artery (ALCAPA), obstructive cardiac lesions, borderline ventricle).
  - As a bridge to diagnosis, recovery, VAD support, or transplantation.
- Intractable arrythmia.

Pulmonary

- Pulmonary infection. Viral pneumonia is the most common cause of respiratory failure in children beyond the neonatal period.
- Acute respiratory distress syndrome/acute lung injury.
- Refractory asthma.
- Aspiration.

- Neonatal lung disease:
  - Primary PH.
  - Congenital diaphragmatic hernia.
  - Meconium aspiration.
  - Hyaline membrane disease (infant respiratory distress syndrome).

Others
- Septic shock.
- Drowning.
- Hypothermic arrest.
- Arrest of unknown cause: bridge to diagnosis and resuscitation.
  - ECMO support in cardiac arrest (E-CPR) can be offered for witnessed cardiac arrest with ongoing resuscitation attempt where conventional measures have failed. Caution should be exercised in unwitnessed arrest situations.

Technical aspects of ECMO

Various configurations exist to provide pulmonary-alone or cardiopulmonary support. Regardless of configuration, the basic principle of ECMO combines a centrifugal pump, oxygenator, sweep gas exchanger, and heater–cooler and optional haemofiltration device in complete circuit with the patient.

Venoarterial support

(Also see Chapter 8.) VA ECMO supports both the cardiac and pulmonary systems and is warranted where both gas exchange and cardiac output are inadequate. Blood is extracted from the venous system, oxygenated, and returned to the arterial system via a centrifugal pump.

VA ECMO should be considered in patients with inadequate cardiac output to maintain tissue perfusion despite maximal inotropic therapy.

Venovenous support

(Also see Chapter 8.) VV ECMO can be employed to support the pulmonary system alone in paediatric patients with potentially reversible causes of respiratory failure. Blood is extracted from the venous system, oxygenated, and returned to the venous system via a centrifugal pump. Concomitant cardiac dysfunction warrants consideration of VA ECMO as cardiac output is not supported in a VV configuration. Older children with irreversible pathology such as cystic fibrosis may also be candidates as a bridge to lung transplantation.

VV ECMO should be considered in patients with:
- Oxygenation index >35–40 in neonates and >25 in older children.
- Severe hypoxic respiratory failure demonstrated by PaO_2/FiO_2 ratios <60–80.
- Severe hypercapnic respiratory failure demonstrated by sustained respiratory acidosis.

Patients will have reached maximal ventilation therapy including appropriate application of high-frequency oscillatory ventilation, prone positioning, and inhaled NO therapy.

Other configurations

VA ECMO with left heart drainage

LA venting is recommended in cardiac ECMO for poor ventricular function to optimize recovery. As ECMO flow is established, afterload increases which may negate any ejection from the poorly functioning LV. A poorly contractile left heart is unable to empty collateral return effectively. Consequently, left heart distension occurs resulting in pulmonary oedema and limited myocardial recovery due to increased wall tension, compromised coronary flow, and subendocardial ischaemia.

Options for management

- Ideally, a left heart vent should be routinely placed and incorporated into the venous return limb:
  - Central cannulation: direct placement via LAA or right superior pulmonary vein, LV apex is another option; in the context of previous cardiac surgery, LV apex can be approached via left thoracotomy.
  - Peripheral cannulation: percutaneous insertion via femoral vein across PFO/ASD under fluoroscopy/TOE guidance.
- A balloon/blade atrial septostomy with placement of a stent is performed. This decompresses the left heart into the negatively pressurized RA.
- Inotropic support allows some ejection to empty to left heart. This must be balanced with resting of the myocardium to allow recovery.

VAV ECMO

(Also see Chapter 8.) VAV ECMO may be required in patients with both cardiac and pulmonary failure who are being supported by femoral VA ECMO. In VA ECMO with minimal cardiac ejection, the myocardial and cerebral flow is achieved in a retrograde fashion from the femoral ECMO cannula to the head and neck vessels. As cardiac function recovers, the heart will eject poorly oxygenated blood, due to the concomitant presence of pulmonary failure, preferentially to the upper body, while the lower body is supplied with oxygenated blood via the ECMO circuit. The mixing zone is dependent upon the competing cardiac ejection and can result in differential hypoxia. This phenomenon can also be observed in congenital heart patients with large amounts of collateral returns into the left heart bypassing the lungs.

Patients on femoral VA ECMO should have continuous monitoring of saturations in both upper and lower limbs and cerebral/flank oximetry.

Options for management

- Increase ECMO flow to drive mixing zone retrograde to ascending aorta. This may be limited by cannula size and may be detrimental to cardiac recovery.
- Optimize ventilation to improve oxygenation of pulmonary venous return. This may be limited by barotrauma and oxygen toxicity concerns.
- VAV configuration (see Chapter 8): additional arterial inflow cannula via right IJ vein to deliver oxygenated blood returning to the RA and thereby improving saturations of ejected blood from left heart. Alternatively, hybrid combination of FA inflow and Avalon cannula can be used.
- Conversion to central cannulation.

Conversion of ECMO configuration

A changing clinical picture may require a reconfiguration or conversion of ECMO. Patients on VV ECMO may develop hypotension and inadequate perfusion requiring a conversion to VA ECMO. Patients on VA ECMO may experience resolution of cardiac dysfunction but persist with hypoxia related to lung injury. The patients should be considered for conversion from VA to VV ECMO to mitigate complications associated with arterial cannulation and to provide longer support on VV ECMO until lungs recover.

Cannulation strategies

Suitable cannula size, site, and safe insertion is critical to achieve adequate support and achieve successful patient outcomes. Strategy depends on the desired mode of ECMO, age/weight of patient, vessel availability, underlying condition, and experience of surgeon.

Choice of cannula

Imaging of vessels pre ECMO can be useful to guide cannula sizing. It is important to note that adequate flow is dependent on both inlet and outlet cannula calibre. The size of cannula is determined based on patient weight (Table 22.2.1). While the larger cannula offers higher potential flow, these are more likely to cause vessel damage, lead to venous obstruction, intermittent cannula obstruction due to vessel wall proximity, and distal flow compromise. The cannula size/weight table is used as a guidance only to achieve the estimated full ECMO flow for the patient size. Smaller cannula should always be made available and used when native vessels are small or fragile and in difficult cannulation to avoid vessel damage or dissection. The modern design of ECMO cannulas is capable of achieving optimal flow at a smaller calibre.

Table 22.2.1 Choice of cannula

Patient size (kg)	Arterial cannula (Fr)	Venous cannula (Fr)
2	8	8–10
3–6	10	10–12
6–8	12	14
8–16	14	17
16–30	17	19
30–40	17	21
>40	21	25

VV ECMO

- The classic configuration of VV ECMO includes two venous cannulas: bilateral common femoral or femoral–right IJ. Direct open cannulation or Seldinger technique are both possible. Guidance can be with TOE or fluoroscopy. The separation distance between the tips of these two cannulas is important to minimize recirculation of the oxygenated blood.

- A bicaval double lumen cannula can be inserted into the right IJ permitting venous outflow to the oxygenator from the RA and IVC and oxygenated outflow into the RA through a single site. The oxygenated return is directed toward the tricuspid valve orifice to maximize forward flow and avoid recirculation. VV ECMO cannulation can be achieved with a fully percutaneous method under ultrasound guidance. While the benefits of a single IJ cannula include facilitating ambulation of patients, a wired reinforced bicaval design cannula is associated with a higher risk of caval and cardiac perforation.

VA ECMO

Central configuration

Central cannulation is accessed via median sternotomy. Cannulas are placed into the RA and ascending aorta. Central cannulation will be the technique most familiar and reproducible to surgeons due to the routine of placing patients onto CPB.

- Central cannulation may be most appropriate in post-cardiotomy patients requiring ECMO. Cannulas placed during CPB can be used if cardiac dysfunction necessitating ECMO is present at separation from bypass. In patients requiring ECMO due to instability in the postoperative period, re-entry through the sternotomy may be the easiest route.
- Central cannulation can also be achieved rapidly via innominate artery when there is a Gore-Tex shunt *in situ*, such as following reconstruction of the hypoplastic arch or after the Norwood procedure.
- Central cannulation is the preferred route for patients requiring ECLS for sepsis as higher flows can be achieved secondary to larger vessels and cannula calibre.
- Central cannulation is not feasible in children who require emergent ECMO and who have had prior cardiac surgery.
- A disadvantage of central cannulation is the requirement to keep the chest open, exposing the patient to infection, bleeding, sedation, and paralysis.

Peripheral configuration

Neck cannulation

Paediatric patients can be cannulated in the neck for VA and VV ECMO. See Fig. 22.2.1 and Fig. 22.2.2 for technical aspects.

- Cervical cannulation is the primary modality of peripheral ECMO in neonates and infants.
- Higher risk of cerebral events is reported in older children >2–3 years old. Central cannulation should be considered instead, or femoral cannulation in bigger children.
- Patency of bilateral carotid arteries and jugular veins can be established quickly by bedside neck ultrasound scanning.
- If the clinical situation allows, pre-ECMO cross-section cerebral imaging for baseline and assessment of the circle of Willis can be helpful. In neonates, cranial ultrasound should suffice. Bilateral near-infrared spectroscopy can suggest cerebral flow compromise and indicate a change in strategy is required.

- Benefits of neck cannulation include avoidance of sternotomy and its risks of bleeding and infection. In urgent situations, neck cannulation can be rapid and CPR can be continued during cannulation.
- TTE may be used to guide and check cannula position.
- CXR post cannulation to confirm good cannula position (Fig. 22.2.2).
- Upon decannulation, vessels can usually be repaired to re-establish ipsilateral antegrade cerebral flow.

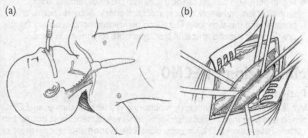

Fig. 22.2.1 (a) The patient is positioned, and anatomy identified for dissection. (b) The vessels are isolated. Caution is required regarding the vagus nerve running between the vessels.

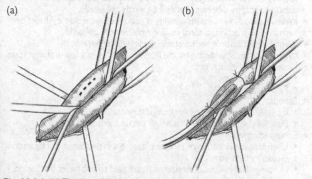

Fig. 22.2.2 (a) The dotted lines indicate the direction of the arteriotomy. (b) Arterial cannulation is performed first, approximately 2.5 cm of advancement into the carotid artery. The cannula is secured, and the process repeated in the same manner for venous cannulation. Venous cannulation can be more challenging. Advancement of 6–7 cm is correct for most neonates. CXR and echocardiography should be used to confirm position and status of LA distension.

Femoral cannulation

In older children weighing >15–20 kg, VA ECMO can be achieved via femoral vessels. While vessel calibre may be amenable to cannulation with adequate size cannulation to achieve flows, caution must be taken to avoid limb ischaemia due to occlusive cannula size.

Distal limb perfusion can be achieved by various methods:
- Avoid direct cannulation of the vessel by a side graft anastomosis to the femoral artery allowing bidirectional flow to the limb and body. Control of flow into the limb can be difficult to monitor and control, resulting in hyperperfusion. Leak via graft wall could be problematic—this could be mitigated by advancing the arterial cannula to the end of the prosthetic graft, just above the femoral arteriotomy.
- A limb perfusion cannula can be placed into the distal femoral artery, superficial femoral artery, or posterior tibial artery. Accurate perfusion is possible with this technique. Distal limb perfusion cannula is usually feasible only in larger patients, that is, in teenagers close to young adult size.

Monitoring of ECMO

Patient

While invasive and quantitative monitoring is essential during an ECMO run, the importance of bedside clinical serial assessment must not be forgotten. Patients on ECMO require close observation and management of haemodynamics as well as vigilance for complications related to bleeding and thrombosis (see Complications of ECMO, p. 285).
- Tissue perfusion: cap refill, urine output, serial lactate measures. Monitor lower limb perfusion with pulse oximetry and Doppler ultrasonography where peripheral cannulas are sited.
- Invasive blood pressure monitoring is required: in cardiac dysfunction with loss of ejection, arterial tracing may be non-pulsatile.
- Pump inlet pressures are helpful in guiding management of hypovolaemia. Shuddering of the lines may occur in a low-volume state.
- Mixed venous saturations:
  - Oxygen delivery.
  - Recirculation in VV.
- Bloods:
  - Coagulation profile (see Anticoagulation, p. 283).
  - Platelet consumption: indicative of circuit thrombus.
- Echocardiography:
  - Useful for confirmation of cannula placement in peripheral configurations.
  - Guide to fluid status.
  - In non-pulsatile flow, attention must be paid to left heart distension.
  - Establishing any underlying diagnosis and temporal changes.
- Detection of intracranial complications during ECMO therapy:
  - Near-infrared spectroscopy.
  - Transcranial ultrasonography.

ECMO circuit
- Flow (L/min): maintain adequate cardiac output. Flow can be adjusted by changing the revolutions per minute (rpm).
- Inlet and outlet pressures: helpful in guiding fluid status.
- Pre- and post-membrane pressures: elevated transmembrane gradient may indicate oxygenator compromise.
- Emboli count: where air emboli are noted, check all access ports and taps of circuit and patient (e.g. central line).

Flow rates

VA ECMO

- Individual patients require clinical evaluation to determine the ideal rate based on perfusion parameters. The following calculations provide a baseline guide for commencing ECMO:
- Patients <10 kg: 100–150 mL/kg/min.
- Patients >10 kg: 2.5–3.5 L/m²/min.

Consider higher flows in patients with septic shock, parallel circulation (single-ventricle physiology), and extracardiac shunts. A systemic–PA shunt such as modified Blalock–Taussig shunt is not usually clipped or ligated.

VV ECMO

- Patients <10 kg: 70–150 mL/kg/min.
- Patients >10 kg: 1.8–3.5 L/m²/min.

Anticoagulation

Haemorrhagic and thromboembolic complications remain the major cause of mortality and morbidity in ECLS. Blood contact with artificial surfaces of the circuit, pump, and oxygenator initiate the clotting and inflammatory cascades in an unpredictable manner. Plasma proteins become denatured during ECMO, increasing plasma viscosity and haemolysis occurs secondary to shear stress, cavitation, turbulence, and osmotic forces. Patients frequently have multifactorial coagulopathies related to underlying pathophysiology.

Important factors of pro-haemorrhagic status:
- Excessive heparin use.
- Consumption of coagulation factors.
- Low fibrinogen levels.
- Thrombocytopenia.
- Platelet dysfunction.
- Hyperfibrinolysis.

Important factors of pro-thrombotic status:
- Inadequate use of heparin.
- Acquired thrombin deficiency.
- Consumption of protein C and protein S.
- Consumption of tissue factor pathway inhibitor.
- Endothelial dysfunction.
- HIT.
- Blood stasis in chambers and venous system.

Unfractionated heparin (UFH) is the most commonly used anticoagulant used in paediatric ECMO, although UFH has an unpredictable response in newborns and children. UFH has a short half-life and is reversible with administration of protamine sulphate. UFH is given as a bolus (50–100 units/kg of body weight) at ECLS cannulation and is then infused continuously during ECMO support under tight control of anticoagulation monitoring.

Alternative anticoagulation includes direct thrombin inhibition (e.g. bivalirudin), factor Xa inhibitors (rivaroxaban, argatroban), and nafamostat mesilate. No large-scale studies on these alternatives are available in the paediatric population. Their use may be indicated in children with HIT and heparin resistance.

Monitoring of anticoagulation

Individual ECMO centres will have protocol-driven monitoring of anticoagulation depending on availability of testing panels. Quantitative tests should be utilized in combination with the clinical picture. Most clotting laboratories assays are chromatography based: elevated plasma bilirubin, plasma free haemoglobin, and triglycerides will affect the accuracy of results.

The following tests are applicable in ECMO but not universally available:

- ACT: this is a readily available quick bedside test. It is the most commonly used parameter in CPB. ACT is affected by many factors such as platelet function, fibrinogen and factor levels, temperature, and haemodilution status. An ACT of 180–220 is typically targeted in the non-bleeding ECMO patient.
- Anti-Xa activity: plasma anti-Xa indirectly measures the activity of heparins. It is commonly used as the primary monitoring tool in ECMO, although controversy exists due to the poorly defined therapeutic range. Anti-Xa below therapeutic range may be due to inadequate heparin or patient antithrombin deficiency.
- Antithrombin (AT) level: heparin effect is due to binding of heparin to AT which results in a many-fold increase in the anticoagulant activity of AT. Adequate AT is required for effect of heparin. A relative deficiency, and lower activity of AT is seen in the neonate and infant population. AT concentrate replacement is indicated when reduced effect of UFH is evident.
- aPTT: aPTT is reportedly less reliable in the neonatal and paediatric population when evaluating UFH status.
- aPTT plasma: measures aPTT after neutralization of heparin.
- Platelet count: should be maintained at a minimum of 80,000 cells/mm³. The decision to transfuse platelets is based on the count alongside clinical assessment of bleeding status.
- Fibrinogen level: maintain at a minimal level of 100 g/dL. Fibrinogen concentrate or cryoprecipitates can be administered at subtherapeutic levels.
- Viscoelastic tests (TEG): evaluate whole-blood coagulation and fibrinolysis. These are relatively new tests and their application is not yet fully established. Time to fibrin formation, kinetics, clot strength and stability, and function of platelets are evaluated.

Principles of clinical activity

- Perform an initial screening following initiation of ECMO to assess baseline coagulation status: consider multifactorial coagulopathy (liver compromise, factor deficiency, sepsis).
- Priming of the ECMO circuit will depend on urgency. In children, a combination of banked blood and colloids is preferable with UFH additive at 50–100 units per unit of packed red cells. Heparin–albumin coated priming tubing is used in certain units to reduce blood–plastic interface.
- Blood products such as platelets, FFP, or cryoprecipitate can be administered if significant coagulopathy exists prior to ECMO initiation. During an ECMO run, the decision to transfuse packed red cells, platelets, fresh frozen plasma, fibrinogen concentrate, or cryoprecipitate is based on laboratory data with accurate correlation of clinical assessment of coagulation status.

- Close observation of all components of the circuit (tubing, connectors, oxygenator, pump head) are required to monitor for clot or fibrin build-up. Monitor transmembrane pressure gradients which may indicate clot formation not visible to the eye.
- Rigorous monitoring of patients for clinical indicators of haemorrhagic or thrombotic sequelae.

Complications of ECMO

- Haemorrhagic events (cerebral, GI, pulmonary, surgical site).
- Thrombotic events.
- Infection.
- Limb ischaemia: in femoral ECMO due to occlusion of the femoral artery—this is mitigated with the use of graft anastomosis to allow bidirectional perfusion or distal limb cannula flow.
- Stroke:
  - Embolic or haemorrhagic.
  - In neck cannulation: consider imaging of the circle of Willis to confirm patency. Avoid neck cannulation in children >2–3 years.
- Massive air embolus.
- Disseminated intravascular coagulation.

Weaning from ECMO

On resolution of underlying physiology, the child will need to be safely trialled and weaned from ECMO.

Prior to weaning ensure:
- The processes and pathology leading to ECMO have been addressed adequately.
- Pulmonary function and cardiac function have been adequately assessed with ECHO, parameters of perfusion, CXR, and check of lung compliance.
- Inotropy is running to an adequate level to support weaning process.
- Patient is on inhaled NO at 20 parts per million.
- Fluid/blood boluses/emergency drugs are available.
- Full ventilatory support and titration of sweep gas accordingly.
- Arterial blood gases should be checked every 5–10 minutes during wean. Echocardiography may be useful to assess cardiac function when separated from ECMO.

Two techniques are reported:
- Once the ECMO is weaned to minimal flow 200 mL/min, a bridge is placed into the circuit between the inflow and outflow pipes. The cannulas are left *in situ* and clamped, resulting in separation from ECMO. The pump continues to circulate volume through the bridge to prevent stasis. Intermittently, the cannulas are unclamped to flush through to prevent clots. In case of a failed wean, the clamps are simply removed and full ECMO circulation reinitiated. After a successful trial period of separation, the child can be decannulated.

- Retrograde flow trial. The rpm speed is reduced to the point where native cardiac ejection overwhelms the pump vacuum. The child begins to eject into the aortic cannula creating retrograde flow. If the child is unable to generate flow >70 mL the trial should be abandoned. In case of a failed wean, the rpm speed is turned up to achieve adequate antegrade flow to re-establish ECMO. After a successful trial period, the child can be decannulated.

Coming off ECMO urgently

In rare situations, one may need to come off ECMO emergently, such as major haemorrhage from accidental decannulation, circuit rupture or leak, or air in the circuit between oxygenator and patient.

- Call for help (theatre team). Do not panic. Continuation of ECMO could be detrimental and lead to exsanguination, Control haemorrhage, cease ECMO, and resuscitate, before re-establishing ECMO.
- Clamp the arterial cannula then the venous cannula, and open the bridge if present.
- Local compression to control bleeding.
- Hand ventilate or optimize ventilator setting.
- Resuscitate with CPR, inotropes, and blood transfusion as necessary.

Outcomes of ECMO

- The use of ECMO has significantly increased over recent years: 68,693 neonatal and paediatric ECLS events have been reported to the Extracorporeal Life Support Organization international registry.
- Short-term survival rates of ECMO are dependent on underlying diagnosis, severity of illness, type of support, duration of support, comorbidities, and complications.
- Survival to discharge is lower for cardiac support with VA ECMO at 43% for neonates and 52% for paediatric compared to 73% and 59% for pulmonary VV support.
- E-CPR carries a 42% survival to discharge for both neonatal and paediatric populations.

Cardiac ECMO and outcomes

Factors reportedly associated with mortality among ECMO recipients in the cardiac population include E-CPR, single-ventricle physiology, lower body weight, prematurity, pre-ECMO acidosis, increased time to diagnosis of residual lesions, and longer time between intubation and initiation of ECMO. The majority of survivors separated from ECMO at <8 days. Early initiation of VA ECMO in cardiac patients and early address of residual lesions may improve outcomes.

The single-ventricle population

ECMO support of this group of patients remains uncommon but is increasing. The unique anatomy and physiology of this population demands thought in regard to cannulation, circuit flow, systemic thrombotic risk, and resting ventilation. Previous opinion was of poor outcomes in this group of patients, but recent data from the Extracorporeal Life Support Organization registry suggest ECMO is a viable option in the single-ventricle population.

Paediatric heart transplant: specific considerations

Heart transplantation remains the most effective therapy in paediatric patients with end-stage heart disease not amenable to conventional surgery. Besides many challenges that can be overcome in terms of unique anatomy, physiology, and technical demands, the shortage of paediatric donors remains the key limiting factor. Despite all these challenges, heart transplantation offers the most durable solution in paediatric patients, after exhausting all available repair options. Currently, with improved surgical outcome, immunotherapy, and long-term surveillance, median post-transplant survival surpasses 15 years in children and 22 years in infants (data from ISHLT).

The first successful human-to-human heart transplant operation (by Christian Barnard on 3 December 1967) was preceded by many pioneers, notably James Hardy (first human heart transplant, chimpanzee donor, 1964); Norman Shumway and Richard Lower (Stanford); Vladimir Demikhov (Moscow); and Charles Guthrie and Alexis Carrel (Nobel Prize in Physiology or Medicine, 1912).

The first paediatric heart transplant operation followed shortly after.

Pioneers in paediatric heart transplantation

- Adrian Kantrowitz (1967, New York: neonatal Ebstein anomaly, survived 6.5 hours).
- Denton Cooley (1968, Houston: 5-year-old, endocardial fibroelastosis, survived 8 days; 2-month-old, complete AV septal defect, survived 14 hours).
- Magdi Yacoub (1984, London: 10-day-old neonate, survived 18 days).
- Eric Rose (1984, New York: 4-year-old, single ventricle, survived late).
- Leonard Bailey (Loma Linda, 1985: neonate, survived late).

Early attempts

Although 'baby Fae' captured the headlines in 1984 by receiving a baboon heart, the first paediatric human heart transplantation took place 3 days after Barnard's success. After many years of intensive research, Adrian Kantrowitz carried out the first paediatric heart transplant in a 20-day old neonate with severe Ebstein anomaly (6 December 1967). Unfortunately, the baby died some 6 hours later, and the procedure was declared a 'failure'. Prior to the discovery of cyclosporine A (1976), there was little progress due to acute allograft rejection.

Successful transplantation

On 9 June 1984, the first successful paediatric heart transplant procedure was performed in Columbia University, New York. The recipient was a 4-year-old boy with a single ventricle, who lived until adulthood after a second heart transplant. Sadly, he died in his sleep during the first week of medical school. In Loma Linda, after baby Fae (survived 20 days), Leonard Bailey performed the first successful newborn-to-newborn transplant on 20 November 1985 in a patient with hypoplastic left heart syndrome. This marked the inception of a paediatric heart transplant programme. The first neonatal transplant recipient was still alive 33 years post transplantation in a late report (2019).

Unique characteristic of paediatric heart transplantation

Paediatric heart transplantation is unique from that for acquired heart disease in adults. Congenital heart disease affects 1 in 120 (0.8%) live births, and constitutes approximately 40% of heart transplantation in paediatric population. More than half of infant recipients have congenital heart lesions.

- Size of recipient is diverse in the paediatric population, ranging from a teenager with young adult size to a tiny newborn.
- Unique anatomy that is rarely seen in acquired heart disease and include higher proportion of left SVC, situs inversus, dextrocardia, heterotaxy, and arch anomalies.
- Pulmonary vascular disease, malnourishment, and sensitization are all more common in paediatric patients. Therefore, heart transplantation presents with specific challenges in the paediatric population.
- On the other hand, paediatric patients benefit from their immature immune system, and, using this advantage, the ABO-incompatible (ABOi) heart transplantation was introduced.

Another important distinction from the adult population, who primarily presented with cardiac (pump) failure, is a paediatric cohort with preserved cardiac function. These patients have circulatory failure as their primary reason for transplantation following Glenn/Fontan failure or multifocal obstructive disease. They form an 'unconventional' group who need a heart transplant.

Specific challenges in paediatric heart transplantation

Besides anatomical and technical demands, the availability of a suitable donor is probably the greatest challenge in paediatric heart transplantation. In end-stage congenital heart disease, patients usually present with a gradual decline rather than acute cardiac decompensation. Therefore, the urgency on the waiting list is under-prioritized, further adding to the waiting time. Excess waiting time increases waiting list mortality. Specific challenges in paediatric patients include:

- Shortage of donors especially in small recipients (particularly <10 kg).
- Lack of clinical prioritization: absence of overt HF as in failing Fontan circulation.
- Sensitized patients: presence of HLA antibodies due to previous blood transfusion or homograft materials.
- Elevated PVR secondary to left heart disease, diastolic dysfunction, or borderline left heart structure as in Shone's complex.
- Multiple significant collateral load in cyanotic patients.
- Anatomical challenges: bilateral SVC, dextrocardia, transposed great vessels, heterotaxy.
- Technical challenges include multiple previous sternotomies, extensive collaterals in cyanotic patients, occluded peripheral vessels for bypass, previous stent or shunts, and additional reconstruction required for arch of pulmonary arteries

Primary transplantation (or conventional surgery)

Although heart transplantation was offered as a primary treatment option for complex congenital heart lesions in the early era, this is rare nowadays. Transplantation is usually reserved for after palliative or repair procedures which have failed to improve the patients, and hence is termed a 'rescue therapy'. Nevertheless, late survival appears to be more encouraging in patients who have had a primary transplant procedure for complex univentricular heart.

The first successful neonatal transplantation recipient who had hypoplastic left heart syndrome was still alive 33 years later with current ongoing follow-up. With reported long-term follow-up of neonatal heart transplantation that exceeded 64% survival at 20 years and 55% at 25 years, late outcome surpassed that of conventional palliation for hypoplastic left heart syndrome. The shortage in the donor pool for the paediatric population precludes heart transplantation as a primary therapeutic option, which is reserved for when conventional surgery is unfavourable.

Common pathologies

The two most common groups of pathologies referred for consideration or evaluation for transplant are *cardiomyopathy* and *congenital heart disease*. In infants, congenital heart disease is the more common indication for transplantation than cardiomyopathy. This differs in children over 1 year old where cardiomyopathy is the most common indication. Cardiac tumours and retransplantation form very small groups.

Cardiomyopathy

* Dilated cardiomyopathy: idiopathic (66%); acute or post myocarditis (16%); neuromuscular disorder (e.g. Duchenne and Becker dystrophy) (9%); Barth syndrome; familial cardiomyopathy (5%); inborn error of metabolism (1%); autoimmune disease; toxins such as chemotherapy; nutritional cause: vitamin D deficiency, carnitine (amino acid) deficiency; thyrotoxicosis.
* Hypertrophic cardiomyopathy: idiopathic (most common), familial, inborn errors of metabolism (Pompe disease, mitochondrial disease), Noonan syndrome.
* Restrictive cardiomyopathy.
* Tachycardia / arrhythmia induced cardiomyopathy.

The incidence of cardiomyopathy is significantly higher in the infant population. DCM is the most common form (approximately 50–75% of all cardiomyopathies) and presents earlier in childhood. Forty per cent of paediatric DCM cases either die or need a transplant within 5 years of diagnosis.

Hypertrophic cardiomyopathy is the second largest group (40% of cardiomyopathies). Although presenting later than DCM, hypertrophic cardiomyopathy has a similar long-term outcome with a mortality rate 2 years after diagnosis of 12.7% versus 13.6% for DCM.

Other forms of cardiomyopathy, that is, restrictive and arrhythmia-induced cardiomyopathy, are rare (<5%) in the paediatric population. Restrictive cardiomyopathy is particularly problematic due to early development of PVR and its consequences related to early graft failure.

Congenital heart lesions

Rescue therapy following conventional surgery:
- Biventricular repair: Shone's complex, borderline left heart, endocardial fibroelastosis.
- Univentricular palliation: failing single ventricle following arteriopulmonary shunts, Glenn or Fontan procedures; protein-losing enteropathy (PLE), more rarely for plastic bronchitis.

Heart transplantation as *primary therapy* can be considered in the following:
- Hypoplastic left heart syndrome with (1) tricuspid, that is, systemic atrioventricular valve that is severely dysplastic and regurgitant or (2) poor ventricular function.
- Other single ventricle disease with (1) poor ventricular function or (2) severely stenotic or regurgitant atrioventricular valve.
- Pulmonary atresia with intact septum and RV-dependent coronary circulation with aorto-coronary atresia or significant proximal coronary stenosis.
- Pulmonary atresia with intact septum, sinusoids in RV myocardium, with reduced LV function and/or sign of myocardial ischaemia but patent proximal coronaries.
- Pulmonary atresia with intact septum with severe tricuspid regurgitation and massive (wall-to-wall) RV dilatation.
- Single ventricle with heterotaxy and total anomalous pulmonary venous drainage.
- Most severe form of Ebstein anomaly in neonates.

Cardiac tumours

- Benign: multifocal and non-resectable intracardiac tumour.
- Primary cardiac malignancy (e.g. sarcoma) that is confined to the heart.

Paediatric waiting list

Waiting list mortality

The size of the donor pool remains at best stagnant if not reduced, while more candidates are added onto the waiting list. MCS in paediatric patients has improved and allowed more children to wait longer. Due to the shortage of donor hearts, time and mortality on waiting list are higher; the issue is more pronounced for the paediatric population. The mortality rate on the waiting list among paediatric candidate under 5 years old is 15–20% by 12 months after listing. Congenital heart disease patients are also more likely than those with cardiomyopathy to die on the waiting list (nearly one-third) prior to transplantation.

The law

There is a regional discrepancy of donor availability that could be due to culture, faith, belief, and public awareness. In order to increase organ donation, the law has changed in the UK. From May 2020, organ donation in England has changed to an 'opt out' system after Parliament approved 'Max and Keira's law': All adults are now presumed organ donors in England unless they've registered to opt out or informed their family. The law does not apply to (1) those under 18 years old; (2) those who lack mental capacity, and therefore cannot opt out; and (3) visitors or those with less than 12 months residency in England before death. The new law, however, may not improve the paediatric waiting list, as it applies only to adults.

Strategies to increase the paediatric donor pool

In order to broaden the donor pool for children, oversized donors are already used for paediatric patients, as well as ABOi donors. In order to further broaden the donor pool, size matching using criteria other than weight has been evaluated (see Special considerations, p. xxx). Awareness among public and intensive care units continues to play a pivotal role to increase donors for paediatric recipient. The rate of organ donation among infants is ten times lower than older age groups. A lower organ donor recruitment rate could be due to unfamiliarity among paediatric practitioners or difficulty in the diagnosis of brainstem death in young patients.

Special considerations

Oversize donor

In the paediatric population, the use of an oversized donor has been shown to be safe: the strategy will widen the donor pool and reduce time on the waiting list. The 10-year survival has been shown to be comparable between oversize and conventional size matching.

Donor versus recipient size

Current practice on the paediatric waiting list is to match recipient and donor based on weight (donor weight 0.6–3.0 times that of the recipient has not been shown to be associated with adverse outcomes). In general, an oversized donor with weight up to three times that of the recipient can be accepted, although some centres reported safe use of 'extreme' mismatched heart that is over three times the recipient weight. Older children (>10 years old or >20 kg) usually can accept a heart from the adult donor pool. Newer assessment methods to match include using height versus estimated cardiac dimension (by echocardiography) to assess for a suitable donor otherwise not matched by conventional weight method.

Potential issues with oversizing

The use of an oversized donor heart is associated with a higher rate of delayed sternal closure.

Other issues that have been linked to oversized donor hearts include (1) hypertension in recipient, (2) early overperfusion and potential cerebral injury, (3) lobar collapse, and (4) RV compression/failure following sternal closure. Many of these issues are rare in practice including 'big heart syndrome' (neurological complication manifesting as post-transplant seizure due to overperfusion and reflex cerebral vasoconstriction).

Technical considerations

To fit in a bigger heart, technical considerations include (1) opening the pleural space; (2) left pericardiectomy above phrenic nerve, rarely bilateral;

(3) reduction of donor atrial size; and (4) relaxing incisions on diaphragmatic surface

Cautions in oversizing

Careful considerations are required in the following settings: (1) very small neonate who has tiny intrathoracic space, and (2) history of multiple re-sternotomies or known to have severe adhesions. In patients with densely cemented adhesions, the pericardial space is tight and pleural spaces may be densely adherent and could not be opened to fit in the donor heart.

When there is concern that a donor heart may not fit, further assessments could aid in the decision of the implanting surgeon whether to accept the offer: (1) cardiothoracic ratio on chest radiographs, (2) echocardiographic assessment (intercaval distance, between SVC/RA and IVC/RA junctions and LV end-diastolic dimension), and (3) feedback from the procuring surgeon after measuring the width and length of the donor heart.

Marginal donor

A significant proportion of paediatric patients awaiting heart transplantation die on the waiting list. The mortality is higher in younger recipients where donors are scarce. On the other hand, offers are turned down in a significant proportion of potential donors (one-third of all donors). Potential donors with impaired ventricular function (EF <50%), on high-dose or multiple inotropes, with functional valvar regurgitation are often turned down. These marginal hearts could be considered as donors.

- Depressed donor heart function could be reversible, such as myocardial dysfunction associated with brain death or in the setting of sepsis.
- Use of donor hearts with mildly impaired (LVEF 45–54%) and moderate-severely depressed (<45%) and/or segmental wall motion abnormalities resulted in comparable post-transplant survival outcomes with donor hearts with normal LVEF (≥55%).
- History of CPR should not prelude a donor.
- Use of vasopressors and inotropes are not contraindications.
- Elective post-bypass ECMO following implantation may be considered to support cardiac recovery.

ISHLT guidelines recommend refusal of donor heart with EF less than 40%.

ABO incompatibility (ABOi transplantation)

ABOi heart transplantation was first performed in infants (late 1990s, Canada). ABOi transplantation is usually contraindicated due to hyperacute rejection: anti-A or anti-B antibodies attack the donor's antigen on vascular endothelial cells, activate the complements, and cause vascular thrombosis. ABO compatible only donor pool would result in excessive wait time and mortality especially for children in O-group.

Immunological basis

The immune system in infants is still immature. In the first few months of life, infants have only maternal antibodies. Anti-A or -B antibodies (isohaemagglutinins) to blood group antigens develop gradually from 6 to 24 months of age due to gastrointestinal colonization of microorganisms. The complement attack system is also not fully mature yet. When an ABOi donor heart is implanted, hyperacute rejection does not occur due to absent or lack of anti-A or -B antibodies.

Interestingly, antibody levels remain absent or very low late after ABOi transplantation in most patients, suggestive of development of long-term tolerance towards the donor's ABH antigen. This immune tolerance (B-cell tolerance) allows excellent long-term graft survival and freedom from antibody-mediated rejection.

ABOi listing is institution based. Currently, UNOS recommends primary ABOi listing for those under 2 years old and low isohaemagglutinin level 1:4 or less.

• Check for detectable anti-A or -B levels in plasma.
• If positive, quantify the level of antibodies by haemodilution (called 'isohaemagglutinin titre'). The plasma is diluted until no antibody is detected (1:16 titre has a higher level of antibodies than 1:4).
• Repeat titre periodically. Immediate repeat test on donor heart offer. If titre is high, discuss with surgeon/cardiologist.
• Intraoperative complete whole body exchange transfusion is commenced until titre is less than 1:4.
• Repeat titre regularly prior to release of cross-clamp and reperfuse heart only after titre level fall. Repeat titre at regular interval after donor heart reperfusion.

Older children can be considered based on urgency (oldest ABOi recipient was 8.8 years old) and higher titre of 1:16 or greater is possible and does not exclude ABOi transplantation (up to 1:256 has been reported successfully).

ABOi listing and transplantation outcome

ABOi transplantation shortens the waiting time (by 20–25%) and reduces mortality (from >50% to <10% in infants). Although ABOi listed patients are younger, with higher urgency status and risks (more mechanical ventilation, congenital heart disease), post-transplant survival, graft rejection, and vasculopathy rates are not inferior in ABOi recipients.

Blood transfusion during and after ABOi transplantation

(See Table 22.3.1.)

Blood group A has A-antigen on erythrocytes (and platelets) and anti-B antibodies in plasma. Group B has B-antigen and anti-A.

Group O has no antigen, but both anti-A and anti-B in plasma, therefore avoid giving O plasma or platelet (as platelet preparation from O blood comes with antibodies).

Blood group AB has both antigens but no anti-A or anti-B antibodies in plasma. Therefore, use AB plasma product or platelet only for A, B, and AB recipients. In an O recipient, product from the AB group or the donor heart's blood group can be used.

For red cell transfusion, use O red cells or recipient's blood group.

Sensitization in paediatric recipients

Allosensitization in paediatric recipients is an important issue that limits the availability of a matching donor and has an important impact on graft longevity. This refers to immunological sensitization due to preformed antibodies against HLA and occasionally non-HLA.

Table 22.3.1 Compatible typing of blood products for transfusion during and after ABOi heart transplantation

ABOi recipient	Donor heart	Blood transfusion	
		Plasma product/ platelet	Red cell concentrate
O	AB	AB	O
	A	AB or A	
	B	AB or B	
A	AB	AB	O or A
	B		
B	AB	AB	O or B
	A		
AB	AB, A, B, or O	AB	AB, A, B, or O

Human leucocyte antigen

HLA is a cell surface protein that differentiates between self and non-self.
- MHC (major histocompatibility complex) is the region on the genome that encodes HLA. In human, the MHC (genes and proteins) is also called HLA and is located on chromosome 6 (>200 genes).
- Most studied HLA genes are A, B, C and D (DP, DQ, DR) and divided into: Class I MHC (A, B, C genes) is expressed on all nucleated cells (HLA-A, HLA-B, and HLA-C); Class II MHC (D genes) is usually expressed by antigen-presenting cells (B-cells, macrophages, dendritic cells, etc.).

Sensitized candidates (defined as PRA >10%)

These have preformed antibodies against specific donor HLAs (DSAs):
- Candidate's serum is added in wells that contain lymphocyte cells from random population samples: anti-HLA antibodies cause cell lysis. PRA represents the proportion of wells with cell lysis (lymphocytotoxicity assay).
- The initial PRA test screens for sensitized candidates and how often their sera will cross-react with the population. It does not specify which type of anti-HLA.

Sensitized paediatric patients formed about one-quarter of the waiting list, with higher-risk morbidity and mortality both while on the waiting list and post transplantation due to longer waiting times, higher rate of acute allograft rejection and vasculopathy, and reduced survival post transplantation. However, HLA sensitization does not preclude transplant. *If PRA is greater than 10%, the next steps involve:*
- More specific newer assays to assess the type of DSA and its strength of binding (MFI).
- Deciding the presence of which HLA(s) on the donor will be unacceptable (certain DSAs are more detrimental than others, e.g. anti HLA-DQ).

- Determining the calculated PRA: an estimate of the percentage of organ donors with unacceptable HLAs. A calculated PRA of 70% implies only 30% of donors will be compatible. Calculated PRA is computed based on national data of HLA frequencies.
- Interval retesting: antibody levels can fluctuate over time and after sensitizing events (e.g. transfusion). Also retest if negative PRA if risk for sensitization (e.g. on VAD).
- Specific antibodies assay allows virtual cross-matching with donor HLA typing (versus prospective cross-matching).
- Consider desensitization therapy (plasmapheresis, IVIG, rituximab) on waiting list for high calculated PRA (threshold is institutional based, e.g. >50%); consider lower threshold for more urgent patients.
- 'Wait' or 'Take' of a donor heart offer for a sensitized candidate is weighed against clinical urgency: (1) in non-urgent patients, await negative virtual cross-match; and (2) in urgent patients, consider 'lower-risk' positive cross-matching (based on type of DSA and its MFI).
- At the time of donor offer for sensitized patients, discuss with HLA lab expert (whether virtual or prospective cross-match). If cross-match is positive and organ is accepted: perform plasmapheresis and/or whole blood exchange on CPB and intraoperative immunosuppressive agents (methyl-prednisolone pre/post bypass and eculizumab post clamp removal).

Paediatric candidates are at higher risk of sensitization. Humoral sensitization occurs after exposure to non-self antigen such as:
- Blood or platelet transfusion.
- Allograft material (i.e. homograft valve, patch, conduit).
- Previous organ transplant.

Risk groups include Fontan patients, older children, congenital heart disease and multiple prior surgery, and those with VADs.

New DSAs can also form *de novo* post transplantation. Persistent *de novo* DSA can contribute to chronic rejection and allograft vasculopathy.

Pulmonary hypertension

Evaluation of PVR is important in paediatric populations. PVR is a challenging issue in paediatric population due to (1) higher risk of PH in paediatric candidates, (2) challenges in assessment of PVR index (e.g. in Fontan patients), and (3) complex interaction between complex congenital heart disease and pulmonary artery pressure.

The paediatric candidates, especially in a congenital heart disease population, are at higher risk of developing PH due to a number of risk factors:
- Unprotected pulmonary vascular bed: single ventricle with unrestrictive pulmonary blood flow; large left-to-right shunt, such as in complete AV septal defect; pulmonary blood flow at systemic pressure (e.g. common arterial trunk/hemitruncus).
- Chronic left atrial hypertension: left-sided obstructive lesion such as congenital aortic or mitral valve disease, multilevel left heart obstruction (e.g. Shone's complex), borderline left heart structure with endocardial fibroelastosis.
- Additional source of high pulmonary blood flow: major aortopulmonary collaterals.

- Failing Fontan patients.
- Other comorbidities that contribute to PH: prematurity, chronic lung disease, chromosomal anomalies (e.g. trisomy 21).

Irreversible PH is unusual in the paediatric age group as there will have been some form of intervention; nevertheless, children may present late without prior diagnosis. Inappropriate pursuit of a biventricular strategy in border-line left heart may also contribute to development of PH. Eisenmenger syndrome implies fixed PH with reversal of a large intracardiac shunt usually late in adulthood and development of central cyanosis—heart transplantation is precluded and heart–lung transplantation is required.

Cardiac catheterization is required prior to transplantation to assess PVR. However, paediatric PVR index assessment is more challenging due to limited peripheral vascular access with occluded vessels, more difficult assessment with central/BT shunt, or cavopulmonary shunt.

The assessment of PVR index and TPG is particularly difficult and un-reliable in failing Fontan due to low pulmonary flow and loss of hydro-dynamic energy. There may be associated intrapulmonary arteriovenous malformations or microthrombi which further complicate true PVR index assessment.

Assessment of PH incudes (1) PVR: (MPAP − PCWP)/Q_p (Q_p = calculated pulmonary blood flow) and (2) transpulmonary gradient (TPG = MPAP − PCWP).

Criteria for heart transplantation

- PVR index less than 6 Wood units (WU).m^2
- A 50% or greater decrease in PVR index after pulmonary vasodilator.
- MPAP less than 25 mmHg.
- TPG less than 15 mmHg (mPAP − PCWP).

High-risk transplantation with PVR index above the traditional criteria may be offered on institutional basis. A PVR index less than 9 WU.m^2 was not associated with increased post-transplant mortality in recent paediatric study.

Failing univentricular and Fontan physiology

Congenital heart disease with univentricular physiology represents a diverse group of patients with heterogeneous morphology and physiology, at different stages of palliation. Their physiology can differ in terms of pulmonary blood flow, atrial pressure, and volume loading which can lead to chronic elevation of pulmonary arterial or venous pressure and ventricular dysfunction. Primary transplantation as a therapeutic option for congenital heart disease is uncommon and most commonly, they present after failed surgical palliation. Univentricle is the most common diagnosis among congenital heart disease patients who need transplantation.

Waiting list mortality is the highest after first-stage palliation with systemic–PA shunt; consideration should be given to progress them to second-stage palliation with Glenn shunt. The Fontan procedure completes the cavopulmonary connection, creating a total non-pulsatile systemic venous flow return to the pulmonary vascular bed. The original atriopulmonary connection has undergone a number of evolutions in the last four decades, and currently the most common modification is an extracardiac conduit followed by lateral atrial tunnel.

Mechanisms of Fontan failure

Fontan patients represents a unique group of patients needing transplant, as patients can present with (1) pump failure, and/or (2) failure of 'Fontan physiology'. Fontan circulation is non-physiological, as there is decoupling between RV and pulmonary vascular bed with loss of pulsatile phasic flow which results in chronic elevation of systemic venous pressure, pulmonary endothelial dysfunction, ventricular unloading, and low cardiac output. Unfavourable haemodynamics pre Fontan or trigger factors post Fontan such as arrhythmia, further aggravate and accelerate the decline in Fontan circulation.

Therefore, systemic ventricular dysfunction and progressive AV valve regurgitation are suboptimal high-risk substrate to construct a Fontan circuit. With higher risk of early failure after Fontan completion and worse post-transplant survival in Fontan patients (versus Glenn), serious consideration should be given for transplantation prior to stage two palliation.

Early Fontan failure

The contemporary surgical outcome has vastly surpassed that of atriopulmonary connection; as such, rescue cardiac transplant in the setting of early Fontan failure is uncommon. Early mortality (<30%) is low (approximately 1.0–1.6%); nevertheless, early Fontan failure that includes mortality, takedown, revision/re-intervention, or ECMO/VAD can occur in the region of 3–6%.

Failure to wean ventilation and inotropic support after Fontan operation with impaired systemic ventricular function or recurrent arrhythmia despite optimal medical therapy are primary reasons for referral to transplantation. Another rescue option is Fontan takedown, if ventricular function is permissible—the early mortality of takedown is high (approximately 25%). A timely rescue cardiac transplant in the setting of early Fontan failure is a more superior long-term option.

Late Fontan failure

Attrition continues with time in all Fontan patients. Those with atriopulmonary connection and hypoplastic left heart syndrome are at the highest risk. Late failure can present as declining functional capacity (NYHA III/IV), HF, PLE, cyanosis, and plastic bronchitis. Freedom from late Fontan failure at 20 years is 70%. Some 5% of paediatric Fontan patients (<18 years old) require heart transplantation. Mean age at transplantation ranges from 8 to 15 years. Patients may remain stable for a long time before acute decompensation, often triggered by loss of sinus rhythm.

Cardiac catheterization

This is an essential pretransplant assessment but precise evaluation is difficult in the Fontan group. This is due to significant dysfunction despite normal EDP due to inadequate volume loading; underestimation of any gradient along the Fontan pathway due to low cardiac output; and unreliable measurement of pulmonary blood flow and PVR index (non-pulsatile, non-phasic flow, systemic venous obstruction, presence of other sources of pulmonary blood flow including minor and major collaterals, arteriovenous malformations, chronic microemboli).

Specific challenges in transplantation for Fontan patients

Only some 4–7% of Fontan patients ever receive a transplant within 20 years of surgery; undoubtedly, they are among the most challenging and highest-risk transplantation candidates. The following is a list of factors associated with the difficulties in undertaking transplantation in this group:

- Under-recognized PH due to difficulty in assessing PVR index in pre-transplant catheter.
- High transplant mortality risk due to comorbidities: severe malnourishment associated with PLE, liver disease, coagulopathy, renal dysfunction—among transplants for congenital heart disease, Fontan patients had an eightfold increase in mortality.
- Technical complexities: multiple prior operations, collaterals and bleeding, extensive PA reconstruction, longer bypass and donor ischaemia time.
- High risk of sensitization, need of cross-matching, limited donor pool; higher risk of acute rejection.
- Under-prioritization on waiting list.
- Associated liver cirrhosis requires careful hepatic assessment and heart transplantation alone may not be adequate.

Due to these challenges, early listing should be considered for Fontan patients. Prompt listing should be considered in the setting of early Fontan failure.

Protein-losing enteropathy and plastic bronchitis

PLE is an indication in 20–40% of Fontan patients receiving heart transplantation, hence it needs special mention. Chronic systemic venous and lymphatic congestion in Fontan patients leads to lymphatic channels rupture into the GI lumen and leak of serum protein. However, the mechanism of PLE and why some 5–15% of Fontan patients develop PLE while others do not remain to be understood, and a link between level of systemic venous pressure and the development of PLE has not been demonstrated. PLE can develop as early as 2 months post Fontan but usually occurs years later. Severe hypoalbuminemia is the main issue, and diagnosis is made by low serum albumin (<3.5 g/dL or total protein <5.5 g/dL), and elevated alpha-1-antitrypsin in stool samples. PLE is suspected when Fontan patients present with diarrhoea, oedema leading to weight gain, abdominal distension, and occasionally GI bleeding. Pleural effusion can be present resulting in breathlessness.

Severe hypoproteinaemia leads to severe malnutrition and immune compromise prior to transplantation with low immunoglobulin levels (IgG, IgA, IgM) and CD4 counts. PLE, without any intervention, carries a risk of infection with mortality as high as 49% after 5 years of diagnosis. This is also reflected by high waiting list mortality, which is almost twice as high with PLE compared to Fontan patients without PLE (21 versus 12%).

However, post-transplant survival is comparable to Fontan patients without PLE. Transplantation is considered for PLE refractory to standard medical therapy (including diet with high protein, medium-chain triglycerides, diuretics, heparin, steroid, bowel rest, total parenteral nutrition) and fenestration of Fontan pathway. Enteric-coated steroid improves PLE and outcome. Heart transplantation remains the most effective treatment for PLE, which provides a 100% long-term cure in all transplantation survivors.

Plastic bronchitis

This is much rarer than PLE. The hallmark of the disease is the formation of thick, mucofibrinous casts in the tracheobronchial tree, which is expectorated on coughing or visualized on bronchoscopy. The development of plastic bronchitis is inadequately understood; like PLE, it reflects a sequela of chronic elevation of systemic venous pressure and low cardiac output in Fontan physiology, with contribution from inflammatory process. Symptoms range from mild cough and breathlessness to severe respiratory distress when the airway is severely obstructed. Plastic bronchitis has a high mortality of 30% and life-threatening airway obstruction requires emergency clearance with rigid bronchoscopy. Medical therapies include high-molecular-weight heparin, bronchodilator, tissue plasminogen activator, sildenafil, and steroid. Catheter or surgical intervention including atrial pacing, thoracic duct ligation, fenestration of Fontan, and conversion of Fontan has resulted in variable degrees of resolution of plastic bronchitis. Unlike PLE, plastic bronchitis is a rare indication for transplantation in Fontan, perhaps reflecting its much lower incidence. Transplantation mortality is higher, but a new heart results in early and durable resolution of plastic bronchitis in all transplantation survivors, with comparable long-term survival with non-Fontan patients.

Ex vivo cardiac perfusion

Ex vivo cardiac perfusion is an organ preservation system which keeps the donor heart perfused in a warm beating state after procurement (Organ Care System (OCS) Heart, TransMedics, Andover, MA, USA). Currently, the system is suitable to support bigger donor hearts from older teenagers onwards due to instrumentation size. Normothermic donor heart perfusion has been shown to be non-inferior to standard cold storage and allows (1) extension of cold ischaemia time, which is relevant in the context of transplantation for failing Fontan and other complex congenital heart disease; and (2) assessment of marginal donor heart and DCD heart.

Donation after circulatory death

The first successful DCD heart transplantation was carried out in paediatric population in 2004 (DN Campbell, Denver). Despite a successful series of three paediatric patients in Denver, DCD transplantation did not take off widely until in recent years in adult heart transplantation. Far fewer DCD procurements were reported in paediatric registries. The long-term post-transplant survival with DCD hearts remains to be defined. The use of DCD hearts could help increase the donor pool for paediatric candidates.

Special considerations in heart transplantation

CHAPTER

Special considerations
in heart
transplantation

Adult patients with congenital heart disease

Adult patients with congenital heart disease

Overview

The prevalence of all congenital heart disease (CHD) is 0.5–0.8% of live births. With drastic improvements in management over the past four decades, particularly palliative procedures of the more complex congenital anomalies, these patients are now surviving into adulthood and presenting with late complications, including HF. A recent population study suggested approximately 1000 adults are living in the UK (population 66 million) with single-ventricle physiology. Many of these patients will require advanced failure management, including transplantation.

HF in adult congenital heart disease (ACHD) is frequently due to structural abnormalities and as such is less amenable than acquired pathologies to pharmacological preservation of the ventricle. An increasing number of young adult patients are presenting to the advanced HF and transplant team and CHD now accounts for approximately 3% of adult cardiac transplantation, with the number of ACHD recipients having increased by 40% over the past two decades.

This expanding group brings unique challenges in the shape of highly complex surgical histories, varied physiology, unusual anatomy, and limited mechanical support options. The worldwide literature reports that cardiac transplantation (and, at times, multiorgan transplantation) is an effective strategy to improve survival and quality of life in a carefully selected group of ACHD patients. These patients carry a higher 1-year postoperative mortality than other indications for transplantation. The success of transplantation for the ACHD group requires multidisciplinary involvement of transplant and congenital heart surgeons, advanced HF and ACHD cardiologists, hepatologists, intensivists, and allied professionals in the transplant assessment and perioperative clinical care.

Considering the rarity of such cases and anatomical challenges, early referral to an advanced HF team for assessment, and ultimately heart transplantation must be undertaken in a centre with an adequate volume of ACHD practice.

Outcomes of transplantation

ACHD recipients carry a high mortality risk in the first year following transplantation. A diagnosis of ACHD confers additional risk with post-transplant 1-year mortality being 16–19% in ACHD recipients versus 6–9% in adults with other diagnoses. Higher incidence of primary graft failure, renal failure, multiorgan failure, and stroke in ACHD patients contributes to early mortality. In-hospital mortality is even higher for those with single-ventricle physiology (8% in biventricular vs 23% in single-ventricle ACHD patients).

Prognosis for those who survive the first year is favourable, with significantly better long-term survival than all other pathologies. The median survival conditioned to 1-year survival is better for ACHD than any other pretransplant diagnoses.

Factors that may contribute to poor early results in ACHD patients include:
- Increased risk of acute rejection due to sensitization from previous blood product transfusion and use of homograft materials in palliative procedures.
- Longer graft ischaemia and CPB times. This is related to factors associated with multiple previous sternotomies, structural anomalies requiring reconstruction, and challenges of haemostasis due to coagulopathy and surgical bleeding.
- Concomitant organ failure—commonly hepatic involvement in the Fontan patient which contributes to turbulent postoperative course in single organ transplant or may require heart–liver transplantation.
- Increased risk of infection due to protein-losing enteropathy.
- PH—this can be challenging to diagnose preoperatively, resulting in RV compromise in the donor heart or the need for higher-risk heart–lung transplantation. PVR >4 Wood units is an independent risk factor for death post transplantation in ACHD recipients.
- Centre volume is associated with post-transplant survival in patients undergoing ACHD transplantation. Low-volume centres perform poorly compared to high-volume centres.

Waiting list criteria and outcomes

Waiting list criteria

ACHD patients may not fit the routine criteria for transplantation despite their deteriorating condition.

Further consideration must be given to additional criteria specific to the failing ACHD patient:
- Refractory arrhythmia (more than one hospital admission over last 3 months with haemodynamic instability or associated with kidney or liver dysfunction).
- ACHD patients with no option for conventional escalation of therapy who are unsuitable for inotropes and/or VAD with one of the following:
  - Bilirubin and transaminases greater than twice normal levels.
  - Deteriorating renal function (eGFR <50 mL/min/1.73 m², or 20% reduction from baseline).
  - Requirement for dialysis/continuous venovenous haemofiltration for fluid or electrolyte management.
  - Recurrent admissions (greater than three in preceding 3 months) with episodes of right HF or protein-losing enteropathy requiring ascites drainage.

Waiting list mortality

Waiting list mortality is similar for ACHD and non-ACHD, although death from HF and sudden cardiac death is more likely in ACHD. Despite this, there is a lower use of ICDs and MCS. While on the waiting list, close clinical observation should highlight patients who could benefit from an ICD given the prevalence of sudden death.

The use of MCS has previously been reported as a risk factor for increased waiting list mortality in ACHD patients. This, along with the technical challenges of device implantation in the congenital heart has deterred the use of MCS as a bridge to transplant. A more contemporary evaluation of the INTERMACS database of 126 ACHD patients supported with mechanical circulatory devices on the waiting list reports a positive outcome for 71% at 6 months (21% successfully bridged to transplantation and 50% remain alive on VAD). Use of MCS is increasing in ACHD and consideration should be given to device employment for waiting list patients anticipated to have an extended wait or clinical deterioration. Recent reports describe individual ACHD cases in which VA ECMO, axillary IABP, and durable and temporary VADs have been successfully employed for bridging.

Time on the waiting list

ACHD patients wait longer on the list than non-CHD HF patients. Suggested reasons for this include:

* High prevalence of elevated panel reactive antibodies, limiting the donor pool and requiring a negative prospective cross-match.
* The perceived need to find an ideal donor with adequate up-sizing to tolerate occult PH.
* The desire to reduce ischaemic time by limiting distance of donor organ transport. This is overcome in some UK centres with the use of the Organ Care System (OCS) Heart (Transmedics, Andover, MA, USA) which allows transport with a beating heart and can limit warm ischaemic time.
* A higher proportion of ACHD patients will require heart–lung or heart–liver transplantation.
* Waiting list status criteria may be more appropriate and designed for non-ACHD patients.

Common aetiologies

Underlying pathologies in ACHD vary greatly on the spectrum of complexity and diagnostics are rarely straightforward requiring description of situs, cardiac orientation, atrial arrangement, intracardiac anomalies, ventricular and valve arrangements, and any shunt defects.

Two distinct groups exist: those with single-ventricle physiology (i.e. Fontan circulation) and those with two ventricles.

For simplicity, common aetiologies found in ACHD patients undergoing heart transplantation have been divided into three broad groups according to the number of functional ventricles.

Biventricular

* Dextro-transposition of great arteries (d-TGA) patients with corrective surgery undertaken before the era of arterial switch operation (before the 1990s). These patients had atrial inversion procedures (Senning or Mustard) in childhood. This configuration results in a sub-systemic right morphological ventricle, which is less robust than the morphological LV resulting in early sub-systemic HF.
* Congenitally corrected transposition of great arteries (ccTGA). This configuration results in a sub-systemic ventricle of right morphology, with a tricuspid valve as the sub-systemic AV valve but with normal sequential pulmonary and systemic systems. The morphology of

the RV and valve in the high pressure left-sided system leads to early failure. These patients may not have undergone surgery, or may have undergone extensive corrective surgery or palliation including the Fontan operation.
- Eisenmenger's syndrome resulting from any uncorrected shunt defect (ASD, VSD, or rarely patent ductus arteriosus). Rarely seen in the current era of transplantation due to improved detection and management, and require combined heart–lung transplant.
- Ebstein's anomaly of the tricuspid valve.

Univentricular

In the adult population, these patients will have undergone palliation staging to achieve a Fontan circulation. Previous surgery is ubiquitous and extensive (see pp. 296–297).
- Hypoplastic left heart syndrome.
- Double outlet RV.
- Double inlet LV.
- Tricuspid or mitral atresia.

Can be either univentricular or biventricular
- Complete atrioventricular septal defect (CAVSD). Number of ventricles and subsequent management depends on whether balanced or unbalanced.

Indications for transplant assessment

Consider earlier discussion with transplant services to allow time for serial assessment. These patients are highly unique in anatomy and treatment history and do not make for a straightforward assessment or listing decision.

Transplant assessment for heart failure

Recognizing HF in the ACHD patient is imperative to permit early referral before complications occur which elevate risk, or contraindicate transplantation. Patients may have lived with the classic symptoms of HF for many years. Baseline expectations, younger age, and lifelong adaptations may mask deterioration of normal parameters and symptomatology. Profound circulatory dysfunction may exist before patients seek help. With this in mind, clinicians must interrogate closely any 'hidden' functional changes which may reflect underlying declining function. To avoid late detection, it may be prudent to undertake frequent and regular haemodynamic assessment via catheterization or CPX in asymptomatic patients.

Transplant assessment for other reasons

Unlike most acquired HF, cardiac transplantation may be considered in ACHD with preserved ventricular function due to the idiosyncratic presentations related to Fontan circulation; patients with debilitating protein-losing enteropathy or plastic bronchitis should be referred for discussion.

Transplantation or further intervention

Atriopulmonary connection Fontan patients with refractory arrhythmia may benefit from Fontan conversion. Similarly, those with sub-systemic AV valve regurgitation may benefit from valve replacement. When such potential interventions exist, the decision between further corrective surgery or listing for transplantation should be undertaken as part of a transplant assessment and multidisciplinary team discussion between congenital and transplant services.

Indications for transplantation

Indications with impaired ventricular function

- Patients with stage D HF refractory to therapy who will not benefit from surgical, interventional, or electrophysiological intervention.
- Patients with stage C HF associated with reactive PH and potential risk of developing fixed irreversible elevation of PVR that could preclude OHT in the future.
- Patients with stage C HF and severe limitation of exercise and activity.

Indications with preserved ventricular function

- Patients with associated near-sudden death or life-threatening arrhythmias refractory to all therapeutic modalities.
- Patients with symptomatic cyanosis that is not amenable to surgical correction.
- Patients with protein-losing enteropathy/plastic bronchitis despite optimal medical and surgical therapy.

Contraindications and special considerations

Traditional contraindications to cardiac transplantation apply to ACHD patients. Additionally, there are ACHD-specific considerations which may be a single absolute contraindication or, more commonly, multiple relative contraindications amass to collectively elevate risk and render a patient untransplantable.

Pulmonary hypertension

- PH is common in this group and is aetiologically different from non-CHD patients. Elevated left heart pressure may be causative, but pulmonary venous irregularities and other left-sided mechanical obstruction, cyanosis, pulmonary over-circulation via collateral flow, shunting, and intrinsic lung disease are frequently present. Patients with established PH require heart and lung transplantation.
- ACHD patients require cautious evaluation and interpretation of pulmonary haemodynamic data including transpulmonary gradient. The quantitative diagnosis is not straightforward due to presence of shunts and collateral flow. RV pressures may be high due to outflow obstruction mimicking a PH picture.

- In addition, the low cardiac output underestimates PVR. Occult PH in these patients can be unmasked following transplantation, with subsequent RV failure of the implanted heart.
- Given the clear challenges in diagnostics, attention should be paid to history including pattern of disease, duration of unprotected pulmonary circulation in infancy, and any extended periods of cyanosis. Qualitative and quantitative data in combination will permit a better understanding of individual situations.
- Pharmacological reversibility of PH is an incremental risk factor but does not preclude cardiac transplantation. Preoperative risk management with pulmonary vasodilators and anticipatory measures of donor RV support, including inhaled NO, milrinone, and RVAD, should be considered.
- In some instances, mechanical unloading of the systemic ventricle may reduce PVR and should be considered.

High levels of sensitization

- ACHD patients presenting for transplant assessment have commonly undergone multiple surgeries with exposure to blood products and homograft material resulting in a high prevalence of sensitization. Strategies to minimize exposure and subsequent sensitization are limited:
  - High PRA level >10% is associated with poorer outcomes post transplantation.
  - Anti-HLA antibodies are associated with worse long-term graft survival.
  - Presence of DSAs is associated with cell-mediated and antibody-mediated rejection and graft vasculopathy.
- Desensitization therapy can be considered in patients with calculated PRA levels >50% although absolute values for initiating desensitization prior to transplantation are unit dependent. Desensitization strategies aim to mitigate risk by perioperative reduction of circulating antibodies and cessation of production. Such deletion of immunological memory is a multi-therapy approach with variable reported success: plasmapheresis, IVIG, anti-B-cell therapies (rituximab), and proteasome inhibitors (bortezomib).

The single-ventricle patient

The single-ventricle patient presents an idiosyncratic set of challenges in peri-transplant management. Patients will likely have undergone palliative staging to reach partial or complete Fontan physiology (Fig. 23.1 and Fig. 23.2).

The Fontan circulation results in non-pulsatile venous return to the PAs via cavopulmonary connections with subsequent adverse physiological consequences:

- High venous pressures leading to liver cirrhosis, protein-losing enteropathy, and plastic bronchitis. These idiosyncratic pathologies can persist long after transplantation and significantly complicate recovery.
- The reduction of hepatic flow to one lung or both lungs in cavopulmonary arrangements results in pulmonary arteriovenous malformations and subsequent chronic cyanosis which can persist postoperatively necessitating angiographic coiling.

- Chronic cyanosis leads to aortopulmonary collaterals.
- The assessment of pulmonary pressures can be hampered by non-pulsatility, collateral flow, and arteriovenous malformations. RV dysfunction in the donor heart is commonly encountered in Fontan patients as high pulmonary pressures are unmasked.

Poorer outcomes are reported in Fontan patients undergoing transplantation, likely due to the additive consequences of prolonged and challenging surgery, longer ischaemic times, and extensive comorbid disease: liver disease, coagulopathy, occult PH, immune dysfunction, renal impairment, and hypoalbuminemia.

Fontan patients presenting for transplantation may be in the unusual position of preserved ventricular function, but be classified as Fontan failure due to protein-losing enteropathy, plastic bronchitis, cyanosis, or intractable arrhythmia. In the presence of poor ventricular function, transplantation may be the only option, but further repair is an attractive option for those with relatively preserved ventricular function in whom failure can be attributed to residual structural defect such as valve regurgitation.

Consideration should be given to Fontan conversion for those patients with poor function and arrhythmia in the setting of the now outdated atriopulmonary connection as good results are reported as an alternative to transplantation.

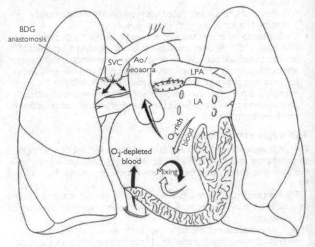

Fig. 23.1 Partial Fontan circulation. The SVC is anastomosed to the right PA as a bidirectional Glenn shunt (BDG) and provides pulmonary flow. Deoxygenated IVC return and oxygenated pulmonary venous return mix in the common atrium and provide systemic flow via the single ventricle.

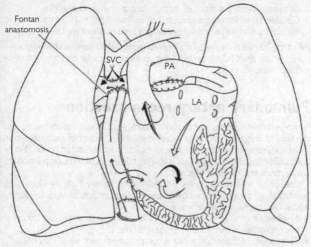

Fontan anastomosis

SVC

PA

LA

Fig. 23.2 Complete Fontan circulation. In addition to the bidirectional Glenn shunt demonstrated in Fig. 23.1, the IVC is anastomosed to the PA as shown. A fenestration remains between the Fontan conduit and the RA to allow offloading. All deoxygenated venous return is now directed to pulmonary flow in a non-pulsatile passive system.

Surgical risk

- ACHD patients frequently have an extensive surgical history with multiple sternotomies. Re-entry to the chest requires planning to allow safe access. Peripheral CPB may be needed prior to sternotomy, or indeed during, in the event of unmanageable injury to a great vessel or ventricle. The extra time for re-entry must be considered to minimize ischaemic time. *Ex vivo* perfusion of the donor organ may be an important strategy to limit total ischaemic time (see Chapter 14).
- Reconstruction, particularly of the PA, is commonly required to permit implantation (see Pulmonary artery reconstruction, p. 314). Reconstruction of the PA at the time of transplantation may be associated with higher mortality in Fontan patients. Patients with heterotaxy or situs inversus may need baffling of left-sided systemic venous return to the donor RA necessitating longer IVC/SVC harvesting. With removal of baffles and caval connections, limited native tissue remains and donor tissue or xenograft pericardium may be required. This adds time to the preimplantation stage. The retrieval team need to be aware if extra tissue is required.
- Aortopulmonary collaterals occur secondary to chronic cyanosis. When damaged, these cause extensive haemorrhage. The increased venous return to the LA can render the surgical field challenging when commencing implantation and maintaining adequate systemic pressures

on bypass in the presence of large collaterals can be challenging. Consideration should be given to coil occlusion pre transplantation or in the postoperative period if high-output cardiac failure persists.

All of the above factors result in prolongation of ischaemic and operative times. Acute graft failure remains the commonest cause of early mortality in these patients.

Pulmonary artery reconstruction

Single-ventricle patients commonly require great vessel reconstruction at the time of implantation, most frequently the PAs. Extent of reconstruction is dependent upon whether there is complete discontinuation of the PAs or partial absence of the vessel wall following takedown of the cavopulmonary connections and removal of stents.

Choice of material includes on-the-shelf materials such as Gore-Tex, polytetrafluoroethylene, or bovine pericardium or jugular vein, or donor tissue: PAs, aorta, and pericardium.

- The benefit of on-the-shelf materials is that reconstruction can occur prior to organ arrival to limit ischaemic time.
- The benefit of donor materials is better haemostasis which may be preferable in these patients with high risk for coagulopathy and bleeding.

The surgeon must be aware of the anatomic variety, reconstruction materials available, and technique options.

Partial PA reconstruction

Limited reconstruction is required following take down of the cavopulmonary anastomoses. A single- or double-patch repair can be performed to complete PA continuity (Fig. 23.3).

Complete PA reconstruction

Hilum-to-hilum reconstruction is required. This can occur due to PA stents *in situ* requiring removal of the majority of vessel (Fig. 23.4a), or less frequently with previous intentional surgical discontinuation due to classical and antiquated Glenn and Fontan arrangements.

Hilum-to-hilum reconstruction is possible utilizing Gore-Tex conduits, donor PAs, or donor descending aorta. The conduit is fashioned to anastomose to both PAs in an interpositional end-to-end technique and an aperture created to allow anastomosis with the graft main PA (Fig. 23.4b–d).

Transplant assessment

ACHD patients required the follow additional considerations to the routine transplant assessment.

History and examination

- Cardiac diagnosis: close attention to anatomy and physiology.
- Symptoms and signs of associated liver, kidney, and pulmonary disease.

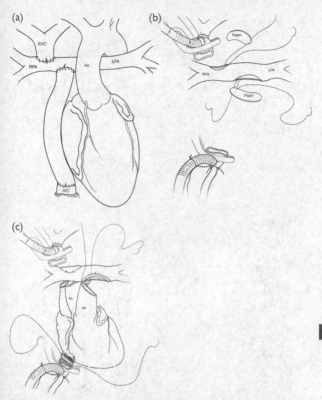

Fig. 23.3 Series demonstrates an extracardiac Fontan and bidirectional Glenn configuration (a), which is frequently encountered in single-ventricle patients presenting for transplantation. The cavopulmonary anastomoses are taken down, and a two-patch technique is used to reconstruct the PAs (b). Cannulas are seen in the IVC and SVC to allow bicaval venous drainage for CPB. An aperture is then opened into the patch to allow the donor heart to be implanted (c). LPA, left pulmonary artery; RPA, right pulmonary artery.

- Current status: dyspnoea, palpitations, exercise tolerance, ascites, changes in bowel habit (protein-losing enteropathy), weight loss or gain, peripheral oedema. Temporal change in symptoms and exercise tolerance since last review. Pay close attention to masked symptoms (see Indications for transplantation, p. 268).
- Surgical history: number of sternotomies, intra- and extracardiac catheter and surgical interventions, baffle stenting, previous use of groin vessels, and history of MCS. Increasing number of sternotomies has been associated with higher risk of mortality.
- Social history: establish support network.

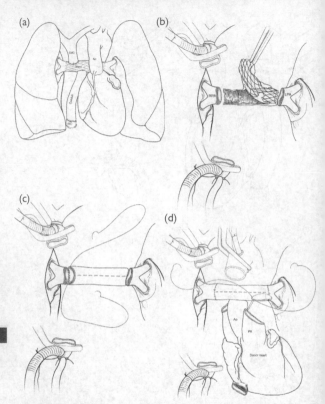

Fig. 23.4 Series demonstrates management of PA discontinuation due to the presence of a hilum-to-hilum stent within the PA in the context of complete Fontan circulation (a). Stent removal at time of transplantation results in PA disruption leaving only partial back wall of the vessel (b). Cannulas are seen in the IVC and SVC to allow bicaval venous drainage for CPB. Following removal, hilum-to-hilum reconstruction is performed in this case using a Gore-Tex conduit (c). An aperture is then created in the conduit to allow the donor heart to be implanted (d). Native aorta is shown with cross-clamp *in situ*. Note the donor PA is trimmed in a bevelled fashion in order to avoid kinking or distortion.

Investigations

To establish criteria fulfilment, planning, and feasibility for transplantation. In addition, investigations should evaluate the presence of residual lesions or repairable structural anomalies common in ACHD which are contributing to the HF picture. Management of such lesions can alter the clinical course and potentially extend time to transplantation.

- Cardiopulmonary catheter data.
- CT: cardiac diagnosis and anatomy. Important to confirm adequacy of pulmonary venous drainage which can be addressed at time of transplantation. Examine proximity of vessels and heart to posterior sternum in planning for re-entry of the chest.
- Echocardiography/MRI: assess structural pathologies which may be amenable to repair or replacement. Confirm valve regurgitation, conduit and baffle patency, and leak. Intervention on valves/stenoses/leaks may be performed transcatheter and can improve symptoms and prolong time to transplantation.
- ECG: consider ambulatory 24-hour ECG if history of palpitations. Electrophysiological studies may be appropriate to determine if arrhythmia intervention is possible to extend time to transplantation.
- Venogram/Doppler studies: patency of access points for CPB and anastomoses.
- CPX: formal exercise testing.
- Liver assessment: liver disease is common due to high venous pressures and significantly increases morbidity and post-transplant mortality. A MELD-XI score should be calculated and discussion with hepatologists as part of the multidisciplinary team. Some centres may consider liver disease as a contraindication for heart transplantation, while others will consider heart–liver transplantation.
  - Transient elastography (Fibroscan) for cirrhosis.
  - CT for monitoring of lesions (hepatocellular carcinoma) with or without biopsy.
  - Liver biochemistry and synthetic function is a late indicator of liver compromise.
  - Hepatitis C: ACHD patients have a higher prevalence of hepatitis C due to transfusion prior to routine screening in 1992.
  - Hepatic venous wedge pressure.

Perioperative considerations

- Surgical planning is critical. Perusal of investigations and previous operative notes is essential to avoid unexpected anatomy. Close liaison with the donor team is critical to reduce ischaemic period.
- A surgical team including both congenital and adult surgeons may be optimal.
- *Ex vivo* donor heart perfusion can mitigate the total ischaemic time and has been used in cases requiring extensive reconstruction prior to implant. One perfusion system is the OCS Heart. This system provides normothermic blood perfusion at near physiological perfusion parameters.
- Redo sternotomy precautions:
  - External defibrillator pads.
  - Ice on the head for cooling.
  - Blood and heparin in the operating room with a primed circuit.
  - CT imaging displayed in the operating room may be helpful.
  - Carbon dioxide suffusion of operative field to reduce impact of air embolism.
  - Team aware of CPB plan in event of inadvertent thoracic injury.

- Blood loss can be significant before CPB is established due to redo surgery, aortopulmonary collaterals, and concomitant hepatic dysfunction:
  - Consider where access is possible due to previous surgery and which vessels will be required for CPB.
  - Concentrated recombinant factor replacement should be available.
  - Unmasking of elevated pulmonary pressures can occur post implantation.
  - Routine use of pulmonary vasodilators in this group of patients: inhaled NO/isoprenaline/milrinone.
  - Early deployment of RV support if required.
- Hypotension and low systemic resistance are common during CPB, especially in Fontan circulation due to vasoplegia. Use vasopressin for low SVR. This can persist into the postoperative period requiring vasoconstrictors including vasopressin, methylene blue, and vitamin B_{12} infusions.

Patient selection criteria and bridging support for lung transplantation

Indications for referral to a transplant centre

General indication

Introduction

Lung transplantation has been shown to prolong patient survival and improve quality of life but is dependent upon appropriate timing of referral and activation on the transplant waiting list to minimize pre-transplant mortality. In 2017, 2478 lung transplants were performed (1860 of these were bilateral) in the USA across 26 centres contributing to 14,000 living lung transplant patients in the US at that time. Conversely, the ISHLT registry reported 4554 adult lung transplants performed in 2016 worldwide.

Recipients with restrictive lung disease (group D) comprised the highest volume at 1407 (57%), followed by obstructive lung disease (group A, 27.1%), suppurative lung disease (group C, 10.7%), and PH (group B, 5.1%). The timing of referral for transplantation, surgical plan, and when to activate patients on the waiting list vary for these lung diseases as different parameters within these disease groups are indicators of the appropriate time to move forward with listing for transplant.

Indications for referral to a transplant centre

General indications

It is important to understand the distinction between indications for referral for transplant and indications for transplant (i.e. to activate on the waiting list and proceed with transplant surgery as soon as a suitable donor is identified). Guidelines for lung transplant candidacy (>50% death within 2 years without a transplant, >80% likelihood of survival at least 90 days after transplant, and >80% likelihood of survival for at least 5 years concerning patients' non-pulmonary medical conditions) generally focus on listing and not indications for referral. Patients with end-stage lung disease generally have a progressive disease with some degree of clinical deterioration over time. Ideally, patients should be listed as soon as their lung disease becomes life-threatening and substantially affects their quality of life. However, as their disease progresses, patients may become too deconditioned or too sick to survive the lung transplantation process. In these instances, patients may miss the opportunity to undergo a lung transplant. This period between the development of an indication for listing and progression to a point where it may be too late to perform lung transplantation is referred to as the 'transplant window.'

Over time, early referral for transplant has become the recommended approach to patients with end-stage lung disease. Many patients who meet criteria for referral will be too early for listing. However, it is essential to recognize that referral does not necessarily lead to a full evaluation or listing. Instead, early referral gives individuals with end-stage lung disease and their care team access to transplant-specific expertise of a lung-transplant centre. This allows for management and optimization of medical conditions, patient education, improved physical conditioning (preferably in a formal pulmonary rehabilitation setting), and solidification of psychosocial factors within the variable rates of symptom progression across these disease groups. Patients are typically surprised by the complexity and variety of the issues (both medical and non-medical) involved in lung transplantation, and early referral provides the opportunity for patients and their caregivers to acclimate and learn what is required throughout their transplant journey.

When a patient is referred for transplant, a composite of testing (pulmonary function testing (PFT), ambulatory and exercise oxygen requirements, arterial blood gas) is necessary to determine the severity of disease as resting oxygen saturation and flow rate do not always adequately capture the degree of pulmonary disease. Some patients may be more advanced than originally appreciated while other patients initially felt to be in their transplant window can prolong their time to transplant with tailored therapies. The patient's recent trajectory can also be an important predictor of clinical demise. Early referral can save patient lives for those with rapid deterioration, but even for those with a slower disease progression, early referral has advantages to improve survival outcomes by allowing the transplant team time to address the host of issues involved. Please refer to Box 24.1 for a list of contraindications to lung transplantation.

Box 24.1 Absolute contraindications to lung transplantation

- Active or recent history of malignancy. Programmes vary as to an acceptable duration of disease-free interval and their willingness to proceed with lung transplantation but the disease-free interval typically ranges between 2 and 5 years based on programmes' risk assessment and experience. Early-stage active malignancies may be amenable to successful lung transplantation (e.g. lung cancer radiographic stage 1, breast cancer stage 1, prostate cancer Gleason score ≤6).
- Major uncorrectable non-pulmonary organ dysfunction (cardiac, kidney, liver) unless combined multivisceral transplantation can be considered.
- Significant multivessel CAD not amenable to revascularization with percutaneous pre-transplant or bypass during transplant surgery.
- Severe chest wall or spinal deformity.
- Acute severe sepsis.
- Untreatable pulmonary infection or intolerance to requisite antimicrobial therapy to treat pulmonary infection.
- Active *Mycobacterium tuberculosis* infection.
- Uncorrectable bleeding disorder.
- Significant obesity (BMI >35 kg/m²); weight distribution primarily across torso can also be problematic at lower BMIs as well.
- Substance abuse or dependence (e.g. ethanol, tobacco, marijuana, cocaine, methamphetamine, or other illicit substances).
- Medical non-compliance.
- Lack of suitable caregiver plan.

Specific aspects of different disease processes

Obstructive lung disease (group A)

See Table 24.1.

Prior to the lung allocation score (LAS) in the USA, transplant for severe chronic obstructive pulmonary disease (COPD) was associated with an improvement in the quality of life more than improved survival. Even under the LAS or composite allocation score (CAS) systems, the timing of referral and transplant to maximize the lifespan of patients with severe obstruction can be challenging. One needs to balance the overall indolent course of the disease with the potential complications of transplantation.

Utilization of the BODE (incorporating BMI, airway obstruction, dyspnoea, and exercise capacity) index in the decision-making can be helpful as a part of the mortality risk assessment. A BODE score of 7–10 has been associated with a 4-year mortality risk of 80% whereas a BODE score of 5–6 has been associated with 4-year mortality risk of 50–60%, suggesting that stratifying COPD patients by BODE score is a helpful adjunct as part of the decision process of when to refer and list for transplantation. Lahzami et al. evaluated COPD patients by BODE index and found improved survival outcome for patients with a BODE score of 7–10. Patients with a BODE score of 5–6 did not achieve a survival benefit; however, they did achieve an improved quality of life following transplantation. A subset of COPD patients may be functionally limited by severe hyperinflation, which is not fully captured in the BODE scoring model. Although the assessment of patients by the BODE index is helpful in most cases, it should be incorporated into a composite approach to evaluate patients' candidacy for transplantation.

Assuming optimization of medical therapy and functional status, other indications that should prompt referral to a transplant centre include an increased frequency of pulmonary exacerbations, patients who are not candidates for lung volume reduction surgery, spirometry revealing a forced expiratory volume in 1 second (FEV_1) <30%, and those who manifest evidence of hypercarbia on blood gas sampling.

Table 24.1 Indications for referral and listing for patients with obstructive lung disease

Indications for referral	Indications for activation on the transplant waiting list
Progressive disease despite maximal medical therapy, including pulmonary rehabilitation and domiciliary oxygen	BODE index ≥7
	FEV_1 <15–20% of predicted
Patient is not a candidate for lung volume reduction	Three or more exacerbations in the last 12 months
BODE index 5–6	One very severe exacerbation with acute hypercarbic respiratory failure
$PaCO_2$ >50 mmHg or 6.6 kPa and/or PaO_2 <60 mmHg or 8 kPa	Moderate to severe PH
FEV_1 <25–30% of predicted	

Pulmonary vascular disease (group B)
See Table 24.2.

Timing of referral of patients with PH is also challenging. The increased number of medical options for management of PH has improved the potential for response to treatment depending on the underlying pathophysiology. It is therefore recommended that patients undergo a trial of medical therapy (phosphodiesterase inhibitor, endothelin receptor antagonist, or prostacyclin analogue) before committing to lung transplantation particularly in patients with idiopathic pulmonary arterial hypertension.

The aetiology of primary pulmonary vascular disease is often unknown, and this contributes to uncertainty regarding response to therapy and the rate of symptom progression. These patients should be followed closely and those manifesting NYHA class III or IV symptoms, rapidly progressive disease, presyncopal/syncopal symptoms, need for IV prostacyclin therapy, or suspected pulmonary veno-occlusive disease/pulmonary capillary haemangiomatosis should be referred to a transplant centre for evaluation and monitoring to minimize mortality. Since this patient population can manifest sudden, expected deterioration of symptoms following extended periods of stability, it is particularly beneficial to refer these patients for transplant consultation earlier on in their disease rather than later to avoid missing an opportunity for transplant.

Table 24.2 Indications for referral and listing for patients with pulmonary vascular disease

Indications for referral	Indications for activation on the transplant waiting list
NYHA class III or IV symptoms despite maximal medical therapy, including prostanoids, endothelin receptor antagonists, and phosphodiesterase inhibitors	NYHA class III or IV symptoms after a 3-month trial of maximal medical therapy
	CI <2 L/min/m²
	Mean RA pressure >15 mmHg
The need for IV agents	Six-minute walk test <350 m
Known or suspected veno-occlusive disease or capillary haemangiomatosis	Haemoptysis
	Pericardial effusion
	Development of signs of right HF (renal insufficiency, increased serum bilirubin, recurrent ascites)

Cystic fibrosis (CF) (group C)
See Table 24.3.

Recent initiatives within the CF community have drastically altered prior guidelines for referral of CF patients. Historically, the timing of referral was recommended when patients were manifesting signs of very advanced lung disease based on severely reduced spirometry, increased number of exacerbations, declining clinical status, pneumothorax, and life-threatening haemoptysis. Now, these indications are more associated with timing for listing for transplant as the referral for consideration of lung transplantation is strongly encouraged to occur much sooner.

The CF Foundation now contends that the above guidelines are not aggressive enough to effectively manage the scope of issues faced by CF patients and instead recommends the following:

1. Routine clinician-led discussion of disease trajectory and treatment options. This may include a discussion of lung transplantation.
2. As soon as spirometry reveals a FEV₁ <50% of predicted volume, team-based discussion regarding lung transplantation should occur. Additional heightened concern should be maintained for patients with rapidly progressive disease or CF-related complications. Early referral may be considered in such patients, which include:

    a. Relative FEV$_1$ decline of >20% in 12 months.
    b. CF exacerbation requiring the use of non-invasive positive pressure ventilation.
    c. BMI <18 kg/m^2 (or BMI <5th percentile for children).
    d. Increased frequency of pulmonary exacerbations (more than two exacerbations per year requiring IV antibiotics or one exacerbation requiring positive pressure ventilation).
    e. Massive haemoptysis requiring ICU admission or bronchial artery embolization.
    f. Pneumothorax.
3. For patients with FEV$_1$ <40%, referral should be initiated for the following reasons:
    a. All patients <18 years of age.
    b. Six-minute walk test <400 m.
    c. Room air hypoxia (SpO$_2$ <88% or PaO$_2$ <55 mmHg, at rest or with exertion; at sea level). Or if supplemental oxygen is required.
    d. Hypercapnia (PaCO$_2$ >50 mmHg, confirmed on arterial blood gas).
    e. PH (PA systolic pressure > 50 mmHg on echocardiogram or evidence of RV dysfunction in the absence of a tricuspid regurgitant jet).
    f. BMI <18 kg/m^2.
4. Referral for all patients with an FEV$_1$ <30% of predicted.
5. Use of up-to-date CF-specific transplant resources.
6. Development of partnerships between CF and transplant centres.
7. Identify psychosocial and physical concerns regarding lung transplantation and address these as part of the transition process to transplantation.
8. Pre-emptive optimization of modifiable barriers to transplantation (nutrition, functional status, diabetes, medical compliance, mental health, substance use, psychosocial concerns).
9. Special consideration for early referral of female patients (due to sex disparate waiting list mortality) and those with short stature defined as <162 cm or 5'3" (due to difficulty in finding a suitably matched donor).
10. Special consultation with transplant centres for patients with micro-organisms that pose a risk for transplantation (non-tuberculous mycobacteria, *Burkholderia cepacia* complex, *Scedosporium*).

For a more comprehensive list of the CF Foundation recommendations on the timing of referral for lung transplantation, please refer to their 2019 publication in the *Journal of Cystic Fibrosis*. Also note that newer therapies for CF are being introduced and will likely significantly curtail the need for lung transplantation in patients with the appropriate underlying genetic mutations. Specifically, elexacaftor–tezacaftor–ivacaftor is a newly approved triple-combination cystic fibrosis transmembrane conductance regulator (CFTR) modulating therapy that contains two correctors and a potentiator of the CFTR channel. This drug was found to be efficacious in patients with CF with Phe508del-minimal function genotypes, in whom previous CFTR modulator regimens were ineffective. CFTR modulators will likely have utility for CF patients both prior to lung transplantation (in postponing or potentially eliminating need for transplant) and after transplantation (to manage significant sinus and/or GI symptoms).

Table 24.3 Indications for referral and listing for patients with CF

Indications for referral	Indications for activation on the transplant waiting list
FEV_1 <30% of predicted	With hypoxia (PaO_2 <8 kPa or <60 mmHg)
FEV_1 <40% with markers of increased disease severity:	With hypercapnia ($PaCO_2$ >6.6 kPa or >50 mmHg)
1. Age <18 years	Long-term non-invasive ventilation therapy
2. Room air hypoxia	PH
3. Hypercapnia	Frequent hospitalization
4. Six-minute walk test <400 m	Rapid lung function decline
5. PH	WHO functional class IV
6. BMI <18 kg/m²	
FEV_1 <50% or decline in FEV_1 >20% in 12 months	
FEV_1 <50% and disease-related complication:	
1. Increased frequency or severity of exacerbation	
2. Haemoptysis	
3. Pneumothorax	
4. Need for positive pressure ventilation	

Restrictive lung disease/interstitial lung disease (ILD) (group D)
See Table 24.4.

Patients with restrictive lung disease have the worst 5-year survival of lung groups at 50–55%. Restrictive lung disease patients include idiopathic pulmonary fibrosis, usual interstitial pneumonitis, non-specific interstitial pneumonitis, hypersensitivity pneumonitis, rheumatoid lung disease and connective tissue diseases (scleroderma, lupus, polymyositis, dermatomyositis, mixed connective disorders). Given the potential for accelerated decline in these diseases, early referral is emphasized based on symptoms, oxygen requirements, PFT, and biopsy results if obtained.

Patients with ILD should be referred for lung transplantation following the development of shortness of breath or limitation in their activity that is a result of their lung disease. Any patient with ILD who requires supplemental oxygen should be referred for transplantation as well as those with abnormal PFT defined as a reduction in the forced vital capacity (FVC) <80% of predicted or diffusion capacity of the lung for carbon monoxide (DLCO) to <40% of predicted.

A referral is also recommended whenever a biopsy reveals histopathological evidence of usual interstitial pneumonitis or non-specific interstitial pneumonitis irrespective of oxygen requirements and PFT. Recently, the advent of antifibrotic agents, nintedanib and pirfenidone, has somewhat altered the current treatment of patients with usual interstitial pneumonitis. However, it is unknown what effect, if any, these agents have on the indication for referral and activation on the waiting list.

Those patients with inflammatory ILD are appropriate to consider for medical therapy and may experience stabilization or improvement in their symptoms, oxygen requirements, or PFTs. Those who do not respond or decline after an initial response should then be referred for transplantation.

Table 24.4 Indications for referral and listing for patients with restrictive lung disease

Indications for referral	Indications for activation on the transplant waiting list
Histopathological or radiographic evidence of usual interstitial pneumonitis or fibrosing non-specific interstitial pneumonitis, regardless of lung function	Decline in FVC ≥5–10% in 6 months
	Decline in DLCO ≥15% in 6 months
FVC <80% predicted	Desaturation to <88% or distance <250 m on 6-minute-walk test or >50 m decline in 6-minute-walk distance over a 6-month period.
DLCO <40% predicted	
Dyspnoea or functional limitation attributable to lung disease	PH on right heart catheterization or two-dimensional echocardiography.
Any oxygen requirement, even if only during exertion	Hospitalization because of respiratory decline, pneumothorax, or acute exacerbation
For inflammatory ILD, failure to improve dyspnoea, oxygen requirement, and/or lung function after a clinically indicated trial of medical therapy	

Indications for transplantation/activation on the waiting list

Obstructive lung disease (group A)

Patients with severe obstructive lung disease should be considered for listing for transplantation if they experience an increase in the frequency of exacerbations to greater than three in 1 year or if they have an admission for management of acute hypercarbic respiratory failure. Patients with three or more exacerbations in 1 year had a hazard ratio of 4.13 for death at 5-year follow-up, compared to patients with fewer number of exacerbations. As stated previously, the BODE index can be a useful guide for referral and listing with a BODE index ≥7 conferring a survival benefit to patients with severe COPD.

Spirometry in isolation is not a useful parameter for listing in patients with COPD but a decline in FEV_1 to <20% is commonly associated with significant disease progression to warrant consideration of listing. Patients with severe COPD who require higher rates of oxygen supplementation often have accompanying secondary PH. In those COPD patients with moderate to severe PH, listing should occur regardless of their FEV_1. Hypercarbia also predicts mortality among COPD patients and should be carefully scrutinized when present.

Pulmonary vascular disease (group B)

Patients with pulmonary vascular disease should be listed for transplantation if they have not responded to combined pulmonary vasodilator therapy, including a prostanoid for at least 3 months and are symptomatic with NYHA class III or IV symptoms.

Patients with early signs of right HF (CI <2.0 or RA pressure >15 mmHg on right heart catheterization) should be listed for transplantation before they experience further disease progression. Those with evidence of advanced failure (development of ascites, elevated bilirubin, elevated BNP, or decreased forward flow with elevated creatinine) should be urgently listed if otherwise functional and felt to be good candidates. However, careful consideration of whether to proceed should be performed as these patients are at high risk for perioperative mortality and overall poor outcome.

Cystic fibrosis (group C)

Despite multiple attempts to develop predictive models of mortality risk for CF patients based on a variety of patient characteristics, 'change in lung function over time' continues to be the single best predictor to guide timing to list for transplantation. Reliance on FEV_1 alone, however, can be deleterious and attention must be paid to other aspects in the CF population as patients with FEV_1 <30% may experience increased mortality if spirometry alone is followed. The risk of death among female patients with FEV_1 values between 20% and 30% is reported as high as 56%, as compared with 38% among male patients. Development of increased severity and frequency of CF exacerbations, haemoptysis, pneumothorax, or non-tuberculous mycobacterial pulmonary infection may all be indicators of a rapid decline, and these patients need to be closely monitored. Those with hypercarbia (arterial PCO_2 >50 mmHg), need for non-invasive positive pressure ventilation, or secondary PH should be strongly considered for immediate activation on the transplant waiting list regardless of their FEV_1. Female CF patients should be monitored closely, given their increased mortality risk. A lower threshold for listing should be considered if they begin to manifest early signs of chronic respiratory failure or increased difficulties with respiratory infections.

Resistant micro-organisms may be considered as relative contraindications to transplant. Burkholderia cenocepacia is typically avoided given its association with increased mortality following transplant. Other infections such as *Mycobacterium abscessus* or pan-resistant organisms (e.g. *Pseudomonas*, *Achromobacter*) can present significant challenges for successful transplant surgery. Patients with multidrug or pan-resistant pulmonary infections must be thoroughly evaluated with a vigorous multidisciplinary approach involving infectious disease, transplant surgery, and pulmonology teams to review past cultures and susceptibilities, chest imaging, and proposed surgical plan. A patient's condition, presence of parenchymal cavities, or significant pleural disease may determine the willingness to proceed with transplantation in the face of these resistant organisms. A patient bridged on ECLS with large cystic cavities adjacent to the pleura is at high risk for bleeding and soiling of the pleural space during explantation of the lungs, and these should be considered as to whether the patient is appropriate for transplantation. Patients with resistant organisms and significant pulmonary architectural abnormalities are generally best served by a referral to a large transplant centre to manage these aspects of their disease.

Interstitial lung disease (group D)

Given the high mortality rate of patients with ILD, early referral for transplantation and frequent monitoring is recommended. Signs of disease progression manifested by an increase in oxygen requirement or decline in PFT (FVC decline >10% or diffusion capacity decline >15%) should prompt consideration of listing for transplantation. Development of secondary PH or hospitalization for management of acute exacerbation of ILD should also trigger activation on the waiting list. In general, the potential for rapid disease progression should lead to frequent, close follow-up of ILD patients with anticipation for listing when manifesting any of the above-mentioned signs.

Maintenance of adequate nutritional status and conditioning are essential for all transplant candidates, but these are particularly crucial for ILD patients. Frailty is common in ILD patients (due to the age of disease onset, pulmonary cachexia, and accumulation of other medical comorbidities) and correlates with poor outcomes following transplant surgery. It is imperative that patients with ILD be referred early for transplantation as well as to pulmonary rehabilitation at the time of their diagnosis to either maintain or improve their functional status in anticipation of transplantation. ILD patients are at risk for pulmonary cachexia, given the catabolic nature of their disease, which can be exacerbated by an exercise programme or antifibrotic drug therapies. An early and aggressive comprehensive treatment programme to address both nutrition and conditioning may be the key factors of ILD treatment to bridge these patients to transplantation successfully. Patients who are robust physically can be safely transitioned to transplantation despite rapid progression of their disease whereas those with frailty and malnutrition assume a much higher and potentially prohibitive risk.

Pre-transplant evaluation

Pulmonary evaluation

The pulmonary evaluation serves three purposes. The first is to determine whether the pulmonary disease has progressed to the point that justifies transplantation. The second objective is to identify complications of the disease that may or may not be amenable to tailored therapies that may ameliorate the lung disease. For example, the CT scan and ventilation/perfusion (V/Q) scan may identify COPD patients who may be candidates for lung volume reduction surgery. Finally, the pre-transplant evaluation is useful for operative planning.

- PFT: PFTs are used to assess disease severity. FEV_1 is an important determinant of indication for waiting list activation in patients with CF and COPD. FVC and DLCO serve a similar purpose in patients with restrictive lung disease. Additionally, FVC is used in the calculation of the LAS. Finally, the total lung capacity (TLC) is important in determining the size match for potential donor lungs.
- Arterial blood gas: the degree of hypoxaemia or hypercapnia is determined. These are used to titrate supplemental oxygen requirements as well as the utility of non-invasive positive pressure ventilation. Hypoxaemia and hypercapnia are used to determine indications for activation on the waiting list.
- VQ: the main purpose of the V/Q scan is to determine the laterality in patients who are listed for single-lung transplantation. Additionally, in programmes that perform bilateral sequential lung transplantation off pump, the perfusion scan guides the operative team by identifying which side to transplant first.

- Six-minute walk test: like blood gases and PFTs, the 6-minute walk test is an important determinant of disease severity and is used as an indication for activation in certain disease processed (e.g. distance <250 m in patients with restrictive lung disease). It can also serve as a crude assessment of functional status and deconditioning.
- CT imaging: in patients with CF, the CT scan is important in identifying the degree of infection and cavitary lung lesions, which may aid in operative planning. In patients with obstructive and restrictive lung, who are predisposed to lung malignancy, a CT scan is important to rule out lung cancer.

Cardiac evaluation

The cardiac evaluation is integral to the pretransplant evaluation. It is very important to assess the cardiac function of the transplant candidate and their ability to undergo the immense stress of lung transplantation. Furthermore, it is important to identify modifiable heart disease, such as CAD, which needs addressing before lung transplantation. Non-modifiable heart disease is important, and a determination needs to be made as to whether this would constitute a contraindication for lung transplantation. Finally, it is important to determine the presence of PH and the condition of the right heart. Irreversible severe right heart dysfunction is a contraindication for lung transplantation, and the patient may be better served with combined heart–lung transplantation instead.

- Left heart catheterization: the main purpose of the left heart catheterization is to rule out significant coronary disease. Identification of important CAD will prompt a discussion of how to address it. Options include medical management and PCI. Combined coronary artery grafting at the time of transplantation is used as well in selected patients. In some institutions, imaging with CT coronary angiography is used. If an important lesion is identified, then traditional coronary angiography is indicated for intervention.
- Right heart catheterization: this is used to determine right-sided heart pressure, including RA pressure, PCWP, and PA pressure. These values are used to compute the LAS or CAS. They are also important in stratifying the severity of disease in patients with secondary PH. This test is mandatory in patients with pulmonary vascular disease.
- Echocardiogram: determination of cardiac function is important in determining the ability of a patient to undergo lung transplantation, especially in patients with PH. Mild left or right heart dysfunction is acceptable but raises the possibility of intraoperative cardiopulmonary support in programmes that use it selectively. In patients with severe heart right heart dysfunction, it is important to determine whether the lung transplantation may reverse this, or whether the patient should undergo a heart–lung transplant instead.
- Cardiac MRI in selected patients (sarcoidosis; stress MRI in certain cases with CAD).
- ECG.

Gastrointestinal evaluation

The GI evaluation focuses on the assessment of upper GI function and the likelihood of aspiration. Patients with oesophageal dysmotility are at increased risk for post-transplant complications from gastro-oesophageal reflux and aspiration. Those with systemic sclerosis or mixed connective tissue disease may have significant gastro-oesophageal dysfunction that can present across a wide spectrum of symptoms and clinical findings. Given the role of chronic aspiration and gastro-oesophageal reflux in the development of chronic lung allograft dysfunction (CLAD), it may be advantageous to identify these problems preoperatively so that they can be addressed. Early fundoplication may reduce the incidence of CLAD in this population. In patients with CF, GI abnormalities and delayed gastric emptying are common. Identification of these issues helps delineate a nutrition strategy that may or may not incorporate direct enteral access, whether by gastrostomy or jejunostomy. Finally, patients with scleroderma and other connective tissue disorders are at risk for significant oesophageal motility problems. Upper GI evaluation is very important to identify patients who would need modification and tailored therapy to address the oesophageal dysmotility in the post-transplant period. Each transplant centre's experience with scleroderma and scleroderma-like patients will dictate their willingness to accept these patients for transplantation. Some centres have achieved very acceptable outcomes with this patient subset, but symptomatic patients with air-fluid levels in a patulous, immotile oesophagus are at high risk to do poorly outside of experienced centres.

- Barium oesophagram.
- Oesophageal manometry and 24-hour pH monitoring.
- Speech therapy assessment for oropharyngeal dysphagia (consider fibreoptic endoscopic evaluation of swallowing).
- Solid gastric emptying in patients with symptoms or history of gastroparesis.

Nutritional evaluation

This evaluation is preferably undertaken by a dietician with experience in managing lung transplant patients. Malnutrition is common in patients with CF and restrictive lung disease. Malnutrition should be addressed with a diet plan, oral dietary supplements, and enteric nutrition in some cases. Occasionally, activation on the waiting list is delayed until the malnutrition is addressed. If possible, it is best to avoid transplantation of patients who are extremely underweight (BMI <18.5 kg/m^2) or extremely overweight (BMI >35 kg/m^2). Outcomes in these patients are significantly worse, and it is preferable to address the weight before listing.

Hepatic evaluation

- Ultrasound of the liver in patients <50 years of age.
- CT imaging to assess liver, vasculature, rule out malignancy >50 years of age.
- Consider Fibroscan of liver or transjugular liver biopsy with pressure measurements in a subset of patients with increased risk for liver disease (e.g. CF, hepatitis C, etc.).

Renal evaluation

- Serum creatinine and eGFR generally adequate (creatinine clearance >50 mL/min is considered acceptable for lung transplantation).
- Consider measured GFR in patients with chronic kidney disease to establish creatinine clearance >50 mL/min.
- Screen for significant proteinuria with urinalysis (may need 24-hour urine collection/nephrology referral if significant).

Infectious evaluation

- Hepatitis serologies.
- HSV, VZV, CMV, EBV serologies.
- HIV screen.
- Toxoplasmosis.
- Syphilis testing (rapid plasma reagin/*Treponema* screen).
- Sputum for bacteria, acid-fast bacilli, fungal stain, and culture.

Immunological evaluation

- HLA screen to evaluate for preformed PRAs.

Functional status/frailty

- Varies by centre (regular participation in pulmonary rehabilitation strongly recommended).

Cancer screening

- Colonoscopy for patients >50 years of age (endoscopic preferred; virtual colonoscopy may be considered in certain conditions).
- Mammogram, pelvic exam.
- Prostatic serum antigen.

Clinical management after listing

General guidelines for patients on the list

Once patients have completed their evaluation and have met their transplant centre's criteria, they can be activated on the waiting list. Time on the waiting list until undergoing transplantation varies by centre and may be impacted by blood type, HLA sensitization, extremes of chest cavity size, and stature. To optimize patient outcome following transplantation, it is imperative patients achieve and maintain adequate nutrition and conditioning. All patients should be active in a regular exercise programme up until the time of transplantation. In centres where patients have relocated to participate in their pulmonary rehabilitation, this approach has the advantage of having trained therapists to actively assess patients' clinical status while on the waiting list to avoid surprises at the transplant surgery involving patients who have significantly deteriorated since they were last seen.

Patients should generally be evaluated every 4–12 weeks while on the waiting list by the transplant team to ensure stability and determine if there are any clinical status changes (increased oxygen requirements, decreased walk distance, worsening hypercarbia) that would warrant an adjustment of the allocation score or sequence on the waiting list. If patients are on the waiting list for 6 months, certain tests including blood work and right heart catheterization may need updating to avoid a default entry that could negatively impact the allocation score.

The deteriorating patient

For patients who are deteriorating on the waiting list, every attempt should be made to identify any aetiology for the decline that may respond to therapy. Their sequence on the waiting list may need to be modified. For example, their allocation score should be recalculated to see if they should be prioritized on the waiting list. If unable to remain in the outpatient setting, hospitalization can provide a setting to stabilize and assess frequently to determine suitability for transplantation. Occasionally, oxygen requirements exceed flow rates that can be delivered outside the hospital and an admission to the hospital provides an opportunity to remain functional, improve their clinical status, and still safely undergo transplant surgery. These patients should be carefully assessed as it has been shown that those with rapidly increasing allocation scores immediately prior to transplantation have worsened survival following transplantation. In these instances, the large change in clinical status or allocation score may be a surrogate marker that the mortality risk outweighs survival benefit which warrants a thoughtful assessment of the decision whether to move forward with transplantation as much as is possible.

ICU management

For those inpatients who develop worsened hypercarbic and/or hypoxaemic respiratory failure that necessitates management in the ICU and are felt to remain suitable transplant candidates, an early discussion by the team to determine the extent of interventions that will be offered is prudent for effective management. Some patients may require increased oxygen delivery (via high-flow device), intubation with mechanical ventilation, tracheotomy placement, or ECMO cannulation. All of these interventions increase the level of risk for transplantation and potential for worsened outcome. Although ECMO (most commonly VV ECMO but also VA ECMO in certain patients with right HF) has become an acceptable and effective strategy to bridge unstable and declining patients, it is preferable that the patient be ambulatory or at a minimum off sedation and neurologically intact. Sedation and ECMO support can hide a multitude of unstable conditions for successful transplantation. Each centre should establish criteria in these instances for which they feel they can achieve a good outcome for these deteriorating patients to not only guide medical care and clinical decision-making but also to provide clear communication to patients and their families and appropriately manage their expectations.

Special considerations

Single- versus double-lung transplantation

In patients with suppurative lung disease or severe PH, a bilateral lung transplant is mandatory to ameliorate the disease effectively. However, in patients with restrictive lung disease and COPD, single orthotopic lung transplantation (SOLT) is considered an appropriate transplantation approach.

Improved survival in patients receiving bilateral orthotopic lung transplantation (BOLT) has been demonstrated in multiple retrospective studies. Studies employing the registry of the ISHLT have likewise supported this finding. Being retrospective in nature, these findings may be affected by selection bias. A study by Thabut et al. showed that in patients with pulmonary fibrosis, this survival advantage might be related to baseline differences between the groups, and correcting for these differences may nullify the mortality benefit in favour of BOLT. Moreover, they concluded that while single-lung transplantation confers short-term survival benefit but long-term harm, and bilateral transplantation confers short-term harm but long-term survival benefit.

The balance between short-term risk versus harm and the desire for the optimal good long-term survival is the underlying tenet that drives the decision between SOLT and BOLT. Multiple criteria have been proposed as a means to define the group of patients where overall short-term risk profile favours SOLT, such as advanced age. Based on these studies, it would seem that with increasing donor age and frailty, the lower perioperative mortality of a single-lung transplant may outweigh the advantage of better long-term survival. Gulack et al. found that bilateral lung transplantation was associated with improved long-term survival in older patients with idiopathic pulmonary fibrosis, except in patients with reduced functional status. Villavicencio et al. found that bilateral lung transplantation does not confer a survival advantage in patients >70 years old. However, they recommended against the use of single-lung transplantation in patients with PA pressure >30 mmHg and LAS >45.

Recognizing that there are no definitive data on the subject, the decision to offer single-lung transplantation has varied from centre to centre. At our institutions, we offer bilateral lung transplantation to all patients with CF, suppurative lung disease, and pulmonary vascular disease. Bilateral lung transplantation is our preferred strategy for patients with restrictive and obstructive lung diseases. However, we will offer single lung transplantation for some elderly patients >65 years of age, especially if they have reduced functional capacity, significant comorbidities, CAD, or previous chest surgery. We would generally avoid single-lung transplantation in patients with significant secondary PH (mean PA pressure >40 mmHg), since registry data suggest that BOLT may be a preferred option in these patients.

Highly sensitized patients

Patients with class I or class II PRAs are considered sensitized. The typical approach is to avoid donors with the same antigen–antibody profile as the recipient given the risk for graft dysfunction. Several considerations of PRAs are important in determining their significance, including their MFI and presence on 1:16 dilution, which correlates with strength. Whether they are class I (present on all cells) or class II (only present on immune cells) is also important in determining their significance. Most often, patients either do not have these antibodies or have reasonably low levels such that avoiding donors with the corresponding antigens will not result in a prolonged time on the waiting list. Some patients, however, do have very high PRA levels (>80–90%) and when combined with their blood type and stature, can result in very long wait times.

Attempts at 'desensitization' (a reduction in the antibody burden) prior to transplantation by plasmapheresis (PLEX) and medications have not shown consistent results thus far. Examples of medication used for desensitization include proteasome inhibitors (e.g. carfilzomib, bortezomib) to impact the plasma cells which produce antibodies and rituximab to affect B lymphocytes. Positive results have been seen in the administration of PLEX, proteasome inhibitors, and rituximab in highly sensitized patients following transplantation in patients with a negative or even positive cross-match.

Retransplantation

Patients who develop CLAD may be considered for retransplantation. According to the 2017 Organ Procurement and Transplantation Network Annual Data Report, retransplantation comprised 3.2% of all lung transplants. Those with obstructive CLAD tend to have a slower rate of disease progression and overall better prognosis, including for retransplantation than patients with restrictive CLAD.

Each transplant centre has its own guidelines regarding retransplantation (some will avoid retransplantation altogether and others perform multiple operations in the same patient). Centres that perform retransplantation adhere to their basic criteria of candidacy for the initial transplantation. In general, obstructive CLAD, long duration following prior transplant surgery, absence of antibody sensitization, and absence of significant chronic kidney disease all confer a better prognosis with retransplantation. Even with these more favourable characteristics, programmes and patients should expect a retransplantation to potentially be more challenging than their prior transplant surgery due to the likelihood of pleural adhesions and bleeding as well as the risk of worsened kidney function.

Multiorgan transplant

Heart–lung transplantation

The majority of patients with end-stage lung disease will benefit from isolated lung transplantation and preservation of the native heart. Even the majority of patients with some degree of cardiac dysfunction will not require cardiac transplantation, and cardiac dysfunction is likely to improve after lung transplantation. However, there are rare situations where combined heart–lung transplantation is unavoidable. These include the following:

- Patients with PH secondary to CHD and irreparable congenital defects.
- Patients with acquired heart disease (CAD, valvular heart disease), who are being considered for cardiac transplantation, and who have irreversible PH:
  - In these patients, assessment with a heart catheterization should be performed. Pulmonary arterial hypertension and elevated PVR (defined as a PVR >5 Wood units, a PVR index >6, or a transpulmonary pressure gradient 16–20 mmHg) should be considered contraindications for isolated cardiac transplantation. Vasodilator therapy may be used to reduce PVR. However, this is typically limited by the precipitation of systemic hypertension. In these cases, heart–lung transplantation should be considered, as the incidence of RV failure after isolated cardiac transplantation is very high.
- Patients with end-stage lung disease, complicated by PH and irreversible RV or biventricular dysfunction:
  - The majority of these patients with RV dysfunction will benefit from lung transplantation only. However, there is a subset of patients where RV dysfunction is irreversible and may not improve with lung transplantation alone. This is a very difficult group to define. In some programmes, lung transplantation is offered for all patients with pulmonary arterial hypertension, and RV dysfunction, with heart–lung transplantation, offered only to patients with significant LV dysfunction (defined as EF <40%, CI <2.2 L/min/m², with or without PCWP <15 mmHg).

- In patients with PH, chronic pressure or volume overload imposed on the RV initially promotes compensatory mechanisms. This is characterized by elevated PA pressure, elevated PVR, and elevated RA pressure, and a preserved ventricular function. With time, and with prolonged exposure to overload, the ventricle transitions from a compensated to a decompensated phase characterized by myocyte loss and scarring. In the decompensating phase, as PVR and RA pressure remain elevated, RV function declines and forward flow of blood into the PA is decreased. Cardiac output subsequently declines, followed by a reduction in PA pressure. Declining PA pressure in the setting of high PVR is an ominous clinical finding, heart–lung transplantation should at least be considered.

Combined kidney and lung transplantation

Deterioration in kidney function is common in SOT recipients. The aetiology is multifactorial, but the unavoidable use of CNIs is most likely to blame. It has been shown that kidney function declines rapidly in the first month after transplantation, declines slightly in the first year after that, and stabilizes up to 10 years. GFR is used to stratify kidney function, with a GFR of <50 mL/min/1.73 m² used as a threshold for determining the risk of adverse outcomes. However, a study of the UNOS database shows that some of these adverse outcomes can be ameliorated by receiving a kidney transplantation. In this study by Osho et al. of the lung recipients listed for kidney transplantation after receiving a lung allograft, 56% were not on dialysis. Time to listing was approximately 80 months. Patients who received a kidney transplant had better survival than those who did not. Given the high morbidity and mortality following lung transplantation in patients who develop end-stage renal disease in the first year following their transplant surgery, an increasing attractive option is utilizing living donor kidney transplantation. Those candidates noted to have marginal renal function prior to their lung transplant may benefit from identifying a living donor kidney to provide an option to proceed with isolated living donor kidney transplantation following their lung transplant if end-stage renal dysfunction develops and chronic hemodialysis is required.

Combined liver and lung transplantation

Certain diseases, such as CF and alpha-1-antitrypsin deficiency, will have combined lung and liver dysfunction. In these patients, lung dysfunction is typically more severe. Combined liver and lung transplants have been reported mainly in UNOS database publication and small case series. Patients with combined liver and lung dysfunction should meet disease-specific criteria for activation for both lung and liver transplantation. However, caution should be exercised in patients with very advanced liver disease (albumin <2.0 g/dL, INR >1.8, or the presence of severe ascites or encephalopathy). However, many patients with less advanced liver disease may be considered for combined lung and liver transplantation. The decision to proceed with concomitant transplantation during the same operation is influenced by many aspects. These include concern about the progression of organ dysfunction after single-organ transplantation, the rate of decline of lung or liver dysfunction, concern for coagulopathy due to the liver disease, and time on the waiting list for patients with unfavourable characteristics (high PRA levels, short stature).

De-listing

Removal from the waiting list may be one of the most difficult decisions undertaken by a lung transplant team. However, it is inevitable that some patients on the list will progress or develop new problems that render them unsuitable for lung transplantation. Patients on the waiting list should be followed regularly to screen for the development of issues, progression of disease, and contraindications for lung transplantation. The development of any of the contraindications from Box 24.1 (see p. 321) should prompt removal from the waiting list. Perhaps one of the most difficult decisions to make is to determine the level of deconditioning that should prompt removal of the waiting list. The decision should be made by taking into consideration input from all members of the team, including physicians, physiotherapists, nurses, and dietician.

Lung donor selection and management

Introduction

As lung acceptance rates from donors stand at <20%, there is a stark contrast with the demand for transplantation. As a result, much work has been done on widening donor lung selection and acceptance criteria to safely use less than ideal (marginal) lungs.

Current criteria for ideal lung donors include a donor age <55 years, PaO_2 >300 mmHg (40 kPa), no smoking history, and a clear bronchoscopy and CXR. Finding a donor that meets all of these criteria is rare in the modern era but accepting lungs with extended criteria can lead to excellent and equivalent outcomes.

Donor care

Donor lung functional criteria can be improved through careful and active donor management by the team caring for the patient. This can optimize donation criteria, increase conversion rates, and support better long-term outcomes after transplantation.

As brain death and the catecholamine surge lead to haemodynamic instability, the activation of inflammatory pathways, and endocrine dysfunction, the quality and function of donated lungs can be affected significantly. The sympathetic storm leads to increased pulmonary capillary pressures and disruption of the alveolar–capillary membrane. The loss of protein-rich fluid into the alveoli can cause hypoxaemia and prolong this phase of high-permeability pulmonary oedema.

To mitigate against these effects, several strategies can be employed in intensive care to maximize the yield of lungs from suitable donors.

The beneficial effects of employing lung protective ventilation strategies (tidal volume 6–8 mL/kg predicted body weight, PEEP 8–10 cmH_2O) and careful fluid balance to avoid the neurogenic pulmonary oedema associated with increased capillary permeability are important. Ventilation should aim to maintain a PaO_2 ≥10 kPa and a pH >7.25.

Optimal intensive care management of the lung donor ahead of retrieval should also include:
- Administration of methylprednisolone (15 mg/kg).
- IV crystalloid maintenance fluid to maintain Na^+ <150 mmol/L and urine output between 0.5 and 2.0 mL/kg/hour.
- Vasopressin (0.5–4 units/hour) to treat diabetes insipidus.
- An insulin infusion to keep blood sugar at 4–10 mmol/L.
- The use of antiembolic stockings and low-molecular-weight heparin to prevent thromboembolic issues. Subclinical microemboli are quite commonly encountered in donor lungs at retrieval and can be flushed out of the PA during retrograde perfusion of the lungs through the pulmonary veins.

Criteria for lung decline

Transplant surgeons and physicians must maintain broad acceptance criteria to avoid discounting potentially transplantable organs that could benefit those on the waiting list. The usual exclusion criteria for donation of any

organ always apply but certain donors are clearly unsuitable for lung procurement and can be declined.

These include:

- Donors with a PaO_2 <25 kPa (187 mmHg) on an FiO_2 of 1.0 and
  PEEP of 8 cmH_2O after rigorous attempts have been made to recruit
  atelectatic segments, clear the airways of secretions, and endotracheal
  tube malposition has been excluded.
- Where a clear and irreversible cause for hypoxaemia has been
  established such as bilateral significant pulmonary contusion or other
  trauma, documented aspiration with gross airway contamination which
  cannot be cleared, or CXR evidence of major pulmonary consolidation.

In the presence of a PaO_2 <25 kPa on an FiO_2 of 1.0 and PEEP of 8 cmH_2O
and unilateral CXR changes only, the possibility of single-lung transplantation should be considered (pulmonary venous sampling during organ
retrieval is recommended as this may demonstrate good function in the
unaffected lung making it suitable for donation despite concerning systemic
blood gases).

Ex vivo lung perfusion (EVLP) where available should always be considered before declining organs where potential exists to recondition the
lungs to transplantable status. Situations where EVLP would be beneficial
will include those with a PO_2 <40 kPa (FiO_2 100% PEEP 8 cmH_2O). Lungs
showing pulmonary oedema clinically or radiologically, those with persistent
atelectasis despite optimal recruitment manoeuvres, or excessive purulent
secretions are especially suitable. Trauma lungs (e.g. multiple transfusions,
lung contusion, 'hanging' cause of death) and logistical reasons are also very
reasonable indications for considering the use of this technology.

Surgical assessment at the donor hospital

After reviewing the age, previous medical history, behavioural history, and
travel history, further tests are required: standard clinical blood tests, blood
group determination, infectious disease screening, and review of CXRs or
CT scans. A standardized blood gas analysis will reveal, determined while
ventilating on an FiO_2 of 100% and a minimum PEEP of 8 cmH_2O, whether
the gas exchange is adequate (PO_2 >35 mmHg). Appropriate recruitment
manoeuvres and bronchoscopy should be undertaken before evaluating
function. Donor and recipient can then be matched on blood group, height,
sex, total lung volume, and antibody status. The latter can be a direct cross-
match or the more often used virtual cross-match.

Lung donor acceptance criteria

Inherent donor characteristics may influence the quality of the lungs and
potentially impact recipient outcome. In general, but not exclusively, ventilation of the donor should be for <10 days. The presence of a tracheostomy
does not preclude lung donation.

There are a number of characteristics that should be considered by the
retrieval and implanting surgeons:

Cause of death

Donor death by asphyxiation or drowning should not automatically exclude transplantation provided airway contamination with marine flora and algae or parenchymal injury have been excluded. However, aspiration of seawater can induce a direct lung injury and so one should be cautious in this scenario.

Donors arise from suicidal hanging where occlusion of the airway is combined with carotid artery obstruction. The former will cause pulmonary oedema which can be neurogenic or due to high negative intrathoracic pressures. Inspiration against the occluded upper airway causes a fall in intrathoracic pressure, increased venous return, and increased pulmonary capillary pressure, with a simultaneous fall in pulmonary interstitial pressure resulting in pulmonary oedema. Hypoxia also increases pulmonary capillary vascular resistance increasing hydrostatic pressure and pulmonary capillary permeability. Air trapping may cause parenchymal barotrauma and lung surface bullae and haemorrhage may be evident at inspection on retrieval.

However, studies have shown no effect on the rate of airway dehiscence, rejection, or long-term survival from drowning or asphyxiation donor lungs after transplantation. Ten-year survival curves in >18,000 lung transplant recipients were not influenced by donor cause of death, either when analysed individually or when asphyxiation or drowning was compared with all other causes.

However, alterations in surfactant have been described and so care must be taken in the evaluation of the lungs at retrieval.

Carbon monoxide poisoning is a rare cause of organ donation but should not necessarily lead to rejection of the lungs. In a small series from Cambridge, UK, satisfactory outcomes were achieved. Concomitant smoke inhalation, however, suggests that caution should be taken and bronchoscopy may show airway burns which preclude use for transplantation.

In patients who have sustained severe chest trauma, the lungs may still be utilized for transplantation. Mild to moderate lung contusions are acceptable and do not contraindicate use. CT scanning may be helpful if available to specifically evaluate this. The presence of rib fractures or pneumothorax is not a problem in isolation nor is the presence of a chest drain. Inspection of the lung at retrieval, however, is critical in the final decision-making pathway as parenchymal injury that cannot be easily repaired may be evident.

Age

The mean age of donors in Europe has been increasing. Registry data suggest that donors with ages <18 and >64 years are related to a higher mortality at 1 and 3 years. Donor age up to 70 years for brainstem dead donors (DBD) and 65 years for donors after circulatory death (DCD) are, however, acceptable with good outcomes demonstrated in several series. This can be extended further to 75 years especially if the donor had not smoked for 10 years or was a non-smoker. Donor age criteria can be safely extended, and caution need only be applied if there are compounding risk factors in addition, such as a prolonged ischaemic time.

The interaction between donor and recipient age alone is not an independent factor in determining survival.

Sex and race

Donor and recipient sex and racial combinations have been analysed with diverse results.

Fessart et al. failed to discern a difference in recipient survival after analysis of all gender combinations but other retrospective single-institution studies have demonstrated an increase in survival and decrease in bronchiolitis obliterans syndrome (BOS) for donor–recipient male into female and female into male sex mismatches. Male donor to male recipient combinations had a significant decrease in survival. ISHLT registry review has shown decreased survival in female donors to male recipients. Female donor to female recipient matching though showed a short- and long-term survival benefit.

Race-matched donor/recipients have improved outcomes and African American donors are associated with worse survival irrespective of the race of the recipient. Overall, though, recipient race is not associated with survival variability. No changes in 1-year rejection rates have been associated with race matching.

As the nature of gender interactions between donor and recipient have yet to be fully elucidated, it should not play a major role in donor selection or acceptance.

Donor size

TLC (both predicted and actual) and recipient pathology (e.g. fibrosis or emphysema) are important in considering an appropriate donor-to-recipient match. For double lung transplants, patients with emphysema should be matched to a donor with a TLC of 60–100% of the recipient's TLC. For pulmonary hypertension and CF patients, the predicted TLC of the donor should be 100–120% of the recipient's actual TLC.

Due to the reduced TLC seen in recipients with pulmonary fibrosis, the donor's TLC should be approximately halfway between the recipient's actual TLC and predicted TLC plus 20%.

Generally, it is preferable to slightly oversize rather than undersize.

Experienced surgeons may consider graft volume reduction using techniques such as right middle lobectomy and multiple wedge resections using pericardial strip reinforced staplers.

Very good outcomes comparable to conventional transplants have been described using this technique.

Blood gases and ventilation

On an FiO_2 of 100% and PEEP of 8 cmH_2O, a PaO_2 ≥35 kPa (or a PaO_2 ≥14 kPa with an FiO_2 of 40%) are acceptable for transplantation. The addition of 8 cmH_2O of PEEP is recommended to prevent atelectasis and help minimize neurogenic pulmonary oedema. Initial PaO_2/FiO_2 ratios of <300 mmHg (40 kPa) should not exclude donor organ usage and recruitment techniques should be implemented with intent to transplant alongside the use of bronchoscopy to clear secretions.

Normal ventilatory parameters and normal lung compliance are essential.

Oxygenation (although considered by many to be the most important element in lung donor acceptance) is probably the weakest physiological measure to define and determine the suitability of the lung for transplantation but is frequently used as a critical decision-making parameter.

In a recent Australian study of 93 brainstem dead lung donors, an arterial PO_2/FiO_2 ratio of <300 mmHg (40 kPa) was largely caused by a low ratio in the lower lobes. There were no differences between the recipients receiving donor lungs where the ICU PO_2/FiO_2 ratio was <300 mmHg compared with those ≥300 mmHg in time to extubation, severity of primary graft dysfunction, pulmonary function at 6 and 12 months, and survival at 1 year.

Had a donor PO_2/FiO_2 threshold of 300 mmHg been adhered to, then up to a third of the donor lungs available would have been declined. A ratio of 300 mmHg therefore can be considered very conservative, wastes acceptable donor lungs, and leads to the unnecessary and expensive use of EVLP.

The blood gases should always be evaluated in the context of other donor characteristics, but lungs should not be discarded out of hand in the face of initially poor blood gases. These can very often be improved *in situ* in the donor, may mask a usable single lung, or can be reconditioned with EVLP.

Smoking history

Smoking history is not a concern if lung function and assessment at retrieval is otherwise good.

A smoking history of up to 30 pack-years is perfectly acceptable but if in excess of this then other relevant factors and donor characteristics should be considered in combination to ensure that hazards are not compounded (such as donor age, ischaemic time) as decline might then be appropriate for particular recipients. Donor lungs with a >20 pack-year history are not associated with greater BOS or reduced survival.

Smoking history is associated with a reduced 3-year recipient survival (by 10% compared to non-smoker donors) when compared to non-smoker donor lungs. Patients receiving lungs from donors with a positive smoking history had a lower hazard of death after registration than those who remained on the waiting list. Thus, the transplantation of recipients with smoker lungs remains advantageous as mortality on the waiting list is greater than the added postoperative risk.

However, in the UK experience, recipients whose donors had a smoking history >20 cigarettes/day have a 6-year survival of 20% less than that observed with non-smoker donor lungs (and 10% less than those who had smoked <20 cigarettes/day).

The collapse test at retrieval is important in determining whether significant air trapping is present suggesting chronic obstructive airways disease. If the lungs do not rapidly deflate, they should be declined. EVLP is not appropriate in such situations as this is not a reversible pathology where reconditioning will help.

Bronchoscopy and microbiology

Post-transplantation pneumonia and sepsis are serious concerns to the transplant surgeon. It is critical to gain the expert advice of a transplant microbiologist in most cases to advise on donor culture results where they have been obtained.

Purulent secretions do not automatically preclude lung donation unless there is evidence of inflamed mucosa and contact bleeding on bronchoscopy. Gram stain evaluation of the airways in a single-centre retrospective study found that 12% of donors with a positive Gram stain subsequently developed recipient pneumonia compared to 20% in those with negative Gram stains! This refutes the association of donor Gram stain with recipient pneumonia. In this study, however, donor lungs were not accepted if there was evidence of frank aspiration on bronchoscopy.

Multiple organisms on Gram stain may indicate normal flora and are unlikely to lead to post-transplant infection despite the patient being immunosuppressed. Positive Gram stains in tracheal aspirates usually do not indicate ongoing pneumonia but simply purulent secretions harboured in the upper airways. These are readily removed at bronchoscopy. No specific Gram stain findings are associated with or reflect a risk of poor outcome in recipients. Heavy fungal contamination of the bronchial tree may, however, exclude donation.

Importantly, though, positive cultures from donor BAL specimens may indicate ongoing and clinically significant infection and lead to longer ICU stay and prolonged ventilation in recipients when compared to donors with negative BAL cultures.

Lavage specimens should be taken for culture from all donors to aggressively adapt and refine antibiotic therapy postoperatively. This practice has significantly reduced the incidence of recipient pneumonia.

Prospective analysis of donor airway cultures and bronchial tissue cultures revealed a <1.5% transmission rate of donor organ contamination. With appropriate antibiotic prophylaxis to cover *Pseudomonas* and *Staphylococcus aureus*, the risk of transmission of donor-associated infections is negligible.

CMV mismatches are acceptable unless specified in high-risk recipients.

Radiological imaging

CXRs are a poor indicator of lung donor function or long-term post-implant recipient survival. No studies have ever correlated CXR findings to infections in recipients.

As such, CXR should not be used alone to decline organs. Radiological abnormalities may be transient and signs such as infiltrates do not influence outcome and may often resolve. Borderline blood gases combined with a unilateral abnormality on CXR may mask a usable contralateral lung.

CT scans may have been obtained and are increasingly made available to transplant teams. This can be useful in better resolving lung abnormalities such as nodules, but also in assessing the severity of consolidation as opposed to atelectasis.

Lung contusions from trauma can be evaluated accurately on CT in terms of number and severity. If modest, lungs may still be acceptable for use but may lead to lung decline if severe.

Pleural effusions are usually reactive or inflammatory but can be associated with chest trauma. The presence of an effusion alone is not a reason to decline the lungs, only if the pleural fluid is infected or there is radiological evidence of empyema should microbiological advice on the usability of the lungs be sought.

Ischaemic time

Ischaemic times have traditionally been kept to <6 hours, but more recent studies have suggested that the lung is very resistant to ischaemia and with better organ preservation techniques, ischaemic times can safely be more generous. An ischaemic time of up to 8 hours is acceptable.

Ischaemic time alone therefore should not limit donor retrieval distances or transport times.

Several single-centre studies have demonstrated no effect on survival with preservation >6 hours, but surgeons should be cognisant of the additive effects of adverse donor characteristics where factors such as age or heavy smoking history may combine with a long ischaemic time to increase risk in certain recipients.

A review of >5000 lung transplant recipients showed greater early mortality with cold ischaemic times of 7–8 hours and donors >45 years of age.

Ischaemic times of ≥10 hours have been successfully reported with optimal donors.

Donation after circulatory death

When, after careful assessment of a patient in ICU, it appears that further medical treatment is considered futile, withdrawal of treatment is appropriate. The considerations outlined previously in this chapter for DBD donors apply similarly in this category of donor although the retrieval process is very different.

The donor can be extubated with the intent of allowing death to occur. Respiratory and haemodynamic parameters are observed: blood pressure, pulse frequency, respiration rate, and oxygen saturation are documented at regular intervals. For lung retrievals, the only important parameter is the systolic blood pressure. A systolic blood pressure <70 mmHg cannot be permitted for >1 hour. After this period of warm ischaemia, the lungs are considered non-transplantable and should be declined. After 30 minutes of warm ischaemia the use of EVLP can be considered if available.

Once the donor has been declared dead, a legally defined 10-minute period has to be respected before the actual retrieval procedure can start. Unfortunately, most DCD procedures do not progress to organ retrieval as the donor remains haemodynamically stable beyond the prescribed time limits.

Conclusion

Given the low acceptance rates of donor lungs for transplantation, every effort should be made to increase acceptance, improve function, and therefore utilization. This begins with optimal ICU care of the donor with appropriate management of the catecholamine storm, careful fluid balance to mitigate against neurogenic pulmonary oedema, and lung protective ventilation strategies.

Ideal donors are now a rarity. Surgeons must be prepared to thoroughly evaluate and accept marginal lungs as excellent outcomes in recipients can be obtained.

Donor age can be extended to >65 years and even to 75 years. Donor smoking history is associated with good outcomes after transplantation and is certainly better than the chances of survival on the waiting list.

CXR abnormalities should never be used alone as a reason for decline. Abnormalities may be transient or reversible.

Poor blood gases can be misleading and should not be used to decline lungs out of hand. Excellent outcomes can be obtained from lungs where the donor initially demonstrated hypoxaemia and setting the bar too high can result in the decline of perfectly suitable lungs for transplantation.

Lung recruitment manoeuvres and bronchoscopy are very important in the optimization process. Upper airway secretions are easily cleared and lavage specimens should always be obtained to guide postoperative anti-biotic strategies.

Ischaemic times can safely be prolonged well beyond the traditional 6-hour limit with good results.

In lungs that cannot meet acceptance criteria for transplantation despite careful evaluation and optimization, the use of EVLP shows great promise in reconditioning lungs where there is a reversible pathology.

Lung procurement following donation after brain death and donation after circulatory death

Donation after brain death donor lung procurement

Upon arrival at the procurement site, the team should begin by assessing available imaging, recent blood gases, and measuring the length and width of the prospective donor's chest. Any CT imaging should be examined for any emphysema or nodules that may not have been mentioned previously. Once the candidate donor is deemed suitable, flexible bronchoscopy is performed to evaluate the extent of secretions, to assess for any anatomical variations that may complicate implantation, and to thoroughly suction the airways. Secretions may be copious, but attention is paid to the rate of re-accumulation and whether the lungs contain enteric material.

The lungs are procured via a median sternotomy incision. The pericardial and bilateral pleural spaces are entered and the lungs are visually inspected. Visual inspection should include not only looking for blebs but also areas of diffuse emphysema. During the inspection phase prior to organ harvest, it is important to specify that the settings on the ventilator are appropriate with a PEEP of 8 cmH$_2$O and an FiO$_2$ of 100%. A sustained recruitment manoeuvre of 30 cmH$_2$O for several seconds is made to recruit atelectasis and, upon deflation, both lungs are manually palpated to detect for pathology. Lung deflation should be done by disconnecting the ventilator, which has the effect of allowing the surgeon to accurately assess the compliance of the potential donor lungs.

A central gas should be obtained no sooner than 5 minutes after this 'recruitment manoeuvre'. If performed too quickly, the challenge gas may be artificially low due to donor hypotension during lung manipulation and recruitment. Individual pulmonary vein gases may also be sampled to assess the PaO$_2$ in the individual lobes. A central arterial blood gas with a PaO$_2$ of >300 mmHg is generally deemed suitable. At this point, communication with the implanting team should be made to confirm or abort the transplantation.

Once assessment of the lungs deems them suitable for transplantation, it is generally advisable, if the donor is stable, to proceed with additional dissection. This serves the purpose of reducing the chances for iatrogenic injury at the time of explant. Encircling the aorta and freeing it from the underlying right PA helps to ensure that it is not injured at the time of aortic transection. The aortopulmonary window is dissected, separating the main and right PAs from the aorta, in order to prepare for the aortic cross-clamp. The SVC is dissected circumferentially and a tourniquet loosely passed around it cephalad to the azygous vein. The azygous vein is tied off approximately 0.5–1 cm off of the SVC to prevent stenosis. Dissecting the SVC away from the underlying right PA as it courses under this vessel also ensures that it is not injured later during explant. The trachea is then mobilized by retracting the aorta and PA, incising the superior posterior pericardium along the PA and using a finger to bluntly dissect in the plane around the trachea. If a longer length of trachea is required as is often desired with subsequent EVLP use, the innominate artery can be dissected out and encircled and retracted which will provide ample exposure to the trachea at a more proximal level. Our institutional preference is to avoid dissection in the interatrial groove of the heart (Waterston's or Sondergaard's groove) until right before cross-clamp as this has a tendency to provoke potentially unstable heart arrhythmia.

Once dissection is complete, and cardiac and abdominal harvest teams ready, the patient is systemically heparinized and the main PA cannulated, typically with a 6.5 mm high-flow cannula. If the heart is not being procured then separate aortic cannulation is not necessary. Cannulation of the PA generally occurs a short length distal to the pulmonary valve; cannulating too far distally on the main PA can lead to an uneven flush as the tip of the catheter is directed down one of the two main PAs. Prostaglandin E1 (500 mcg) is directly injected into the main PA using a fine bore needle and should be done prior to cross-clamp as it can induce hypotension. Alternatively, prostaglandin can be administered via the preservation solution by injecting it into the perfusate to ensure its delivery.

Immediately prior to cross-clamping, the SVC tourniquet is then tightened and preparations are made for venting the heart. If the wish is to vent via the LA, the interatrial groove (Waterston's or Sondergaard's groove) is developed and a stab incision made for the purposes of venting. Alternatively, the venting of the LV can occur through the LAA. The cardioplegia and pulmonary perfusate are prepared for infusion, flushed, and de-aired. The right heart is vented via transection of the IVC at the level of the diaphragm. With the heart adequately vented, the aorta is then cross-clamped and the cardiac and pulmonary preservation solutions are initiated. Typically, preservation solution such as Perfadex (XVIVO Perfusion AB, Göteborg, Sweden) is used. Note that cross-clamping is not necessary in instances when the heart is not being procured.

The preservation solution should be administered via gravity. During antegrade perfusion, it is important to first confirm that the flush is running efficiently by communicating with the preservationist. Once that has been established, one must then proceed with placing ice slush into each pleural space to offset the warm blood that tends to collect in this area and impede uniform cooling of the lungs. Focus is then turned back to assessment of the flush which is best done by paying close attention to the rate and colour change of the flush as it exits the LA. Initially bloody, it should quickly dilute and become clear. A full antegrade flush is at least 4 L. The antegrade flush should not be administered with a pressure bag.

With completion of the perfusate, the heart is explanted. This can be performed a number of different ways, but if done in the absence of a heart team, our team generally transects the great vessels, beginning with the PA, then the aorta, and finally both the SVC and IVC. In the presence of a heart team, the successful negotiation of the pulmonary vein cuff is critical. One of the subtleties of this step is realizing that with the heart elevated and on stretch, the pulmonary vein cuff can appear satisfactory, but that it always retracts upon cutting. One must also pay particularly close attention as the heart surgeon cuts along the right pulmonary veins, an area in particular where the cuff can be inadvertently shortened. Should this happen, and it often does, it can be corrected by adding a strip of pericardium to the edge of the vein cuff at the time of back-table preparation. It is therefore critical to procure excess donor pericardium as well for possible vascular reconstruction.

Division of the LA usually begins with the LV elevated out of the chest and a stab incision made halfway between the left inferior pulmonary vein and the AV groove towards the base of the LAA (Fig. 26.1). It is then continued from the inside of the LA to include all four pulmonary vein orifices. The ideal LA cuff includes a rim of LA muscle encircling all four pulmonary vein orifices.

After removal of the cardiac structures, retrograde pulmonary perfusion is carried out by delivering 2 L of perfusate into each of the pulmonary vein orifices. The flow of perfusate out of the PA cuff is important to note. The PAs are also inspected at this time to look for clot that might impede an effective back flush.

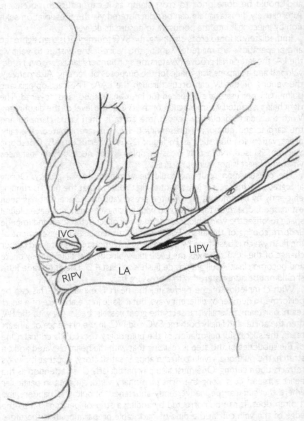

Fig. 26.1 Division of left atrium (LA). LIPV, left inferior pulmonary vein; RIPV, right inferior pulmonary vein

The lungs are then explanted using the following steps. The pericardium is cut sharply down to the hilum bilaterally, removed, and saved. The PA is transected at the level of the pulmonary perfusion cannulation site. The left lung is eviscerated, and inferior pulmonary ligament divided, identifying the thoracic aorta. The right lung is then eviscerated, the inferior ligament divided, and the anterior surface of the oesophagus bluntly dissected (Fig. 26.2). This can be carried up under the lung bloc to free it from posterior mediastinal attachments. With the lung bloc freed posteriorly, the trachea is encircled with instructions to the anaesthesiologist to slowly remove the endotracheal tube. When an adequate transection site on the trachea is identified, the anaesthesiologist is instructed to give a final Valsalva breath of sustained 30 cmH$_2$O pressure for several seconds with the endotracheal tube completely retracted, and the trachea is stapled twice and cut sharply between the two fires. Traction is placed on the bloc inferiorly and the surgeon sharply divides additional soft tissue attachments in the superior mediastinum. The lung bloc is removed from the chest (Fig. 26.3) and placed in a sterile plastic transport bag filled with cold preservation solution (no ice). The lungs are examined briefly prior to bag closure for surgical damage, unexpected pathology, or inadequate margins. The lungs are triple bagged with the outer bags containing ice.

Injuries to the PA can and do occur in general during the time of explant, usually because the right PA, for instance, has not been adequately dissected out during initial dissection. Proximal injuries are not a concern as much of the right PA is sacrificed on the back table but more distal injuries can require technical reconstructions that are readily avoidable if the SVC is separated from the underlying artery. A short atrial cuff is also a common problem, but again readily overcome by simply adding a lip of pericardium to the abbreviated atrial cuff.

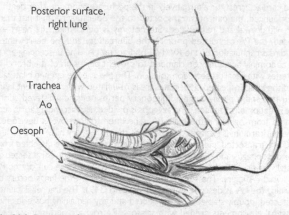

Posterior surface,
right lung

Trachea

Ao

Oesoph

Fig. 26.2 Dissection of posterior aspect of trachea. Oesoph, oesophagus.

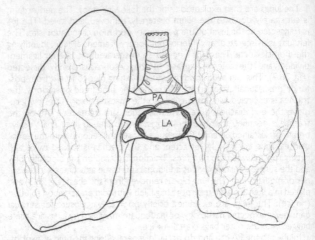

Fig. 26.3 Explanted lungs.

Donation after circulatory death donor lung procurement

The lung procurement operation in the DCD setting differs from the DBD setting in that the dissection prior to explant is generally more limited. In most hospitals, systemic heparin can be administered prior to extubation and cardiac arrest, or alternatively in the perfusate solution. After death is pronounced, the patient is transported to the operating room if not there for withdrawal and reintubated. Sternotomy is performed, the heart exposed, the PA cannulated prior to the bifurcation, and the heart vented by direct cannulation of the RV/IVC and aorta/LA. The descending aorta or abdominal aorta may be clamped to prevent perfusion of the bronchial arteries with renal preservation solution. The pleurae are opened bilaterally and the lungs inspected, atelectatic areas re-inflated with recruitment manoeuvres, and topically cooled. Pulmonary perfusate is administered during the initiation of dissection. The azygous is divided, and ascending aorta separated from right and the main PA. The interatrial groove is developed. The pericardium is excised to the level of the pulmonary hila. The SVC and IVC are transected and the posterior plane of the lungs are dissected from the oesophagus and descending thoracic aorta. The aorta is transected as distally as possible, leaving the ligamentum arteriosum as a cuff on the PA to avoid PA injury. The separation of the heart from the lungs occurs by dividing the LA as described previously (see p. 349). The trachea is bluntly dissected, doubly stapled, and transected and any remaining posterior mediastinal attachments divided with scissors. Retrograde perfusion via each pulmonary vein is performed. The lungs are removed and sterilely packed for transport.

The use of DCD lung donors has increased in recent years due to demonstrated comparable outcomes with DBD donors, although still remains much less common than DBD. It has been theorized that the lungs may tolerate longer ischaemic times because the lungs have a relatively low metabolic demand, and cells and alveoli have a high oxygen concentration, which permits continued aerobic cellular metabolism. The lungs are resilient and tolerate substantial cold storage time, which allows for thorough investigation of the graft on the back table prior to packaging for delivery to the recipient hospital.

The evaluation of DCD lung quality has been assisted by the development of EVLP, described elsewhere in this text (see Chapter 27). Results from abdominal organ transplantation suggest that allograft viability is optimized if perfused with cold flush within 30 minutes of withdrawal of life-sustaining therapy; however, this interval has been demonstrated with successful implantation up to 120 minutes of withdrawal of life-sustaining therapy. Typically, most centres accept 60–90 minutes of warm ischaemic time for lung DCD allografts. Whereas DBD donor criteria are generally widely accepted, several factors add complexity to selection of DCD donors, such as warm ischaemic time, time of extubation, onset of low blood pressure or oxygenation, the administration of heparin pretreatment, and use of EVLP. A meta-analysis pooling five studies reporting on DCD lung transplantation (n = 271) compared with DBD (n = 2369) found no difference in 1-year mortality, either within the studies or in the pooled analysis. There was also no difference in primary graft dysfunction or acute rejection in the pooled analysis.

Ex vivo lung perfusion

Introduction

Lung transplantation is now a well-established treatment for end-stage lung disease with a median survival of >10 years in specific patient groups. There is, however, a critical shortage of suitable donor lungs and a significant attrition among those on the lung transplant waiting list.

The high susceptibility of donor lungs to injury and dysfunction during the time of the donors' demise and before procurement mean that <20% of lungs from multiorgan DBD and as few as 6% of those from DCD are at present deemed suitable for transplantation in the USA and the UK. Despite a year-on-year increase in absolute transplant numbers, an annual waiting list mortality of up to 20% persists.

Ex vivo lung perfusion (EVLP), whether it is mobile or static, has emerged as a promising new technique for evaluating and reconditioning donor lungs that would previously have been regarded as unusable. By increasing the number of lung transplant procedures in individual centres by 15–30%, EVLP is already showing potential to substantially increase the availability of suitable donor lungs. The clinical experience has rapidly evolved over the past decade and with the introduction of portable EVLP, we might now face a new era of lung preservation where EVLP may also improve outcomes from donor lungs already deemed acceptable.

History of ex *vivo* lung perfusion

With the development of the first CPB machines in the 1950s grew an interest in its potential in organ transplantation and various groups came to investigate the effects that perfusion, storage, and preservation had on tissue viability and function. In the case of hearts and lungs, the preserved organs were found to be particularly delicate yet had to be capable of performing at almost full normal function immediately following transplantation. Early attempts at perfusing the lung were almost invariably frustrated by oedema formation and deteriorating function.

Contribution of Steen

Originally designed to enable an improved assessment of lungs from DCD donors, Stig Steen and colleagues in Lund, Sweden, developed the first well-functioning EVLP circuit for clinical use. A fundamental step towards success was the development of Steen Solution, a buffered perfusate solution with two major components. Firstly, a high albumin concentration to create an 'ideal' colloid osmotic pressure (about 30 mmHg) allowing physiological perfusion pressures and flow to be maintained without the development of either tissue oedema or dehydration. Secondly, a high dextran content, which is designed to coat the endothelium and protect it from excessive leucocyte interaction.

The preclinical work was translated by Steen and colleagues in 2000 when they performed the first human lung transplantation using a DCD lung assessed by EVLP and the first successful lung transplantation of an initially unacceptable donor lung reconditioned ex *vivo* in 2005. The Lund group EVLP circuit provided the blueprint for all circuits currently used in clinical centres worldwide. A pump generates a perfusate flow through a leucocyte filter and an oxygenator connected to a heater–cooler unit and gas exchange membrane before entering the lung through a cannula in the PA. Pulmonary venous return is collected in a sterile reservoir either through an open LA or through a closed LA cannula and is then recirculated. A ventilator is connected to the trachea allowing 'protective' ventilation to be carefully started *only* after the lungs have been rewarmed to 32°C and steadily increased while approaching normothermia (Fig. 27.1).

In 2019, around 550 human donor lungs are expected to be transplanted after EVLP reconditioning worldwide. Three main groups (Lund, Toronto (Canada), and Hannover (Germany)) have contributed the research into the physiology and technology to facilitate it and the theory behind their creations differ slightly. The Lund and Toronto groups were the pioneers inventing and spreading the technique of static EVLP around the world

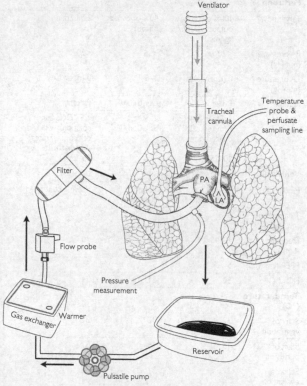

Fig. 27.1 Line diagram of an EVLP circuit. HCU, heater–cooler unit.

and the Hannover group/Organ Care System (OCS) Lung (TransMedics, Andover, MA, USA) have since facilitated a portable adaptation of the EVLP circuit (Table 27.1).

The Lund EVLP protocol is designed to mimic the physiological conditions a transplanted lung will face after reperfusion in the recipient. It serves primarily as a thorough assessment of borderline lungs not meeting standard acceptance criteria to reclaim those demonstrating suitability for clinical transplantation on the *ex vivo* circuit.

Table 27.1 EVLP protocols in clinical lung transplantation

	Lund	Toronto	OCS Lung
Circuit	Static	Static	Portable
Perfusion			
Target flow	100% of cardiac output (70 mL/kg/min)	40% of cardiac output	2.5 L/min
PA pressure (mmHg)	<20	<15	<20
LA pressure (mmHg)	0 (open LA)	3–5	0 (open LA)
Pump	Roller	Centrifugal	Pulsatile
Perfusate	2. Steen Solution with red cell concentrates (Haematocrit 10–15%)	2. Steen Solution	1.5. 'OCS Lung solution'ᵃ with red-cell concentrates (haematocrit 15–25%)
Ventilation			
Mode	Volume controlled	Volume controlled	Volume controlled
Tidal volume (mL/kg)	6–8	7	6
Frequency (bpm)	10–15	7	10
PEEP (cmH$_2$O)	5	5	5
FiO$_2$ (%)	50	21	21
Temperature (°C)			
Start of ventilation	32	32	32
Start of perfusion	15	15	32
Start of evaluation	37	37	37

ᵃ The 'OCS Lung solution' is similar in composition to low-potassium dextran with added glucose, and does not contain any albumin (personal communication, Dr Warnecke, Study Director of the OCS Lung INSPIRE Trial).

Toronto: developing and validating EVLP

Shaf Keshavjee and his colleagues in Toronto have with their extensive contributions changed the landscape of EVLP into a technique to significantly improve transplantation rates. The focus of Keshavjee and Cypel's studies have not been to just evaluate if a graft is usable or not, but to prolong the perfusion times to be able to potentially treat and better recondition injured lungs before transplantation. They have most notably revised the Lund protocol to possibly increase the option of longer-term perfusion with:

- An acellular perfusate to avoid potential detrimental haemolysis.
- A low-flow strategy with only 40% of estimated cardiac output to reduce pulmonary vascular sheer stress and oedema formation.
- A closed circuit with both the PA and LA cannulated creating a positive LA pressure.

In 2011, they presented their landmark results from the HELP trial in *The New England Journal of Medicine* where they showed non-inferiority in severe PGD (grade 3) and 30-day mortality between 20 transplants of initially declined lungs reconditioned with EVLP compared to 116 standard lung transplants performed in their centre. Table 27.2 shows the most pivotal clinical EVLP trials to date.

Portable EVLP

In a pilot study published in *The Lancet* in 2012 followed by a multicentre randomized controlled trial (INSPIRE) in *The Lancet Respiratory Medicine* in 2018, Gregor Warnecke et al. investigated the effect of normothermic preservation and transportation of standard criteria human donor lungs on a portable EVLP system. Standard donor lungs were, instead of being brought to their centres by means of cold preservation on ice, preserved by normothermic perfusion and ventilation on the transportable OCS Lung. These are the first reports of a portable EVLP system used in clinical transplantation, with short-term outcomes non-inferior to controls. Of the randomly assigned 370 patients in the INSPIRE trial, >80% underwent transplantation, roughly divided between perfused lungs and controls. Portable EVLP preserved lungs showed significantly lower rates of severe PGD compared to standard cold preserved lungs after transplantation. A feasibility study (the EXPAND trial) has since shown that portable EVLP can result in a high utilization rate for also extended criteria donor lungs with short and long-term post-transplant clinical outcomes comparable to what we see in standard lung transplants preserved on ice.

The OCS protocol is a hybrid of the Lund and Toronto EVLP protocols. A cellular perfusate based on OCS Lung Solution supplemented with erythrocytes and an open LA is combined with a perfusate flow limited to 2.5 L/min resembling the protective approach developed by the Toronto group. Fig. 27.2 shows the semi-automated EVLP circuits used in the listed clinical trials in Table 27.2.

Table 27.2 Pivotal trials investigating EVLP in clinical lung transplantation

Trial title	Design	Comparison	Location	EVLP protocol	EVLP system	Start date	Primary endpoint	Outcome
HELP trial	Prospective non-randomized controlled trial	EVLP reconditioned donor lungs vs standard criteria donor lungs	Toronto	Toronto	In-house XVIVO circuit	2008	Primary graft dysfunction 72 hours after transplantation	No significant difference in PGD rates or 30-day mortality between EVLP reconditioned (n = 20) and standard criteria transplant lungs (n = 116)
NOVEL Lung trial	Prospective non-randomized controlled multicentre trial	EVLP reconditioned donor lungs vs standard criteria donor lungs	USA	Toronto	XPS	2011	Survival rates and rates of grade 3 PGD at 72 hours with success if and only if the secondary endpoint of survival at 3 years is met	1-year reported results shows no difference in PGD rates or early mortality between EVLP reconditioned (n = 42) and standard criteria transplant lungs (n = 42)
OCS Lung INSPIRE trial	Prospective randomized controlled multicentre trial	OCS preserved standard criteria donor lungs vs standard cold static organ preservation	Germany, Belgium, France, Italy, Spain, UK, USA, Canada, Australia	OCS	OCS Lung	2011	Absence of PGD3 within the first 72 hours after transplant and 30-day survival	Significantly lower incidence of severe PGD rates in the OCS preserved lungs (n = 141) compared to standard cold storage preserved lungs (n = 165). However, significantly higher 30-day mortality in the OCS preserved lung group compared to the control group. Mortality was similar between groups at 1 year

DEVELOP-UK trial	Prospective non-randomized controlled multicentre trial	EVLP reconditioned donor lungs vs standard criteria donor lungs	UK	Lund/Toronto	Vivoline LS1	2012	1-year survival	No significant difference in 1-year survival between EVLP reconditioned (n = 18) and standard criteria transplant lungs (n = 184). Higher rates of severe PGD and more ECMO required in the EVLP group, study stopped
VIENNA trial	Prospective randomized controlled trial	EVLP reconditioned standard donor lungs vs standard cold static organ preservation	Vienna	Toronto	In-house XVIVO circuit	2013	Safety of EVLP in standard criteria lung donors	No significant difference in PGD rates or 30-day mortality between EVLP reconditioned standard lungs (n = 35) and standard cold storage preserved lungs (n = 41)
International EXPAND Lung Pivotal trial	Prospective non-randomized non-controlled multicentre trial	OCS reconditioned extended criteria donor lungs, no controls	USA, Belgium, Germany	OCS	OCS Lung	2013	Composite of patient 30-day survival and PGD grade 3 in the first 72 hours post transplantation	30-day survival in a cohort of 79 transplanted recipients was 98.7%. The utilization rate (number of donor lungs transplanted/number of donor lungs placed on OCS) was 87%

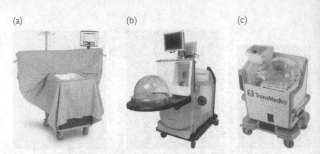

Fig. 27.2 Semi-automated EVLP circuits used in pivotal multicentre trials investigating EVLP in clinical lung transplantation. (a) Vivoline LS1 (Vivoline Medical AB, Lund, Sweden) static EVLP with the Lund EVLP protocol. (b) XPS (XVIVO Perfusion AB, Göteborg, Sweden), static EVLP with the Toronto EVLP protocol. (c) OCS Lung (TransMedics, Andover, MA, USA) portable EVLP with the OCS EVLP protocol.

Criteria for EVLP assessment and reconditioning

As recently described by Cypel and colleagues, the criteria for EVLP assessment and reconditioning can be grouped into four different categories: extended criteria DBD, routine DCD, extended criteria DCD, and logistics (extension of preservation time).

- Extended criteria DBD: this accounts for the majority of EVLP indications. Donor lungs with marginal oxygenation, pulmonary oedema, CXR infiltrates, unacceptable bronchoscopy, pulmonary emboli, pneumonia, or aspiration can meet these criteria. EVLP can be used simply to reassess organ quality or to recondition the lungs by means of antibiotics, thrombolysis, or amelioration of pulmonary oedema by optimal V/Q strategies.
- Routine DCD: these are controlled DCD (Maastricht category 3–5) that present no concerning donor findings prior to or after withdrawal of life-sustaining therapies. Normally the time from withdrawal of treatment to cardiac arrest in this group will be <30 minutes. There is an ongoing discussion in the lung transplant community whether EVLP is essential in this category. While some studies have demonstrated that routine use of EVLP provides improved outcomes by ruling out some organs with an unrecognized lung injury that ultimately would lead to significant PGD, many centres have demonstrated excellent results with routine DCD donors without the use of EVLP. Therefore, EVLP does not appear to be a requirement for DCD lung transplantation, but may aid in these more difficult assessments.
- Extended criteria DCD: these are uncontrolled DCD or controlled DCD with concerning clinical features similar to high-risk DBD or donors with a delayed time to arrest (>60 minutes) after withdrawal of life-sustaining therapies. EVLP has potential to be very helpful in expanding DCD transplants by confirming stable function of these

lungs where very little history or time for assessment is available. If uncontrolled DCD donation would become a safely established procedure it has the potential to completely alter donor graft availability.

• Logistics: EVLP can give an indispensable logistical advantage by extending preservation times from the traditional 6–8 hours to >20 hours of total 'ischaemic time'. Experimental and clinical studies have demonstrated the safety of this approach which has the potential to not only extend the donor pool, but to also bring lung transplantation procedures to a semi-elective operation with multiple benefits for patients and clinicians. Common logistical reasons that could extend donor lung ischaemic time >10–12 hours and prevent standard donor organ use are:
  • Awaited viral studies.
  • HLA compatibility studies.
  • Pathology assessment of indeterminate mass in any donor.
  • Awaited recipient admission.

Decision to transplant EVLP lungs

Most centres use the following combination of acceptance criteria after re-conditioning to decide whether to use the lungs or not. All of the following:
• Any DBD or DCD donor lungs meeting criteria for standard transplant.
• PA pressure <20 mmHg, while achieving target perfusate flow.
• Oxygen capacity shown by deltaPaO$_2$ of >300 mmHg (perfusate LA PaO$_2$ – perfusate PA PaO$_2$)/FiO$_2$.
• Selective pulmonary vein gas >225 mmHg on 100% FiO$_2$ and 5 cmH$_2$O PEEP.
• Stable or improving lung compliance and stable or falling lung resistance.
• No pulmonary oedema build-up in the endotracheal tube.
• Satisfactory assessment on inspection and palpation including bronchoscopic evaluation and deflation test (as a marker of compliance).

Surgical technique

Technically, the procurement of lungs from an EVLP donor follows the standard protocol, apart from the necessity to have a *longer section of trachea and PA* for swift cannulation ex vivo. If a long enough main PA cannot be achieved, due to simultaneous heart procurement, we usually resect a segment of descending aorta which is anastomosed end-to-end to the main PA to facilitate secure cannulation. After anterograde (through the PA) pneumoplegia and retrograde (through pulmonary veins) Perfadex (XVIVO Perfusion AB) flush and graft retrieval, the lungs are either connected to the portable circuit or cool stored as new cold storage devices are now available (LungGuard for example) and transported to the recipient site where EVLP is ready to start in case of static EVLP. The lungs are connected to the machine perfusion by cannulation of the PA and, if using a 'closed atrium technique', by an end-to-end anastomosis between the LA cuff and a venting cannula connected to the reservoir chamber. If an 'open atrium technique' is used, the perfusate from the LA is drained freely and collected by gravity in the reservoir chamber. A temperature probe is placed in the drainage area of the LA cuff as a surrogate for core lung temperature. The flow of perfusion is incremented slowly with a maximum perfusion pressure of 15–20 mmHg and the ventilation started at 32°C once the desired softening of the tissues has been achieved. During EVLP multiple examinations are carried out, even selectively from each pulmonary vein, to assess the function of lungs and lobes separately.

This type of selective evaluation, along with a visual and bronchoscopic assessment, helps guide the decision of whether to accept the lungs for transplantation, to further assess and recondition, or to discard the lungs from clinical use and direct them to a strict research pathway.

Ventilation strategy

The re-warming EVLP lung, having endured the donor's demise, lung procurement, cooling to 4°C, and then slow rewarming towards normothermia, is vulnerable and highly sensitive to hyperventilation. The EVLP ventilation strategy is therefore adapted from that of ARDS lungs.

In brief, mechanical volume-controlled ventilation is initiated when temperature in the perfusate outflow reaches 32°C:

Reconditioning phase

- Intermittent positive pressure ventilation (IPPV) setting.
- Pmax 20 to keep peak airway pressure <20 cmH$_2$O.
- PEEP 5 cmH$_2$O.
- FiO$_2$ to 0.21–0.5.
- Set I:E ratio 1:2 and inspiratory pause at 10%.
- Lund advocates an incremental approach to ventilation, beginning with a minute volume of 1 L/min at 32°C (tidal volume 3 mL/kg) and increasing by 1 L/min for each degree Celsius, finally reaching 6 L/min at 37°C (tidal volume 5–7 mL/kg). Breaths are 50% oxygen given at 5–20 breaths/min with a PEEP of 5 cmH$_2$O.
- Toronto recommends an immediate tidal volume of 7 mL/kg at a rate of 7 breaths/min, 21% oxygen, and with a PEEP of 5 cmH$_2$O.
- If persistent atelectasis, perform a recruitment manoeuvre either by careful hand ventilation or by transiently increasing PEEP from 5 cmH$_2$O in increments up to 10 cmH$_2$O for a few breaths while always keeping airway pressure (Paw) <25 cmH$_2$O.

Evaluation phase

Once rewarming is complete and target perfusion established, the function of the donor lungs undergoing EVLP can be assessed. Once the perfusate is deoxygenated and confirmed on blood gas analysis, perform recruitment manoeuvres as previously described and set the ventilator for evaluation as shown here:

- Increase FiO$_2$ via the ventilator from 21–50% to 100%.
- PEEP can be increased to a maximum of 8 cmH$_2$O for a short period.
- Keep peak airway pressure (Paw) <25 cmH$_2$O.

- Perform blood gas analyses 15 minutes after FiO_2 is increased to 100%.
- A lung deflation test is performed by disconnecting the tracheal tube at the end of inspiration. Remember to first reduce perfusate flow to maximum of 1.5 L/min to avoid tracheal oedema. Recoil of the lungs is evaluated subjectively; global collapse of the lungs is defined as normal.
- If transplant suitability criteria have not been achieved, return to the reconditioning phase.
- If transplant suitability criteria have been achieved, move immediately to cooling phase for organ preservation.
- Before discontinuing ventilation, perform a bronchoscopy for final assessment and toilet. Stop ventilation at 32°C, clamp trachea with lungs partially inflated with 50% FiO_2, and carry on with the transplantation.

Cellular or acellular perfusate?

One of the fundamental questions in EVLP is whether or not to use blood in the circulating perfusate. The Lund and OCS protocols advocate a cellular perfusate, whereas the Toronto technique uses an acellular solution. Comparative animal studies have shown no significant difference in lung performance between the two.

The EVLP logistics are simplified, costs lowered, and ethical conflicts arising from the use of limited blood products in studies of organs that may not be used clinically are prevented by avoiding erythrocyte concentrate. The oxygen supply to the lung cells during EVLP also appears to be sufficiently provided by the ventilator alone without the need of oxygen carriers for parenchymal preservation. A potential benefit of a cellular perfusate is the oxygen binding capacity that erythrocytes provide and its possible advantage during lung evaluation. It has been shown that blood gas analyses during EVLP with an acellular perfusate are unreliable and could disguise oxygenation deficits during assessment, especially in the case of a V/Q mismatch. It is also argued that the presence of red blood cells provides a more physiologically relevant assessment of flow through the pulmonary microvasculature.

EVLP centres or EVLP in every centre?

There is an ongoing debate on how the EVLP service should best be delivered in the future. The Toronto group has shown the feasibility of the 'EVLP centre' approach in a case report with the team in Chicago, USA. To manoeuvre around the restriction on EVLP in the USA outside the NOVEL Lung trial, a pair of unacceptable donor lungs was transported on ice to Toronto for reconditioning and then flown back to Chicago for successful implantation. Thus, concentrating the volume to fewer centres will presumably increase the experience of the EVLP team. The most obvious drawbacks of establishing such specialized EVLP centres are transportation and environmental costs, more complex logistics, and the inevitable prolonged cold ischaemia inflicted on an already injured organ.

By either approach there is witness of less quantifiable benefits with the mere availability of the EVLP technique. In Milan, Italy, they stress how the implementation of EVLP in their low-volume centre has facilitated the safe use of extended criteria donor lungs in recent years and in the UK we have seen a clear increase in the numbers of donors assessed by our retrieval teams since EVLP was put into practice in 2009. Currently, the retrieving surgeon frequently manages to optimize intended EVLP donors, who would previously not have been approached, to reach standard transplant criteria. Initially rejected lungs are therefore now being brought immediately to implantation as often as taken back to our centre for reconditioning, an important 'side effect' of EVLP provision.

Static or portable EVLP?

The optimal method for lung preservation remains unclear. In the process of lung transportation, cold storage at 4–8°C has routinely been used to decrease cellular metabolic activity and preserve lung function. This can, however, compound lung injury due to ischaemia-reperfusion and ATP depletion and increase the risk of PGD. A large registry review in 1999 of 5052 lung transplants, reported higher 30-day mortality with cold ischaemic times exceeding 8 hours. Since the introduction of improved extracellular lung-preservation solutions, ischaemic times of up to 10–12 hours have been safely reported. Cypel and colleagues showed that normothermic EVLP can interrupt hypothermic ischaemic lung injury after 12 hours of cold storage and ameliorate immediate transplant outcomes in a porcine model. What effect shorter periods of cold ischaemia have on graft function and patient survival in lung transplantation is still to be elucidated.

The INSPIRE lung trial showed that in comparison to static cold storage, portable EVLP reduced the amount of PGD. There is still much uncertainty about whether or not the benefits of this approach will balance its considerable costs and logistical hurdles. If it does however, the portable EVLP technique has the potential of leading the way of a new era in lung assessment and organ preservation. This could enable transport of organs over longer distances, opening up many new possibilities for organ allocation and therapeutic intervention. An exciting avenue is its implication for combined transplants where there are now reports of lung–liver transplantation being done liver first with the lung kept on EVLP. Liver first has several technical and physiological advantages, but is only feasible with EVLP. With distance no longer a factor in donor–recipient matching, closer matches could also be achieved. This could decrease rejection and the need for immunosuppression and extend graft lifespan, while increasing access to transplantation for disadvantaged patient populations. Organs could also more easily be routed through specialized facilities, which have been suggested by several groups as a way to make technically challenging assessment, repair, functional augmentation, or banking procedures a clinical reality. Thus, approaches that today would not be seriously considered could become practical and fruitful areas of innovation.

Platform for translational research

The recent success of EVLP in clinical lung transplantation is also contributing significantly to advances in translational research in the lungs. The EVLP circuit has allowed many types of research projects, including pharmacotherapy, stem cell therapy, gene therapy, and organ/tissue engineering. Results obtained using lungs on EVLP have potential to be highly translatable to clinical practice. In theory, EVLP should allow the administration of the most effective medications based on the specific causes of lung injuries while avoiding systemic toxicity. Some notable successes have been reported using this approach.

Antimicrobial treatment

The hazard of respiratory infections in the early post-transplant period is notorious and donor-to-host transmission of bacterial and fungal infections is a known cause of morbidity in the immunosuppressed lung transplant recipient.

With a localized closed circuit, EVLP is ideal for high-dose antimicrobial treatment with no risk of side effects to other organs. Extended criteria donor lungs subjected to the assessment form by nature a subpopulation likely to have a higher microbial load than standard lungs. All clinical EVLP protocols therefore use prophylactic broad-spectrum antibiotics in their perfusate solution. Several studies have shown that EVLP with high dose antimicrobials in the perfusate is associated with an effective reduction of both the bacterial and fungal burden of the donor lung. We empirically use meropenem and amphotericin B, and recommend the addition of a broad-spectrum fungicide to the perfusate. Yeast is a well-known cause of infections in the immunosuppressed post-transplant patient and is frequently cultured in the BAL fluid from these borderline donor lungs.

Thrombolysis for pulmonary embolism

Fibrinolytic treatment may be of highest importance in DCD donors when timely heparin use is not possible. Urokinase administration during EVLP has been shown to reduce PVR and improve oxygenation in a preclinical DCD model by Inci et al. The same group later reported a clinical case where normothermic EVLP was used as a platform to deliver therapeutic thrombolysis (urokinase) in lungs with known massive pulmonary emboli followed by complete clot fragmentation and successful transplantation of the treated lungs.

HCV-infected donors

A growing interest in the use of HCV-infected donors followed from the current epidemic of overdose deaths in the North American donor population. Some geographic areas in the USA report up to 20% of all organ donors being NAAT positive for HCV. Underuse of these organs is particularly relevant given that they are often young with less comorbidity than other donors. However, organs from donors with contagious viral infections are traditionally not offered for transplantation due to a high risk of transmission. In a recent report, using normothermic EVLP as a treatment platform, the Toronto group presented a method for treatment of HCV-infected human donor lungs with physical clearance and light-based therapies that efficiently prevented HCV transmission without deleterious effects on the lung or perfusate solution. This strategy of treating viral infections in a donor organ during preservation could significantly increase the availability of organs for transplantation and encourages further clinical development, especially in an era where available rescue therapies using novel direct-acting antivirals have been shown to be very effective.

Acute lung injury

Interleukin (IL)-8 and other proinflammatory proteins have been suggested by several groups as prognostic markers in lung transplantation indicating severity of donor lung injury. We could in a study of 42 human donor lungs clinically investigated for transplantation demonstrate the potential role of interleukin-1β as a biomarker of EVLP reconditioning and more importantly post-transplant survival. Interestingly, IL-1β levels in the EVLP perfusate correlated with extent of neutrophil adhesion to conditioned pulmonary endothelial cells ($R^2 = 0.33$, $p <0.001$), upregulation of ICAM-1 in donor lung vasculature ($R^2 = 0.68$, $p <0.001$), and upregulation of ICAM-1 ($R^2 = 0.30$, $p = 0.001$) and E-selectin ($R^2 = 0.29$, $p = 0.001$) on conditioned pulmonary endothelial cells, and importantly neutralization of IL-1β in perfusate strongly inhibited neutrophil adhesion to conditioned endothelium (91% reduction, $p = 0.002$). Therapeutic targeting of IL-1β or other proinflammatory components therefore provides one of many exciting opportunities to decrease endothelial activation and potentially reduce the incidence of early graft injury post transplantation. If successful, these principles may expand to other organs experiencing ischaemia-reperfusion injury.

Blood type conversion

In a recent Science publication Wang and colleagues showed that depletion of donor lung A-Ag can be achieved with EVLP treatment. By adding antigen cleaving enzymes to the perfusate they managed to effectively convert group A (ABO-A) donor lungs to group O (ABO-O) universal blood type lungs within 4hr of EVLP. This strategy has great potential to expand ABO-incompatible lung transplantation and lead to improvements in fairness of organ allocation.

Stem cells

Because of a number of evolving technologies, there have been rapid advances in the field of stem cell therapy over the past few years and stem cell therapy has become a potential future for treatment of chronic lung disease. The beneficial effects of mesenchymal stem cells have been confirmed in lungs on EVLP with various types of acute lung injury. In *Escherichia coli*-injured human lungs, for example, tracheal instillation of mesenchymal stem cells during EVLP restored alveolar fluid clearance, reduced inflammation, and exerted antimicrobial activity. It has also been reported that intravascular administration of mesenchymal stem cells in pig lungs on EVLP leads to decreased circulating IL-8 levels, suggesting potential therapeutic effects against ischaemia-reperfusion injury and PGD. Multipotent adult progenitor cells are another promising resource for stem cell therapy with notable anti-inflammatory effects in lungs on EVLP. Mesenchymal stem cells and multipotent adult progenitor cells are able to regenerate damaged tissue with new cells. However, the primary role of stem cell therapy in recovery from acute lung injury appears to be attributed to paracrine signalling from the cells by regulating epithelial and endothelial permeability, thereby enhancing alveolar fluid clearance and lessening the immune response in injured lungs.

Gene therapy

Similar to drug therapy, gene therapy administered during EVLP is also a feasible targeted approach for reconditioning. A pilot study of IL-10 gene transfection using adenovirus infection during EVLP of porcine lungs was reported by the Toronto group with notable success and improved post-transplantation outcomes. This was an encouraging study that foreshadows the potential major impact of gene therapy during EVLP. We must be mindful of viral toxicity, however, as adenoviral vectors can induce inflammation. Non-viral gene delivery methods during EVLP may be valuable alternatives.

Conclusion

As organ perfusion has become one of the 'hot topics' in all fields of transplantation in recent years, EVLP continues to lead its progression. Its application in clinical lung transplantation is spreading rapidly across the globe at the same time as exciting research into new ways to treat and recondition the perfused lung continues. Mapping and targeting the compounded inflammatory insults caused by brain death, aspiration, infection, and reperfusion and limiting oedema formation by haemoconcentration of the perfusate are some of the more promising advancements in recent years. EVLP offers a unique platform tailored to this clinical and investigative work, aiming to find novel ways to increase the donor pool, and to make lung transplantation a reality for more waiting list patients with life-threatening lung disease.

Technical aspects of lung transplantation

Lung transplantation operative technique

There are many methods and techniques for performing a lung transplant operation. Each variation in technique has advantages and disadvantages. The prototypical lung transplant operation is bilateral sequential lung transplantation performed through a bilateral anterior thoracosternotomy. This is the most common way that transplantations are performed in North America and Europe. However, it is by no means the only method or best method. Differences in technique arise because of clinical situations, institutional resources, and surgeon preferences.

In this chapter, we will describe the technical aspects of performing bilateral orthotopic lung transplantation (BOLT), sequentially via a bilateral anterior thoracosternotomy (clamshell incision). During each step, we will discuss variations in technique, and situations where perhaps such variation may be reasonable, or even preferred alternatives to the standard method.

Anaesthetic considerations

After identification of a suitable donor, and confirmation that the donor lungs are of good quality, then the recipient operation is started. The recipient procedure begins with the induction of anaesthesia, obtaining IV access, placement of adequate monitoring, and positioning on the operating table.

Specifics of anaesthesia are discussed in Chapter 37.

Pulmonary hypertension with right heart dysfunction
Patients with severe PH and right heart dysfunction are a particularly risky group during induction. These patients are susceptible to haemodynamic instability during induction that may be catastrophic. If standard anaesthetic induction is undertaken, there is a high probability that the agents will compromise any pre-existing right heart dysfunction to the point of inducing systemic hypotension and even cardiac arrest. The dysfunctional RV is largely dependent on an adequate arterial blood pressure for myocardial perfusion. Even minimal periods of hypotension can induce significant RV ischaemia, further compounding the right heart dysfunction. The result is further dysfunction and the creation of a vicious cycle resulting in cardiac arrest which is extremely difficult to recover and will necessitate 'crashing' on cardiopulmonary bypass or ECLS. This situation is potentially avoidable.

In such patients, a safer strategy is to place adequate central access and monitoring lines prior to induction. Radial arterial line and central access via the IJ vein or femoral vein are placed in the awake patient under local anaesthesia. Care is taken to avoid hypoxia. Placement of the PAC is not necessary at this point and may induce arrhythmias. These arrhythmias are usually inconsequential, but in a patient with a tenuous right heart, they may be detrimental. A vascular sheath may be inserted but the PAC is only floated after the chest is opened. Once adequate vascular access is ensured, anaesthesia induction is performed under invasive haemodynamic monitoring to avoid cardiac depression. When performed in this manner, any instability can be detected early and treated promptly to avoid a spiralling situation and catastrophe at induction.

In cases of extremely severe right heart dysfunction and an unstable patient, it may be prudent to have the femoral areas exposed and ready for initiation of emergent femoral–femoral ECLS. Placement of femoral arterial and venous catheters will expedite the process in case of the need to 'crash on'. Taking it one step further, the patient may be placed on ECMO prior to induction. After placement of adequate venous access and monitoring lines, and prior to induction, the femoral artery and vein are exposed under local anaesthesia. They are cannulated and low-flow ECMO is initiated. This technique has been described with good results. Alternatively, cannulation can be performed percutaneously using a Seldinger technique. Preclosing of the femoral artery using a percutaneous vascular closure device facilitates decannulation without open repair.

Choice of incision

Bilateral anterior thoracosternotomy

This incision, also known as the 'clamshell' incision, is the most commonly used incision for performing a BOLT. The incision provides excellent exposure to the pulmonary hilum, visualization of the phrenic nerves, and access to the heart for central cannulation. Access to the chest wall is good for managing pleural adhesions. However, adhesions in the posterior costophrenic angles may be challenging to manage. The major disadvantage of this incision is the transverse sternal transection and the potential for sternal wound complications.

The skin incision is made starting in the midline at a point two-thirds of the way between the sternum and the xiphoid process. The incision is extended laterally to the point that is one fingerbreadth below the nipple on each side, and then carried slightly superiorly in a curvilinear fashion (Fig. 28.1). In women, the incision is carried along the inframammary folds to avoid incising the breast tissue. The subcutaneous tissue and the pectoral muscles are transected. The thoracic cavity is entered in the fourth or fifth interspace, depending on the size of the cavity. Both internal mammary arteries are ligated and transected. A self-retaining retractor is placed on each side.

Sternal-sparing bilateral/unilateral anterior thoracotomy

For single orthotopic lung transplantation (SOLT) performed without cardiopulmonary support, there is no need to transect the sternum. The operation is performed via an anterolateral thoracotomy or a posterolateral thoracotomy. For the anterolateral thoracotomy, the rib may or may not need to be transected.

For BOLT, a sternal-sparing approach has been described. The operation is performed using bilateral anterolateral thoracotomy incisions; however, the sternum and mammary arteries are not transected. The landmarks are otherwise similar to the 'clamshell' approach.

Sternotomy

Median sternotomy is an option for performing lung transplantation. The incision can be performed rapidly, making it the incision of choice in cases where cardiac arrest happens on induction. It is also easier to close when compared to an anterolateral thoracotomy. The incision is particularly advantageous for women with pendulous breasts. Large breasts may result in significant issues with wound healing for the anterolateral incisions. There

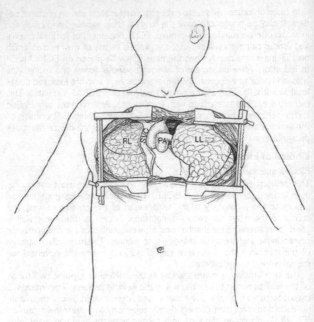

Fig. 28.1 Illustrates the bilateral anterior thoracosternotomy ('clamshell') incision and positioning of the retractor for optimal exposure.

are two main disadvantages. The first is that access to the pulmonary hilum may be difficult, especially on the left, without using intraoperative ECLS. Second, exposure to the lateral and posterior chest wall is limited, and cases with significant intrapleural adhesions may result in a more difficult pneumonectomy and increased bleeding.

Posterolateral thoracotomy

This is the least commonly used incision; however, it is an option for the performance of BOLT or SOLT. Exposure to the pulmonary hilum is excellent through this incision. Its primary disadvantage during BOLT is the need to reposition patients for the second lung. Also, access for central cannulation is more difficult when compared to the anterior approaches. In cases where ECLS is anticipated, especially for a left posterolateral thoracotomy, the femoral area needs to be prepared and draped into the field.

Intraoperative cardiopulmonary support

Regarding intraoperative cardiopulmonary support, there are two schools of thought. In one type of practice, intraoperative cardiopulmonary support is used routinely for all transplants. The second school of thought, which is also the more prevalent, is to use intraoperative cardiopulmonary support only when needed. Each has its own attributes. The former has the advantage of a smoother intraoperative haemodynamic course with minimal hypotension. It also allows controlled low-pressure reperfusion of the lung grafts after implantation. Exposure is also easier, especially for the performance of the left implantation. The advantage of the latter is a reduction of the complications associated with CPB or ECLS, such as bleeding. Both approaches yield acceptable results, and the decision to proceed with one over the other is surgeon or centre dependent.

Technique of intraoperative cardiopulmonary support

Traditionally, intraoperative support was always initiated with full CPB, usually via central cannulation. However, with improvements in technique, ECMO has become an option. With the elimination of a reservoir and an air–blood interface, the intensity of anticoagulation required for ECMO is much less than that required for CPB. Studies comparing intraoperative ECMO to CPB showed a reduction in intraoperative bleeding, transfusion requirements, and ICU length of stay with no difference in 90-day mortality. As a result, ECMO has largely replaced CPB as the default means to provide intraoperative support. However, there remain situations whereby CPB may still be preferred. Therefore, the means of intraoperative support should be selected based on the operative scenario encountered.

In centres where intraoperative support is used selectively, a situation commonly arises where the cardiac function is satisfactory, but lung function is not enough to sustain the patient without some sort of support. This may occur as a result of severe lung disease, or a patient who was bridged with pre-transplant ECMO. Occasionally, this situation arises after implantation of the first lung as a result of PGD affecting the newly transplanted lung. During such situations, single-lung ventilation will result in significant desaturation and substantial hypoxia. Traditionally, these patients were managed by the initiation of CPB. However, if haemodynamic support is not required, and only respiratory support is needed, then there may not be a need for CPB. In such a situation, it may be possible to provide adequate support with VV ECMO. In this situation, femoral–femoral VV ECMO can be initiated to provide intraoperative pulmonary support. Once the lungs are implanted and reperfused, then an attempt at weaning can be performed before closure, or the patient can be transferred to the ICU where weaning can be undertaken there.

If additional cardiac support is needed, then VV ECMO will not suffice. Situations such as known CAD, pre-existing cardiac dysfunction, or inadequate exposure are better managed with CPB or VA ECMO. As mentioned above, VA ECMO is preferred over CPB given the lesser degree of anticoagulation, reduced transfusion requirements, and reduced complications.

There are rare situations where CPB may be the optimal support method in cases where concomitant cardiac surgery is required, especially if it is intracardiac surgery (e.g. lung transplantation in a patient with PH and a repairable congenital cardiac defect). An additional situation where CPB is advantageous is when significant intraoperative bleeding is expected. Certainly, it would seem counterproductive to use CPB over ECMO, and by consequence, a higher level of anticoagulation, in a situation where bleeding is encountered. However, massive blood loss is much better handled by using pump suckers and recirculating the blood through the CPB circuit, rather than putting it through a cell saver and transfusions to maintain an adequate intravascular volume.

Recipient pneumonectomy

- Determining laterality:
  - For transplants planned without the use of extracorporeal support, single-lung ventilation is required, and the contralateral lung will support the patient during the explant pneumonectomy and implantation. The preoperative V/Q scan can be used to determine which lung should be transplanted first. Typically, the lung with the least amount of perfusion is transplanted first, so the functionally better lung can support the patient during single-lung ventilation. For procedures performed with ECLS, the sequence of pneumonectomy is unimportant.
- The phrenic nerve is identified early and protected.
- Dissection and division of the superior pulmonary vein with a vascular stapler.
- Dissection and division of the PA:
  - The PA is dissected and encircled. Care is taken to ensure that the PAC is withdrawn to avoid including it in the staple line. A test clamp of the PA is performed to ensure that the patient tolerates single-lung perfusion. If test clamping is not tolerated, then ECLS is required. This will need to be initiated before completing the pneumonectomy.
  - The truncus anterior branch is isolated and stapled, followed by the remaining artery going to the lower and middle lobes. Transecting the artery at the level of its branches gives more length to perform the anastomosis. Excess length can always be trimmed when preparing the hilum.
  - Once the PA is transected, the ventilation to the ipsilateral lung is ceased. Single-lung ventilation before clamping the main PA causes significant desaturation and should be avoided.
- Incision of the inferior pulmonary ligament.
- Dissection and division of inferior pulmonary vein.
- Dissection and division of the bronchus:
  - The bronchus is transected just proximal to the take-off of the upper lobe bronchus, and the anastomosis is performed at this level. One could transect the lobar bronchi and trim the excess length off subsequently. Bronchial arterial branches and peribronchial lymph nodes will need to be controlled with judicial use of electrocautery, clips, or suture ligation.
- Completion of pneumonectomy:
  - Once the bronchus is transected, the pneumonectomy is completed. Occasionally, adhesions to the chest wall, diaphragm, or mediastinum are encountered. These can be easily incised, and the specimen is sent off to pathology.
- Preparation of the hilum (Fig. 28.2):
  - The next step is to prepare the recipient's hilum for the implantation. If not already performed, the bronchus is trimmed to the point that is just proximal to the take-off of the upper lobe bronchus. Overzealous dissection of the peribronchial tissues should be avoided to maintain the blood supply of the recipient bronchus, and it is not necessary to dissect more than one or two rings for the performance of the anastomosis. During dissection of the posterior mediastinum, bleeding can be encountered from the paraesophageal and subcarinal

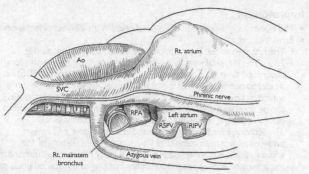

Fig. 28.2 Illustrates preparation of the hilar structures and mobilization of the right main bronchus in preparation for anastomosis. Note the position of the phrenic nerve during mobilization of hilar structures.

lymph nodes. When obtaining haemostasis, care should be taken not to injure the oesophagus or the vagus nerves, which are particularly at risk during this part of the procedure.
* The PA is dissected circumferentially and as far centrally as possible to provide adequate length for the anastomosis. The pulmonary vein stumps are gently retracted, and the pericardium is opened circumferentially to allow space for placement of a vascular clamp.

Donor lung preparation
* The donor lung/s is/are unpacked:
  * The lung block is immersed in cold saline and covered in cold gauze or towels to keep the lungs cool during the preparation.
* Inspection of the lung block for quality or iatrogenic injuries.
* The posterior pericardium is split.
* The LA cuff:
  * The LA Is split exactly down the middle. The atrial cuffs are trimmed to size. Occasionally, especially if the heart was procured for another recipient, the LA cuff may be left too short. This situation is encountered occasionally but is easily corrected by sewing a patch on the atrial cuff. This could be a patch of pericardium from the donor block, or autologous pericardium from the recipient, or bovine pericardium.
* The pulmonary trunk is divided at its bifurcation.
* The tracheobronchial tree is divided.
  * The is usually achieved by double stapling the left mainstem bronchus just distal to the carina. The airway is transected distal to the staple line, and the excess length is trimmed. Care should be taken not to denude the bronchus of the peribronchial tissue and damage its blood supply. Finally, the bronchus is trimmed leaving no more than one cartilaginous ring from the origin of the upper lobe bronchus. This avoids having a long ischaemic donor bronchus and helps to minimize the incidence of anastomotic complications.

Implantation

- The donor lung is placed in the pleural cavity in the correct orientation.
- Bronchial anastomosis:
  - The first step of the implantation is the bronchial anastomosis (Fig. 28.3). This is typically performed with an absorbable suture with a long absorption time. Our preference is to use 4-0 polydioxanone (PDS) on a tapered needle. The anastomosis can be performed as a single running suture technique. Alternatively, the membranous wall of the bronchus can be approximated using a single running suture, and the cartilaginous portion can be approximated with several interrupted sutures.
  The technique for bronchial anastomosis is dependent on surgeon preference, and both techniques yield similar results. Testing of the anastomosis is not always necessary but is easily achieved by submerging the anastomosis in water and ventilating that lung to a sustained pressure of 25 cmH$_2$O. The appearance of air bubbles signifies a defect in the anastomosis which may need reinforcement with additional sutures.
- Pulmonary arterial anastomosis (Fig. 28.4):
  - A vascular clamp is placed on the recipient's proximal PA and the vascular staple line is excised to lay open the stump. The arterial anastomosis is performed with a single continuous suture of 4-0 or 5-0 polypropylene suture. The vascular clamp is left in place until all anastomoses are complete and the lung is ready to be perfused.
- LA anastomosis (Fig. 28.5):
  - The atrial anastomosis is next. A curved vascular clamp is placed on the recipient LA. The vascular staple lines of the two pulmonary veins are excised and the junction incised to provide a LA cuff in preparation for the anastomosis. The anastomosis is performed with a single continuous suture of 4-0 polypropylene. In order to avoid LA thrombosis, every attempt should be made to restore endo-atrial continuity by everting and excluding the atrial cut edges and epicardial fatty tissue. Once the suturing is completed, the sutures are left long and not tied to allow for de-airing.
- Reperfusion and de-airing:
  - Once the anastomoses are completed and verified, the lung can be reperfused and de-aired. The patient is placed in steep Trendelenburg position. The lung is ventilated gently. After a few puffs, the arterial vascular clamp is opened partially, and the lung is reperfused. The atrial clamp is left in place, the atrial suture line is left loose, and the de-airing is performed through the atrial suture line (Fig. 28.5). Once the graft is de-aired, the atrial clamp is removed, and the suture is tied. The pulmonary arterial clamp is then released slowly over 10 minutes. Reperfusion is performed in a controlled fashion to avoid injuring of the graft.
  - Alternatively, retrograde de-airing can be performed to wash the lung preservation solution. Using this technique, the LA clamp is opened first, allowing the blood to flow retrograde and out through the pulmonary arterial suture line, washing out the air and preservation solution. Once adequate de-airing is performed, then antegrade flow can be re-established.
  - After completion and reperfusion of the first lung, attention is turned to the contralateral side. For cases performed on ECLS, attention must be given to ensure reperfusion of the newly transplanted lung. Typically, the flow rate is reduced to ensure pulsatility, creating partial bypass support. PA pulsatility can be monitored by floating a PAC.

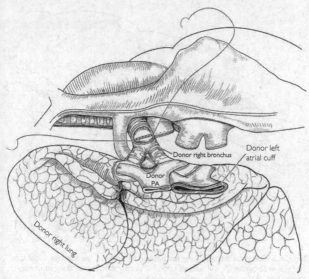

Fig. 28.3 Illustrates the technique of bronchial anastomosis.

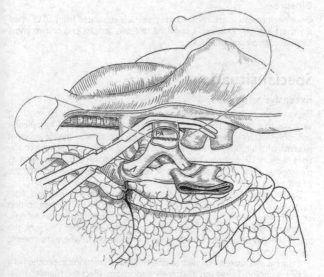

Fig. 28.4 Illustrates the technique for PA anastomosis.

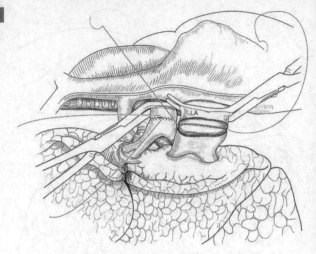

Fig. 28.5 Illustrates the technique for pulmonary vein–LA anastomosis. Note the clamp is kept on the PA and sutures untied in preparation for de-airing following completion of the pulmonary vein anastomosis.

Closure

Once haemostasis is assured and the patient is separated from ECLS, then the chest can be closed. It is standard to leave at least one or two chest tubes in each pleural space.

Special situations

Extensive adhesions

Pleural adhesions are sometimes encountered in patients requiring lung transplantation. These are typically not extensive, and intrapleural adhesiolysis can be performed without much added difficulty. However, in patients with a history of extensive intrapleural surgery, septic lung conditions such as CF or bronchiectasis, or certain disease processes, such as pleuroparenchymal fibroelastosis and coal worker's pneumoconiosis, the adhesions may be significant.

Dealing with such adhesions can be challenging and may increase morbidity. First, it is crucial to gain safe access to the pleural cavity. Identification of the phrenic nerve is important early in the dissection for its protection. In patients who previously underwent lung volume reduction surgery, the staple line may be adherent to the anterior mediastinum where the phrenic nerve is located.

If the hilum is spared from adhesions, the hilar dissection can proceed in a standard fashion. However, if extensive adhesions affect the hilum and dissection is treacherous, then an option is to commence the dissection within the pericardium. The planes within the pericardium are typically unaffected in these cases. The pericardium is opened in the midline, and the vessels are identified within the pericardium. They are dissected from the inside of the pericardium, but it is important to transect the vessels outside the pericardium to obtain adequate lengths to perform the anastomoses.

Retransplantation

Patients who undergo retransplantation can be managed similarly to patients with extensive pleural adhesions. The major difference is that hilar adhesions are more extensive. Furthermore, if the pericardium was accessed during the initial transplantation, then intrapericardial adhesions will make intrapericardial dissection more difficult. It is imperative to have the ability to initiate CPB or ECLS rapidly in case of vascular injury or severe haemodynamic embarrassment. Once the incision is made, the first step is to commence intrapericardial dissection and ensure that there is access to the aorta and RA. This manoeuvre allows for rapid cannulation and initiation of CPB. If intrapericardial adhesions are too extensive, then access to the femoral vessels should be considered. In certain situations, it may be beneficial to initiate ECLS or CPB before commencing the hilar dissection.

Once the recipient pneumonectomy is performed, and the hilum is prepared, then the implantation can proceed in a similar fashion to a first-time lung transplantation.

Postoperative ECLS

Occasionally, postoperative ECLS is needed for respiratory or haemodynamic support. This is most commonly required in patients who develop PGD. Increased FiO_2 may increase the production of free oxygen radicals and, therefore, prolonged exposure to high FiO_2 may exacerbate ischaemia-reperfusion injury and PGD. As such, it is advisable to avoid high FiO_2 and have a low threshold of commencing VV ECMO when the FiO_2 requirements reach 80% or higher. In such situations, VV ECMO is initiated peripherally with bifemoral cannulation, or dual cannulation of the right IJ vein and femoral vein.

On rare occasions, postoperative VA ECMO may be required. This is usually the case in patients with severe PH and RV dysfunction. Postoperative VA ECMO is typically established via dual femoral cannulation. However, if there is any element of PGD, the VAV ECMO should be initiated to avoid upper body and myocardial hypoxia due to Harlequin syndrome.

Critical care management and primary graft dysfunction following lung transplantation

Introduction

Lung transplantation is the gold standard therapy for appropriately selected individuals with end-stage lung disease. Lung transplantation is a durable therapy that offers improvements in overall survival and quality of life for recipients. As a resource-intensive therapy that is in part limited by the availability of suitable donor allografts, outcomes are appropriately highly scrutinized. Excellent multidisciplinary care is a prerequisite to successful outcomes following lung transplantation.

Successful management of the lung transplant recipient in the perioperative period is the culmination of not just postoperative decision-making and care, but rather is the composite outcome of candidate management in the pre-transplant and intraoperative period, donor selection, and intraoperative technique. As such, outcomes after lung transplantation are heavily impacted by the decisions made with respect to the candidate (now recipient), donor lung allograft, and intraoperative technique and management.

As is the case across many disciplines within cardiothoracic surgery, current literature notes that complications occur at a predictable rate, and that centres with excellent outcomes demonstrate a superior ability to both diagnose and manage these early complications. Postoperative care of the lung transplant recipient requires constant vigilance for the early detection and rescue from postoperative complications.

Physiology of the lung transplant recipient

While the approach to the care of the lung transplant recipient must be individually tailored to the recipient's history and indication for transplantation, donor history and associated considerations, and technical factors from the procedure itself, several overarching principles should be considered in the early postoperative period. This early postoperative management centres on fluid balance and ventilation. Adequate tissue perfusion and gas exchange must be preserved despite the need to minimize IV fluid administration, cardiac work, and barotrauma. Selection of sedation, analgesia, and strategies for haemodynamic support are all informed by the need to optimize fluid balance and ventilatory performance in the immediate postoperative setting.

Two physiological considerations are unique to all lung transplant recipients and warrant consideration in the postoperative period. First, the transplant allografts are by convention denervated following implantation, and as such lack the cough reflex that otherwise protects in part the functioning lung from pulmonary infections. This highlights the need for aggressive pulmonary toilet, as well as careful assessment of the swallowing reflex and for the presence of reflux. Second, the mandatory period of ischaemia followed by reperfusion—along with the disruption of the lymphatic drainage of the lung allograft—results in a predisposition to increased vascular permeability and susceptibility to oedema. The management of fluid balance as such requires attention to the minimization of the development of pulmonary oedema despite this increased vascular permeability.

Medical histories of both the donor and recipient bear consideration in individualizing the approach to postoperative management. Candidates— now recipients—differ significantly in their underlying aetiology of lung disease, which may necessitate changes to their postoperative management. Lung transplant recipients with CF may require ongoing antibiotic therapy tailored to the microbiome of their (explanted) lungs, while those with vascular indications may require more aggressive management of PA pressures in the early postoperative phase. Donors, likewise, increasingly are accepted despite histories of pneumonia or potentially transmissible disease. Antibiotic therapy for the recipient can similarly be tailored to culture data from the donor taken at the time of procurement. As donors with a history of hepatitis C—usually absent evidence of viraemia—are increasingly considered for use in lung transplantation, institution-specific protocols for the use of direct-acting antivirals should be employed to decrease the risk of disease transmission to the recipient.

Like other cardiothoracic procedures, mechanical support may be individually tailored to the recipient depending on the degree of haemodynamic support required to tolerate the procedure and the need for concomitant cardiac procedures. Lung transplantation may be performed with inotropic support without mechanical support, with an IABP, on VV or VA ECMO, or on full CPB. Each strategy carries advantages and disadvantages with respect to the degree of haemodynamic (or ventilatory) support provided, the propensity towards bleeding and coagulopathy, and the degree of expected systemic inflammatory response. The appropriate selection of these strategies to perform lung transplantation safely is described in Chapter 28. The recipient's postoperative physiology may therefore likewise be impacted by the choice of MCS to perform the procedure.

Postoperative considerations

Sedation and analgesia

Lung transplantation is a necessarily invasive procedure. The degree of postoperative pain may be impacted by the incision selected to attain adequate exposure to the thorax. Bilateral lung transplantation may be safely performed via median sternotomy or by bilateral anterior thoracosternotomy (clamshell incision) or thoracotomies ('sternal sparing'). In concordance with an overarching desire to optimize ventilatory function in the postoperative setting, the selection of an appropriate analgesic strategy should be made to minimize respiratory depression and facilitate pulmonary toilet. Multimodal analgesic strategies can help to decrease the need for narcotic pain medication. The use of an epidural catheter is generally well tolerated from a haemodynamic standpoint and results in less respiratory depression than strategies that rely more on narcotic pain medication. Preoperative placement of an epidural catheter is likewise associated with decreased use of narcotic pain medication and shorter time to extubation than the use of an epidural catheter placed postoperatively. Erector spinae and other blocks may provide analgesia without the small, but real risk of an epidural haematoma from the epidural catheter.

Ventilator management

Barotrauma and high airway pressures may lead to ischaemia of the bronchial mucosa or shearing injury to the alveoli. As such, lung-protective ventilatory strategies are required as soon as the allograft lungs are transitioned on to the ventilator. Adjustment of the FiO_2 as low as possible to attain a PaO_2 >70 mmHg is conventional and may be associated with decreased rates of PGD. Lower tidal volumes—such as to 10–12 mL/kg—will reduce peak airway pressure. Remember that the donor size dictates tidal volume ratios, not necessarily the recipient. Serial blood gas examination is employed to ensure adequate oxygenation and acid–base status, and to facilitate appropriate weaning of supplemental oxygen. Recipients are extubated after a period of haemodynamic and ventilatory stability and having tolerated conventional weaning of pressure support ventilation. Regular bronchoscopy and endotracheal suctioning—in addition to aggressive pulmonary toilet and incentive spirometry—reduce mucus plugging and atelectasis. Early tracheostomy for those recipients unable to promptly wean from the ventilator helps achieve early mobilization and adequate enteral nutrition.

Infection prophylaxis

Standard intraoperative antibiotic prophylaxis following lung transplantation includes empiric broad Gram-negative and Gram-positive coverage (cefepime for Gram-negative coverage, vancomycin for Gram-positive coverage) and fluconazole for *Candida* prophylaxis. Coverage may be tailored—or discontinued—as donor cultures finalize as negative. The need for antifungal prophylaxis may be tailored to observed local rates of invasive candidiasis.

Patients with known pretransplant colonization with antimicrobial pathogens, such as those with CF, are evaluated by transplant infectious disease for development of a customized perioperative antibiotic regimen. The duration of such pathogen-directed antimicrobials should be determined in a multidisciplinary fashion given that complete source control should be obtained at the time of recipient preparatory pneumonectomy.

TMP–SMX 80/360 mg daily is a first-line agent for *Pneumocystis jirovecii* prophylaxis starting 7 days after the transplantation. Nystatin swish and swallow four times daily for the first 6 months post transplantation is standard prophylaxis for oral candidiasis.

Viral prophylaxis is dependent on donor and recipient CMV status. Recipients who are at risk for CMV are treated initially with ganciclovir and transitioned to valganciclovir orally daily. Recipients with prior exposure to CMV are continued on CMV prophylaxis for 12 months post transplantation. Those high risk for CMV disease due to donor CMV IgG positivity without pre-transplant recipient exposure are continued on prophylaxis indefinitely as tolerated. For recipients who are both donor and recipient CMV IgG negative, aciclovir prophylaxis is given IV initially and then at a dose of 400 mg orally twice daily for the first 6 post-transplant months.

Postoperative complications and management

Haemorrhage

Haemorrhage is an uncommon but potentially life-threatening complication of lung transplantation. Extensive adhesiolysis necessitated by prior cardiac or pulmonary surgery may increase the risk of postoperative bleeding, as does the use of mechanical support such as CPB or ECMO. Meticulous haemostasis and correction of undesired coagulopathy is mandatory in the immediate postoperative period.

Airway complications

Airway stenosis, dehiscence, and necrosis are all uncommon complications following lung transplantation. Immediate complications more frequently reflect technical error, while late complications may manifest as a result of tenuous anastomotic perfusion or due to infection. Early failure may require reoperation to revise and correct technical error. Late complications may be better managed with more conservative measures such as dilation and stenting and less frequently require operative intervention.

Primary graft dysfunction

PGD after lung transplantation is the major contributor to both morbidity and early mortality. Prompt diagnostic workup and a high index of suspicion are mandatory to evaluate for alternative causes of respiratory failure, such as vascular torsion, infection, cardiogenic oedema, or hyperacute rejection. These reversible causes must be promptly addressed to correct ventilatory status. The direct mechanistic sequence leading to PGD is not yet elucidated, though retrospective studies suggest that the degree of ischaemic-reperfusion injury contributes significantly. Several factors may decrease the risk of PGD. During the transplant procedure, several manoeuvres may be employed to minimize the extent of reperfusion injury experienced by the allograft. In addition to the use of extracellular preservation solutions, administration of IV methylprednisolone (500 mg) and mannitol (25 mg) prior to reperfusion of both allografts have been shown to reduce the degree of reperfusion injury. Importantly, reperfusion is performed in a controlled fashion over a period of 10–15 minutes when done off of CPB. Similarly, ventilation and lung recruitment should be held until the newly implanted lung has rewarmed. Inhaled NO or other pulmonary vasodilator can used to decrease PVR during the operation. If additional pulmonary vasodilation is thought to be necessary, the patient can be continued on inhaled NO or inhaled epoprostenol after initial stabilization in the ICU and prior to extubation.

Those patients exhibiting severe PGD despite preventive and less invasive rescue manoeuvres are considered for mechanical support with ECMO. Those with peak inspiratory pressures approaching 30 cmH$_2$O and requiring FiO$_2$ >0.60 after excluding other causes for failure are considered candidates for post-transplant ECMO. VV ECMO provides short-term support while lung recovery is anticipated. Support can be initiated at the bedside by way of a single dual-lumen cannula, although many cannulation strategies can be employed as the situation necessitates. Once

ECMO support is established, patients are transitioned to lung-protective ventilatory settings with low pressures and FiO$_2$ of 0.21. Of those patients requiring VV ECMO post transplantation, the vast majority are successfully weaned from support as graft performance improves. Patients are typically weaned from ECMO within 24–72 hours as evidence of pulmonary recovery is observed. Though survival rates of those experiencing PGD continue to improve with advances in ECMO technology, PGD continues to decrease overall survival rates and leads to a decrease in overall graft function once free from ECMO support.

Conclusion

Lung transplantation is a life-saving therapy for candidates with end-stage lung disease. Improvements in donor and candidate selection and care, surgical and anaesthetic technique, critical care management, and immunosuppressive strategies have made lung transplantation safer than ever before. Exceptional care of both the donor and the candidate/recipient at all phases of the transplantation process is critical to the overall outcome of the recipient. In the immediate postoperative period, utmost vigilance is required for the early detection of and rescue of the recipient from a small number of predictable but impactful complications. The ability of the care team to safely recover the lung transplant recipient from the transplant procedure is a critical facet of quality care delivery in thoracic transplantation.

Management of rejection following lung transplantation

Acute cellular rejection

Despite advances in surgical, anaesthetic, surveillance, and transplant immunosuppression strategies, acute lung rejection remains a common post-lung transplant complication seen in lung transplant patients within a year after transplantation. Rejection is often diagnosed on clinical grounds, using a composite of symptoms, lung function, imaging, DSAs, and immunohistological examination of transbronchial lung biopsy specimens by experienced multidisciplinary teams. A third of lung recipients will have an episode of treated rejection within the first year. Further ACR/AMR are major risk factors for early graft loss and CLAD. Registry data from the ISHLT indicate that ACR is responsible for 3.6% of deaths within 30 days after transplantation.

Risk factors for ACR
See Table 30.1.

Table 30.1 Risk factors for ACR

1	Degree of HLA mismatch: HLA-DR, HLA-B, HLA-A, etc.
2	PGD
3	Infections: bacterial, fungal, community-acquired respiratory virus (CARV), CMV
4	Gastro-oesophageal reflux disease
5	Non-compliance with immunosuppression

Aetiology

The immunological mechanisms of lung allograft rejection are complex and multifaceted. From a simplistic perspective, lung allograft transplantation exposes the host immune system to a multitude of damage and pathogen-associated molecular patterns that test the discriminatory ability of the lung innate and adaptive immune response systems. Non-self-major histocompatibility complex patterns from the donor-derived antigens and pathogens are recognized by direct, indirect, and semi-direct pathways of allo-recognition involving the T-cell receptor (TCR)–CD3 complex. This is followed by allo-activation of the T cells in the presence of co-stimulatory signals driving complex adaptive effector immune responses that lead to graft rejection or tolerance. Effective immunosuppression is therefore one of the key strategies for dampening the immune response to the lung allograft to minimize acute rejection of the graft and improve long-term outcomes.

Clinical manifestations and diagnosis

Symptoms of acute rejection are often unreliable and non-specific, including shortness of breath, cough, and low-grade fever. CXR can demonstrate new evolving pleural effusions or persistent effusions and infiltrates. *De novo* DSAs may be detected. Symptoms and signs are more often pronounced in severe acute rejection and help direct appropriate investigations including imaging, bronchoscopy evaluation, and transbronchial biopsies. Routine surveillance transbronchial bronchoscopies also help in identification of ACR in asymptomatic patients particularly in the early post-transplant period.

Laboratory results

There are no pathognomonic markers of ACR on routine blood panels. Their use is limited to help identify adequacy of trough CNI levels (tacrolimus/ciclosporin), infective, haematological, renal, and hepatic abnormalities post transplantation.

Pulmonary imaging

Serial CXRs are routinely obtained for all patients after lung transplantation. The presence of bilateral pulmonary infiltrates or new evolving pleural effusions or persistent pleural effusions are harbingers of acute rejection. High-resolution CT is not always helpful; however, the presence of interlobular septal thickening and bilateral ground-glass changes in the absence of fluid overload/consolidation or atelectasis can be complementary for diagnosis of acute rejection.

Pulmonary function tests

Spirometry is routinely performed post transplantation on the ward, at home, and during follow-up visits after discharge. Our protocol for spirometry is at 2 weeks post transplantation and then bi-weekly until discharge from hospital in a majority of uncomplicated lung transplantations. The spirometer marker of clinical interest in the FEV_1 and a decline of ≥10% from a stable baseline in the absence of confounding factors such as pain/sedation/depression or technical quality control issues should trigger additional investigations. While spirometry is helpful particularly when there are no infection/bronchial anastomotic concerns, specificity for diagnosis of ACR is low.

Bronchoscopy and transbronchial biopsy (TBBX)

Surveillance bronchoscopy and TBBX are critical to histological gold standard confirmation of acute ACR and AMR. This allows examination of the bronchial anastomosis, removal of endobronchial plugs, microbiological confirmation of infections by BAL, and tissue confirmation of acute rejection based on the ISHLT criteria. Bronchoscopy and TBBX protocols vary across transplant centres. Our institutional practice is to perform these at 1 month, 3 months, 6 months, and 12 months routinely with additional bronchoscopies when clinically indicated, often by new-onset decrease in lung function, concerns of infection, or changes in radiology. A minimum of five pieces of well-expanded alveolar parenchyma along with terminal bronchioles is required for reliably diagnosing ACR by dedicated, experienced transplant pathologists after exclusion of acute infection. Acute rejection is characterized by perivascular mononuclear infiltrates with or without endothelialitis. In practice, we provide six to nine good-quality biopsy specimens performed under conscious sedation and fluoroscopic guidance. The ISHLT diagnostic criteria for grading and severity assessment of ACR are provided in Table 30.2.

Emerging biomarkers

Emerging biomarkers for ACR include liquid biopsies, that is, quantification of circulating donor-derived cell-free DNA from the allograft in plasma (ddcfDNA) by next-generation sequencing platforms, and are of immense research interest and awaiting prospective validation. Other markers of future interest include micro-RNA (miRNA) signatures in peripheral blood.

Table 30.2 Pathological grading of ACR

Grade	Meaning	Appearance
A	**Perivascular inflammation**	
0	No	Normal lung parenchyma
1	Minimal	Scattered, infrequent small mononuclear perivascular infiltrates; no eosinophils
2	Mild	More frequent perivascular infiltrates seen at low magnification, eosinophils may be present
3	Moderate	Dense perivascular infiltrates, eosinophils, and neutrophils common. Pathognomonic feature is extension into alveolar septa and air spaces
4	Severe	Diffuse perivascular, interstitial, and air-space infiltrates with pneumocyte damage and features of acute lung injury
B	**Airway-associated inflammation**	
0	None	No evidence of bronchiolar inflammation
1R	Low grade	Single layer of mononuclear cells in bronchiolar submucosa
2R	High grade	Large infiltrates of larger and activated lymphocytes in bronchiolar submucosa, with potential involvement of eosinophils and plasmacytoid cells
X	Ungradable	No bronchiolar tissue

Treatment of ACR

Treatment of ACR is by pulse dose steroids (usually methylprednisolone) and the decision to treat often depends on TBBX histological grading of rejection. Grade A2 (mild rejection) and above are definitely treated. Asymptomatic A1 (minimal rejection) and isolated B grade may not merit treatment and centres vary on their management of asymptomatic minimal rejection. At the least, such patients will need to have close clinical follow-up with lung function and surveillance TBBX at 4–6 weeks.

Our institutional policy to use IV pulse methyl prednisolone (10 mg/kg for 3 days followed by 1 mg/kg on a tapering schedule) within the first 3 months after transplantation, with oral prednisolone pulses 1 mg/kg being used after 3 months. Surveillance lung function and TBBX needs to be repeated at 4–6 weeks after treatment of ACR to identify persistent ACR, which is a risk factor for CLAD progression.

The presence of persistent ACR despite augmentation is a marker of coexistent AMR and should trigger investigations for *de novo* DSAs and immune-histological phenotyping (C4d) of TBBX tissue for AMR. In the first instance, the pulse steroid therapy should be repeated and CNI switch to tacrolimus can be considered if the patient has had two prior steroid augmentations. Other potential treatment considerations are a simultaneous switch to MMF from azathioprine. If there is recurrent/refractory high-grade ACR, antibody depletion-based treatments with rabbit antithymocyte globulin (rATG) or alemtuzumab (anti-CD52) can be considered. Depending on institutional practice, expert centres would consider early total lymphoid nodal irradiation or extracorporeal photopheresis in recurrent ACR to prevent CLAD progression.

Antibody-mediated rejection

The role of AMR in the development of lung allograft rejection has been rapidly growing in the last few years. However, it remains a complex pathological and clinical process.

AMR is associated with different forms of rejection including:
* Hyperacute rejection, a rare but fulminant rejection occurring following reperfusion of the allograft and due to pre-existing anti-HLA antibodies.
  * Candidates for transplantation may have pre-existing anti-HLA antibodies following pregnancy, blood transfusion, or organ transplantation.
* Acute AMR, believed to be consequence of the development of de novo DSAs.
* ACR.
* CLAD.

The presence of pre-existing anti-HLA antibodies prior to transplantation and/or the development of de novo DSAs after transplantation is detected with fluorescent-based solid-phase assay (Luminex bead technology). Generally, multiple levels of testing are performed to evaluate the presence and the specificity of circulating anti-HLA antibodies. The first level uses a pool of different class I and class II antigens assessing the presence or absence of antibodies. The last level of testing will use single HLA antigen beads to determine antibody specificity. A note of caution in the interpretation of anti-HLA antibodies tests: the level and function of circulating anti-HLA antibodies should not be based on the MFI of the assays, because the MFI does not represent the strength or the titre of circulating anti-HLA antibodies. There is no consensus currently on how to measure the strength of circulating DSAs. Further available options to estimate the strength of circulating anti-HLA antibodies includes serial dilution assay, IgG subclasses analysis, and/or C1q binding activity.

Differently from other SOTs, in lung transplantation the lack of specific diagnostic features and the variable relationship between DSAs and clinical presentation pose a challenge in defining the clinical diagnosis and treatment. Clinical manifestations of acute AMR are non-specific. Patients tend to present with general respiratory symptoms: dyspnoea, cough, and hypoxaemia. Radiologically, diffuse pulmonary opacities is the most common finding on CXR. Histopathologically, the presence of capillaritis in lung allograft tissue has been seen occasionally in cases of AMR. C4d deposition has been an inconsistent finding in lung transplant biopsy and its role in the diagnosis has been controversial.

Based on the presence of (1) allograft dysfunction, (2) histopathology, (3) C4d staining, and (4) circulating DSA, AMR is currently divided into clinical and subclinical types: clinical AMR if allograft dysfunction is present, and subclinical if there is not allograft dysfunction. Subcategorization includes 'definitive', in case of all criteria being present; 'probable' in case of three criteria; and 'possible' in case of two criteria.

Treatment of AMR

There is no consensus on the optimal treatment for AMR due to the absence of clinical trials. Based on single-centre experiences, a combination of drugs directed to decrease the circulating anti-HLA antibodies and the production of new DSAs are often used. To date, the optimal regimen for the treatment of pulmonary AMR is unknown.

Agents that are often used include:

- *IVIG*: despite the exact mechanism of action being unknown, IVIG is the foundation of most AMR treatment regimens. IVIG may neutralize DSAs, inhibit complement activity and cytokine gene activation, and downregulate B cells. IVIG is typically dosed at 500–2000 mg/kg.
- *Anti-CD20 monoclonal antibody*: rituximab is able to rapidly bind to CD-20 expressed on pre-B and mature B cells causing cell lysis. Generally, 375 mg/m² of rituximab is administered once a week for 4 weeks. However, the optimal dose and number of cycles are also unclear.
- *Proteasome inhibitors*: bortezomib and carfilzomib. These two drugs are directed against proteasome components, which are required by plasma cells to complete production of proteins, including antibodies. Typically, four doses of 1.3 mg/m² of bortezomib are given. Due to risk of infection and other side effects associated with bortezomib, carfilzomib, a newer proteasome inhibitor, has been recently used for the treatment of AMR along with plasmapheresis and IVIG.
- *Plasmapheresis*: the goal of this therapy is to deplete circulating anti-HLA antibodies and mitigate graft dysfunction by separating and discarding plasma component and replacing it with albumin or fresh frozen plasma. There is no consensus of the number of plasmapheresis sessions required.

Induction agents in lung transplantation

The use of strong immunosuppression in the perioperative or early postoperative period to reduce the initial robust T-cell response against the lung allograft was initially motivated by evidence from other SOTs such as kidney, heart, and liver transplantation. However, due to the lack of significant evidence of a clear benefit and the concerns for increased risk of infection, the use of immunosuppressive strategies for induction varies from institution to institution. The use of induction immunosuppression in the recent era is associated with decreased incidence of BOS and increased survival. Despite it not being considered part of the induction therapy, just before reperfusion of the allograft, high-dose glucocorticoids (methylprednisolone 500 to 1000 mg IV) are administered to reduce the risk of reperfusion injury.

IL2R antagonists

Basiliximab and daclizumab are chimeric monoclonal antibodies that act by binding to activated T-cells expressing CD25, blocking cell activation and proliferation.

- Basiliximab is dosed intraoperatively or immediately after lung transplantation at 20 mg on the first and fourth days after transplantation and present a half-life of 13 days with an effective IL2R saturation of 30 days.
- Daclizumab is used at 1 mg/kg within the first 24 hours post transplantation and then repeated for an additional four doses every 2 weeks. Daclizumab has a half-life of 20–40 days with an effective IL2R saturation of 120 days.

The use of daclizumab compared to depleting agents and/or monoclonal antibodies showed no differences in the rate of acute rejection, freedom from BOS, and 2-year survival.

Infusion of basiliximab prior to implantation led to a lower rejection score during the first year after transplantation compared to infusion after implantation or no induction. However, no change in survival or freedom from BOS was observed.

Lymphocyte-depleting agents

Two T-cell-depleting agents are polyclonal immunoglobulins: horse anti-thymocyte globulin (Atgam) and rATG.

- Atgam is administered IV at a dose of 5–15 mg/kg per day for the first day to 14 days following lung transplantation.
- rATG is used at 1.5 mg/kg IV over 6 hours then two or three additional doses given 24 hours apart.

During infusion, cytokine release syndrome including fever, rigors, rash, and myalgia, and post-infusion leucopenia, thrombocytopenia, immune-complex glomerulonephritis, and serum sickness have been described.

Conflicting results have been observed with the use of these agents as induction agents. The use of rATG as an induction agent showed a reduced incidence of acute rejection and trend towards reduced BOS when compared to no induction. However, these findings were not confirmed in the follow-up study with no change in survival at 8 years. A large randomized controlled multicentre trial evaluating the efficacy of ATG-Fresenius (5 and 9 mg/kg, respectively) compared to no induction failed to show reduction in acute rejection, graft loss, or death in the first year after lung transplantation.

Monoclonal antibodies

Monoclonal antibodies used in the induction phase are Muromonab–CD3 (OKT3) and alemtuzumab. OKT3 was voluntarily withdrawn from the United States market in 2009.

Alemtuzumab is a monoclonal antibody that targets CD52, a cell surface receptor expressed by B and T cells, macrophages, monocytes, and natural killer cells. Alemtuzumab leads to cell depletion including B and T cells through direct cellular and complement-mediated cytotoxicity.

Alemtuzumab is dosed at 30 mg IV over 2 hours. It is associated with a cytokine release syndrome that can be attenuated by pre-emptive administration of acetaminophen 500–1000 mg orally, diphenhydramine 50 mg orally or IV, and methylprednisolone 15 mg/kg about 30 minutes prior to infusion. The T-cell depletion can last up to 3 years after infusion, while B-cell depletion lasts about 3 months.

Use of alemtuzumab is associated with comparable 5-year survival but increased freedom from acute rejection and BOS in comparison with anti-thymoglobulin, daclizumab, and no induction regimens.

Alemtuzumab is associated with an increased risk of opportunistic infections.

In conclusion, all induction agents provide benefits with regard to acute rejection but are more modest in terms of long-term survival. Newer strategies are being used in other SOT recipients with more tailored approaches (i.e. belatacept in living-donor kidney transplant recipients) and hopefully soon will start making recommendations based on more significant evidence.

Maintenance immunosuppression drugs

Protocols

After lung transplantation, a maintenance immunosuppression regimen including three drugs is considered the standard of care. This regimen includes one CNI, tacrolimus or ciclosporin; a corticosteroid, usually prednisone; and a cell cycle inhibitor, mycophenolate or azathioprine.

According to ISHLT registry data, the most common regimen both at 1- and 5-year follow-up is tacrolimus, mycophenolate, and prednisone. mTOR inhibitors, sirolimus and everolimus, have been used as an alternative to a cell cycle inhibitor, or to minimize CNI dosing and more recently as an adjunct agent in the setting of rejection (Table 30.3).

Management of a highly sensitized host

The importance of pre- and post-transplant management of HLA antibodies in transplant candidates remains an important limiting factor to long-term survival.

The development of HLA antibodies may be due to prior pregnancies, connective tissue disease, previous transfusion, or prior organ transplantation. Certain infections and ECMO may lead to cross-reactivity antibodies and thus detectable HLA antibodies prior to transplantation.

Acceptance of a donor with HLA to the recipient's detected HLA antibodies has been associated with episodes of hyperacute rejection, and worse early post-transplant outcomes.

Lung transplant recipients with detectable pre-transplant HLA antibodies demonstrated greater number of ventilator days, worse 30-day mortality, higher rate of post-transplant detectable HLA antibodies, and an increased risk of developing BOS, a presentation of CLAD.

• The most common type of pre-transplant management of HLA antibodies is avoidance of any detectable donor-specific HLA antibodies.

Table 30.3 Maintenance immunosuppression drugs

	Class	Target trough level	Side effects
Tacrolimus	CNI	5–15 ng/mL	Nephrotoxicity, neurotoxicity, hyperglycaemia, hypertension, hyperlipidaemia, hyperkalaemia, hypomagnesaemia
Ciclosporin	CNI	75–200 ng/mL	Nephrotoxicity, neurotoxicity, hyperglycaemia, hypertension, hyperlipidaemia, hyperkalaemia, hypomagnesaemia
Sirolimus Everolimus	mTOR inhibitors	5–15 mg/mL	Decreased wound healing, leucopenia, thrombocytopenia, hypertriglyceridemia, proteinuria, and pneumonitis
Myco phenolate	Cell cycle inhibitor	250–1000 mg twice a day	Leucopenia, thrombocytopenia, and GI disturbances (diarrhoea, abdominal pain, nausea, vomiting)
Azathioprine	Cell cycle inhibitor	2 mg/kg daily	Leucopenia, thrombocytopenia, anaemia, hepatotoxicity, pancreatitis
Prednisone	Corticosteroid	5–20 mg daily	Hypertension, weight gain, hyperlipidaemia, hyperglycaemia and diabetes mellitus, osteoporosis, cataracts, poor wound healing, psychiatric disturbances

- Desensitization strategies for lung transplant candidates with elevated PRAs consist of regimens including IVIG, plasmapheresis, rituximab, carfilzomib, or bortezomib. However, no significant improvements in terms of survival or development of CLAD was noted. A different approach based on clinical risk stratification, presence of DSA anti-HLA antibodies, and organ availability including intraoperative plasma exchange prior to reperfusion of the first graft and followed by a total of five sessions postoperatively, IVIG, and rATG (dosed based on the results of the complement-dependent cytotoxicity cross-match), showed less episodes of acute rejection and similar 1-year and 5-year graft survival when compared to patients with detectable PRAs but negative DSAs and unsensitized patients.

Early detection of DSA has been associated with worse outcomes. Thus, aggressive management of these antibodies may impact longer-term outcomes by removing or decreasing HLA antibodies. Regimens include IVIG, plasmapheresis, rituximab, carfilzomib, and bortezomib. However, there is no significant evidence yet of an appropriate regimen in this scenario. Further studies are necessary to define optimal early regimens to treat the memory HLA response.

Late complications following lung transplantation

Chronic lung allograft dysfunction

Despite improvement in surgical techniques, lung preservation, advances in immunosuppressive regimens, and antimicrobial prophylaxis, the long-term survival following lung transplantation remains limited. After the first year, the main causes of morbidity and mortality are CLAD and infections. CLAD is defined as a persistent decline (≥ 3 weeks) in pulmonary function tests from baseline. There are currently three distinct phenotypes of CLAD: (1) bronchiolitis obliterans syndrome (BOS), (2) neutrophilic reversible allograft dysfunction (NRAD), (3) and restrictive allograft syndrome (RAS). Each phenotype in its pure form has supportive lung physiology, histopathological, radiological, and BAL features. The incidence of CLAD has been estimated at 48% within 5 years and 76% after 10 years.

Bronchiolitis obliterans syndrome

BOS presents with shortness of breath associated with declining obstructive lung physiology (decrease in FEV_1 and in the FEV_1/FVC ratio). It is a diagnosis of exclusion, characterized by progressive irreversible airflow obstruction due to small airway obstruction. CXRs are often normal in BOS; however, CT scans are very sensitive and specific, with airway dilation and gas trapping on expiration. Histological features of BOS suggest injury of the small airways leading to excessive fibroproliferation. Transbronchial biopsies have poor sensitivity for BOS (17%). BOS is classified on the basis of lung function as detailed in Table 31.1. A number of risk factors have been associated with the development of BOS. The single best characterized risk factor is ACR, which is characterized by perivascular infiltration of activated lymphocytes. One or more episodes of moderate to severe acute rejection is a significant risk factor for BOS. Lymphocytic bronchiolitis is also a risk factor for BOS. Although often quoted as a risk factor, evidence of an association between HLA mismatching and BOS is unclear. Allo-independent factors are extremely important with viral, bacterial, and fungal infections and compliance with medication all associated with increased risk of BOS. Other potential risk factors for BOS include older donor age, gastro-oesophageal reflux with aspiration, organizing pneumonia, prolonged allograft ischaemia, and persistent DSAs.

Treatment options for BOS are very limited with no established successful regimen. Most focus on augmentation of immunosuppression to inhibit progression; however, this treatment predisposes to pulmonary infections and can increase mortality. Small, non-controlled case series have suggested conversion from ciclosporin to tacrolimus may result in a slowing of BOS. Other immune-modulating strategies that have been trialled in stabilizing lung function include methotrexate, cyclophosphamide, extracorporeal photopheresis, total lymphoid irradiation, and antilymphocyte antibodies. Montelukast has also been shown to slow the rate of decline in FEV_1 compared with a control group.

Neutrophilic reversible allograft dysfunction

NRAD is a phenotype of CLAD characterized by the presence of excess neutrophils $\geq 15\%$ in BAL in the absence of concurrent infection. Neutrophils secrete chemokines, growth factors, and matrix metalloproteinase, increasing oxidative stress damaging epithelium, and leading to an excess repair process with fibroblast proliferation. Azithromycin is a macrolide antibiotic with

Table 31.1 ISHLT consensus on BOS grading

1993 classification		2002 classification	
BOS 0	FEV₁ 80% or more of baseline	**BOS 0**	FEV₁ >90% of baseline and FEF₂₅₋₇₅ >75% of baseline
		BOS 0p	FEV₁ 81–90% of baseline and/or FEF₂₅₋₇₅ ≤75% of baseline
BOS 1	FEV₁ 66–80% of baseline	**BOS 1**	FEV₁ 66–80% of baseline
BOS 2	FEV₁ 51–65% of baseline	**BOS 2**	FEV₁ 51–65% of baseline
BOS 3	FEV₁ ≤50% of baseline	**BOS 3**	FEV₁ ≤50% of baseline

FEF, forced expiratory flow.

both anti-inflammatory and immune-modulatory properties. It significantly reduces airway neutrophilia and inflammatory cytokines. A pilot study in 2003 by Gerhardt et al. demonstrated significant improvement in FEV_1, with low-dose azithromycin. Response to azithromycin is classified as an FEV_1 increase of ≥10% after 2–3 months of treatment. There was a significant correlation between the initial percentage of BAL neutrophilia and the changes in FEV_1 after 3 months of treatment with azithromycin. Patients with NRAD typically have a good prognosis after diagnosis.

Restrictive allograft syndrome

RAS is a form of CLAD that is defined by the development of restrictive lung physiology (persistent ≥20% decline in FEV_1, concomitant ≥10% decline in TLC). Features on CT scanning consist of interstitial infiltrates with ground-glass opacities and fibrotic changes predominantly in the upper lobes. Histologically, RAS is characterized by extensive fibrosis in the alveoli, with pleuroparenchymal fibroelastosis, and in the interlobular septa. RAS develops in about 25–35% of recipients with CLAD and has a very variable course. In the primary progressive phenotype, RAS is associated with poorer outcomes (Table 31.2). Mixed phenotypes of BOS and RAS may develop with some patients first developing BOS with obstructive decline in FEV_1 and then developing RAS. Risk factors for RAS are similar to that of BOS; they include frequent episodes of acute rejection, lymphocytic bronchiolitis, colonization with *Pseudomonas*, and infection. The fibrotic features of RAS have led to a trial of pirfenidone in patients post transplantation and a single case report suggested some improvement.

Antibody-mediated rejection

DSAs are closely associated with AMR in most SOTs. Until recently, in the lungs, AMR was associated with hyper-acute rejection; however, with improvement in the detection of DSA it is now a recognized cause of CLAD. The clinical manifestations of AMR are identical to other form of allograft injury and are thus not specific. The mechanism of injury in AMR is binding

Table 31.2 Short summary of CLAD phenotypes

Parameter	BOS	NRAD	RAS
Lung function	Obstructive	Obstructive	Restrictive
BAL	Limited inflammation	Inflammatory neutrophilia Raised IL-8 Decreased IL-10	Limited inflammation
Histology	Fibroblast proliferation with obliteration of bronchioles	Inflammation with fibroblast proliferation	Alveolar damage Parenchymal and pleural fibrosis
Radiology	Gas trapping Bronchiectasis Mosaic attenuation	Airway wall thickening Mucus plugging	Ground-glass opacities, peripheral fibrosis, and subpleural consolidation
Prognosis	Variable	Good	Poor
Azithromycin	Variable	Good effect	No effect

of DSA to the graft and subsequent inflammatory damage. In 2016, the ISHLT developed a consensus definition for AMR based on findings in renal and cardiac AMR and case series in lung transplantation. The diagnostic features of AMR include (1) presence of circulating HLA or other DSAs, (2) evidence of histological change and C4d deposition in the allograft, and (3) clinical allograft dysfunction. The treatment of AMR remains empirical, there are no randomized controlled trials or comparison studies of treatment regimens for AMR. Treatment regimens consist of use of high-dose corticosteroids in combination with agents aimed at antibody depletion such as ATG, IVIG, plasmapheresis, anti-CD20 monoclonal antibodies, proteasome inhibitors, and complement inhibition.

Airway complications

The transplanted airways are vulnerable to ischaemia as a result of the bronchial circulation being interrupted at the time of transplantation. The flow to the airways early postoperatively is entirely dependent on back flow from the pulmonary circulation until such time as other blood flow can be established. This can result in ischaemia injury occurring in the airways and the peri-anastomotic site is particularly vulnerable (Fig. 31.1a). The frequency of this injury has been difficult to assess, in part related to the lack of a universally accepted definition—the published literature suggests rates of up to 39%. Ischaemic necrosis of the airway results in scarring and fibrosis that can result in the loss of airway diameter. This cicatrizing process results in airway obstruction secondary to strictures and bronchomalacia resulting in increasing breathlessness (Fig. 31.1b). If the ischaemic strictures are severe, airway intervention with balloon bronchoplasty, cryotherapy, or diathermy may improve airway narrowing (Fig. 31.2). Failure of these interventions associated with increasing symptoms may require airway stenting. There are a variety of bronchial stents available for first-generation airways including self-expanding metallic stents, silicone stents, and biodegradable stents. Long-term complications of bronchial stents are common and include bronchial stasis, granulation tissue, haemoptysis, stent fracture, and airway erosion (Fig. 31.3). The use of uncovered stents is decreasing due to the unacceptably high rate of complications. The outcomes in patients who have airway complications are significantly worse than in patients who do not have this complication, particularly in the presence of *Aspergillus*.

(a)

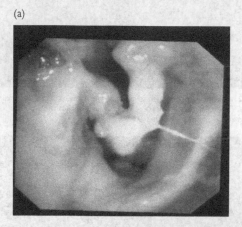

(b)

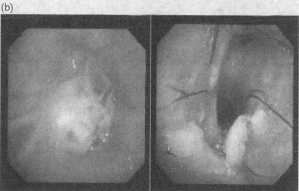

Fig. 31.1 (a) Right main bronchus with severe peri-anastomotic ischaemic necrosis of the airway. (b) Complete occlusion of right main bronchus with granulation tissue, successfully removed by cryotherapy. See plate section.

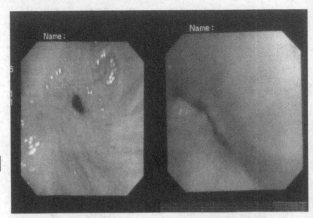

Fig. 31.2 Ischaemic stricture with severe airway narrowing of the right main bronchus. Total dynamic obstruction of right main bronchus secondary to bronchomalacia. See plate section.

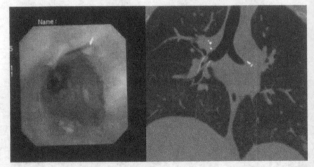

Fig. 31.3 Right main bronchus stent with in-stent bronchial granulation tissue. CT demonstrating in-stent stenosis. See plate section.

Medication-related complications

Many of the long-term complications arise from the necessity for antirejection medication in recipients. Globally, glucocorticoids, CNIs, and cell cycle inhibitors, are the cornerstone of immunosuppressive regimens. Although the intended action is immune suppression, either individually or in concert they can cause significant unwanted side effects.

Cardiovascular

Both glucocorticoids and CNIs can increase the risk of developing hypertension, diabetes mellitus, and renal disease. This is associated with a significantly increased risk of cardiovascular disease. Approximately 90% of patients 3 years post transplantation on ciclosporin-based therapy have at least one new risk factor for cardiovascular disease, either hypertension, hypercholesterolaemia, or new-onset diabetes mellitus. Mortality from cardiovascular disease rises from around 5% at 1 year to 8% at 10 years.

Renal

Many patients may have a degree of pre-existing renal impairment. hypertension and diabetes mellitus are risk factors for chronic kidney disease. CNIs are directly toxic to kidneys and are a cause of renal failure post transplantation. CNI-induced chronic kidney disease arises from a combination of vascular, glomerular, and tubular disease. Dose reduction or withdrawal may ameliorate the effects of CNI-induced chronic kidney disease. In patients without proteinuria, consideration of changing the CNI for an mTOR inhibitor may offer some renal preservation.

Bone marrow suppression

While the immunosuppression targets T cells, the effects of the cell cycle inhibitors in particular are not specific. These medications may cause cytopenia of any of the cell lines, thus leucopenia, thrombocytopaenia, and anaemia may arise. Bone marrow suppression may also arise from antifungals (voriconazole) and antimicrobials (meropenem, co-trimoxazole, and valganciclovir).

Infection

After BOS, infection is the second highest cause of mortality in lung transplant recipients. The lungs interface between the body and the external environment and they are constantly exposed to inhaled pathogens. Following lung transplantation, multiple risk factors exist for infection. Early on, the mucosal defences are compromised with reduction in ciliary function. Patients may also be colonized with pathogenic and multidrug-resistant microbes and there may be donor-derived infections. The loss of the bronchial circulation gives rise to the potential for ischaemia of the proximal airways. Intubation and prolonged critical care and hospital stay expose patients to further risk. Transplant recipients are at increased risk of opportunistic and donor-related infections; the highest risk is in the first 6 months. This correlates with recovery from surgery and the maximum period of immunosuppression.

Bacterial

Post-transplant community-acquired bacterial infections and multidrug-resistant bacterial infections are frequent. Patients transplanted for CF are at higher risk of reacquisition of their previous microbes. Sputum cultures as well as BAL are used to guide antibiotic therapies.

Common respiratory viruses

Influenza, parainfluenza, metapneumovirus, and rhinovirus are common respiratory viruses associated with pulmonary infections in the lung transplant patient. Common respiratory viral infections are also associated with an increased risk of developing CLAD. All patients receiving lung transplants should receive an annual influenza vaccination.

Herpesviruses

HSV-1 (human herpesvirus (HHV)-1), HSV-2 (HHV-2), VZV (HHV-3), HHV-6, and Kaposi's sarcoma-associated herpesvirus (HHV-8) can all complicate transplantation due to immunosuppression. Patient education and regular dermatological surveillance should be initiated to identify active infections. Active cutaneous or mucocutaneous infections provide a disruption to skin defences increasing the risk of bacterial infections. EBV (HHV-4) and CMV (HHV-5) are important viral pathogens in lung transplants. Infection with CMV is one of the most significant causes of morbidity in transplant recipients. CMV may cause leucopenia, thrombocytopaenia, hepatitis, colitis, nephritis, and pneumonitis. CMV may also predispose individuals to bacterial and fungal infection. Most centres offer CMV-positive patients pre-emptive prophylaxis with valganciclovir for an extended period of time.

Fungal

Aspergillus and *Candida* species are the most common fungal infections. Fungal infections have an estimated incidence of 15–35%. *Aspergillus* infection is the most common fungal infection after lung transplantation with an incidence of approximately 6%. The highest risk period is the first 12 months; however, there remains a risk throughout the life of a recipient. The diagnosis of *Aspergillus* is challenging and reliant on imaging with CT, supported by culture and galactomannan assay. Treatment with an azole is often required for protracted periods and will require careful monitoring of the CNI.

Non-tuberculous mycobacteria (NTM)

Active growth of fast-dividing NTM is a relative contraindication to transplantation, the most common NTMs are *Mycobacterium avium intracellulare* (50%) *M. abscessus* (24%), *M. fortuitum* (12%), and *M. immunogenum* (12%). Slow-growing species such as *M. gordonae* have also been shown to be pathogenic, causing 20% of NTM infections. Clinical manifestations are diverse and include pulmonary disease, surgical site infection such as anastomotic and sternotomy infections, lymphadenopathy, and cutaneous manifestations.

Malignancy

Post-transplant recipients are vulnerable to solid organ, cutaneous, and lymphomatous malignancies. PTLD is most common in the first year post transplantation, with skin and then solid organ malignancies increasing over time. At 1 year, the incidence of cancers is approximately 5% rising to 20% at 5 years and 30% at 10 years. Both CNIs and cell cycle inhibitors have been shown to reduce cellular apoptosis, suppress DNA repair, and promote metastasis. In combination, they can promote oncogenic pathways by increasing tumour formation, growth, and spread. They may interfere with immune surveillance responsible for identifying and destroying malignancies. PTLD occurs in up to 5% of patients post transplantation. The risk of PTLD is higher in EBV-naïve recipients which is an oncogenic virus that has a trophism for B cells. Immunosuppression reduces regulatory T-cell activity allowing infected cells to proliferate. Treatment for PTLD involves reduction of immunosuppression burden. In patients with CD20-positive tumours, there should be consideration of single-agent rituximab but for patients with CD20-negative tumours, chemotherapy is usually needed.

Dermatological malignancies

Malignancies of the skin have been estimated to occur in 16% of patients post lung transplantation and account for 61% of all malignancies at 1 year. The risk of skin cancer is increased in older patients with greater sun exposure and in patients with a high burden of immunosuppression. Other risk factors that may predispose to dermatological malignancy include human papillomavirus, underlying skin type, male sex, and duration of immunosuppression. There is also an increased risk in patients on long-term voriconazole.

Lung cancer

Lung transplant recipients are at increased risk of lung malignancy, with an estimated tenfold increased risk compared to the general population of developing bronchogenic carcinoma. Risk factors include the smoking history of both donor and recipient, and environmental and occupational exposures. The prevalence of lung cancer originating from the native lung in single-lung transplants has increased over time and is now estimated to be 9%. Primary bronchogenic carcinoma from transplanted lung has a significantly lower prevalence of <0.4%.

Gastro-oesophageal reflux disease

Gastro-oesophageal reflux disease is very common in patients with end-stage lung disease with an estimated incidence of between 35% and 65%. Post transplantation, the prevalence increases from 30% at 3 months to 50% at 12 months. Multiple studies have shown an association with gastro-oesophageal reflux disease chronic micro-aspiration and BOS. Micro-aspiration reduces surfactant A and D levels, and increases inflammatory cytokines and alveolar neutrophils. Ambulatory pH monitoring is the main investigation. Impedance testing has been shown to be useful in identifying non-acid reflux as well, but no reflux testing clearly demonstrates aspiration. Treatment can be divided into medical and surgical, the use of proton pump inhibitors and H_2 blockers are used to reduce the acid component of reflux. Although proton pump inhibitors reduce acid secretion they may not reduce micro-aspiration. Azithromycin may act as a prokinetic and improve clearance of gastric contents and reduce reflux. Antireflux procedures such as fundoplication have been shown to reduce gastro-oesophageal reflux disease-associated lung injury and improve FEV_1 in some recipients. Studies suggest that early intervention for gastro-oesophageal reflux disease is associated with better outcomes in the long term.

Osteoporosis

Osteoporosis as defined as a bone mineral density <−2.5 SD. Pre-existing bone disease is common in lung transplant recipients with an estimated prevalence of approximately 50%. A significant contribution to this incidence is from prolonged corticosteroid use. Other factors that are associated with bone demineralization include advanced age, reduced BMI, reduced vitamin D levels, and hypogonadism. One-year post transplantation the prevalence increases significantly to 73%. Glucocorticoids reduce osteoblast replication differentiation and apoptosis. Lung transplant recipients should receive screening for osteoporosis prior to transplant with dual-energy X-ray absorptiometry imaging. Unless contraindicated, all patients should receive supplementation of their daily allowance of calcium and vitamin D to ensure an adequate vitamin D status. Bisphosphonates should be added to the regimen, the optimum duration of bisphosphonate treatment has yet to be determined. Concerns over long-term treatment with bisphosphonates causing osteonecrosis of the jaw and atypical femoral fractures require that treatment duration should be reviewed at 3–5 years. If treatment is stopped, risk assessment should be performed at 18 months to 3 years after cessation, or after any new fracture. At this point, reinstatement of therapy should be considered if appropriate.

Neurological complications

CNIs may cause neurological toxicity most commonly associated with higher blood concentrations. Paraesthesia, tremor, and headache are common manifestations and estimated to occur in 20–39% of patients. Posterior reversible encephalopathy syndrome is clinically similar to hypertensive encephalopathy. It causes acute confusion, aphasia, cortical blindness, ataxia, and seizures. The diagnosis is confirmed on MRI with findings of vasogenic oedema. Treatment using a different CNI or withdrawal of CNI altogether generally leads to resolution of symptoms. In the 10 years post transplantation, it is estimated that 92% of patients will encounter neurological problems. These are most common in the first year and often in the perioperative period. Postoperative intracerebral haemorrhage, subarachnoid haemorrhage, and ischaemic strokes can cause significant early morbidity and mortality. Encephalopathy may also arise early post transplantation secondary to drug toxicities, infection, or cerebral hypoxia. Infections with atypical organisms may occur early post transplantation. Neurological complications after lung transplant have an increased mortality at 2 years. There is emerging evidence that recipients may encounter significant neurocognitive deficit, this has been identified at 3 months post transplantation. However, studies looking at this over a longer duration have yet to be performed.

Retransplantation

A very limited number of retransplantations are performed per year and represent <4% of all lung transplants. While survival at 1 year post retransplantation has improved up to 71%, it remains inferior to first transplantations at 86%. The median survival is significantly lower than primary lung transplantation at 2.6 years versus 6.8 years for primary transplantations. However, after allowing for PGD or acute surgical issues, the conditional survival taken at 1 year is 6.3 years. The main indications for retransplantation have been CLAD, airway complications, and end-stage BOS. Patients retransplanted for BOS had an improved survival compared to other indications.

Conclusion

Outcomes from lung transplantation have improved significantly over the last 30 years. However, the burden of immunosuppression necessitated for these outcomes results in a significant incidence of complications. Careful monitoring of patients in specialist lung transplant centres helps to reduce morbidity and mortality and improve both length and quality of life.

Antimicrobial prophylaxis and treatment after lung transplantation

Key recommendations

See Table 32.1.

Table 32.1 Key recommendations for prophylaxis and treatment after lung transplantation

Pre-transplantation colonization management	• Ensure appropriate respiratory cultures from all recipients at regular intervals and consider antimicrobial treatment strategies if clinically indicated • Certain pathogens, namely *Mycobacterium abscessus* complex and *Burkholderia cenocepacia*, need special consideration. Isolation of these pathogens may impact transplant eligibility
Management during operative implantation	• Consider stapling the bronchus prior to explanting the lung • Take care to avoid spillage of secretions during implantation • Irrigate the pleural space with antibacterial solution both after removal of the lung and at the completion of the procedure (such as taurolidine) • Microbiologically sampling of the donor lung: BAL (50 mL of normal saline into a tertiary bronchus and separate swab culture)

Post-trans plantation care	• Patients at high risk, i.e. those with preoperative colonization, need coverage with broad-spectrum antibiotics. Minimizing the duration of antimicrobials is essential to reduce the risk of development of antimicrobial resistance. Nebulized antimicrobials are a useful adjunct. They help deliver appropriate antimicrobials at the anatomic site without the risk of patient developing antimicrobial resistance
	• BAL from the donor and preoperative colonization helps guide antimicrobial management in the immediate perioperative period
	• Avoidance of other healthcare associated infection is also key:
	1. Maintenance of good skin integrity, appropriate management of intravascular catheters
	2. **HOUDINI** is a useful tool to guide urinary catheter management.
	    Haematuria (only requires catheter if in clot retention)
	    Obstruction/retention
	    Urology surgery
	    Damaged skin (open sacral or perineal wound in an incontinent patient)
	    Input/output, fluid monitoring
	    Nursing care end of life/comfort care
	    Immobility, due to physical constraint, e.g. unstable fracture and unable to use bottles/bedpans
	3. Removal of drains at the earliest possible opportunity
	4. Appropriate isolation facilities and adherence to strict infection prevention and control policies

Viral infections in lung transplantation

Viral infection causes specific morbidity and mortality after lung transplantation (Table 32.2). Several viral infections have been associated with long-term morbidity such as CLAD, previously identified as BOS.

Infection with community-acquired respiratory viruses such as influenzae A/B and Paramyxoviridae (e.g. respiratory syncytial virus) occur with seasonal variability and infected episodes range from easily treatable to more persistent infection. The interventions for these infections vary depending on the virus recovered and the currently available treatment regimens. Prevention strategies include yearly influenza vaccination for transplant recipients and their close contacts.

Herpes infection

Most transplant recipients are seropositive for HSV and VZV. Postoperative infections are a consequence of reactivation of previous latent infection. Assessment of serological status of both the donor and the recipient are essential especially for seronegative recipients who are at the greatest risk of developing symptomatic disease.

Cytomegalovirus

Belonging to the beta herpesvirus family, CMV has historically been the number one pathogen occurring after organ transplantation. Interestingly, the incidence of CMV disease (symptoms and active infection—diagnosed by NAAT which identifies CMV replication) is higher in the lung transplant population compared to other solid organs transplanted and is potentially related to the size of the organ and a higher state of immunosuppression.

The symptoms are important to recognize and consist of malaise, myalgia, low-grade temperature, and an end-organ disease such as colitis, oesophagitis, or hepatitis. As well as wanting to avoid the disease for the comfort of the recipients, it is also important to note the link between CMV infection and future allograft dysfunction and so infection prevention is advocated.

Epstein–Barr virus (EBV)

EBV is a gamma herpesvirus (HHV-4) that infects >95% of the world's population. EBV is responsible for a variety of clinical manifestations ranging from an infectious mononucleosis-like syndrome to proliferation of monoclonal lymphocytes leading to high-grade lymphoma. Such clinical entities associated with EBV infection after transplantation are known as PTLD and are mainly the consequence of the lack of cell-mediated immune surveillance of EBV-infected lymphocytes because of immunosuppression.

The main risk factor for the development of EBV-associated PTLD in lung transplant recipients is the serostatus of the donor and the recipient.

EBV D+/R− patients are at the highest risk of developing primary EBV infection which may lead to PTLD. Prevention is a major issue and is managed with reduced immunosuppressive regimens, particularly regimens that avoid the use of lymphocyte-depleting antibodies.

Table 32.2 Viral infection after transplantation

Virus	Prevention	Therapy
HSV-1 and HSV-2 (HHV-1 and HHV 2)	Aciclovir prophylaxis	Mucocutaneous disease: aciclovir, valaciclovir, and famciclovir Disseminated disease: IV aciclovir
VZV (HHV-3)	Aciclovir prophylaxis	Localized disease: aciclovir, valaciclovir and famciclovir Disseminated disease: IV aciclovir
CMV (HHV-5)	D+/R–: CMV mismatch consider prophylaxis with valganciclovir for 3 months D–/R+ and D+/R+: no prophylaxis, weekly surveillance 4 weeks post-transplantation for at least 3 months and treatment when high viral load detected D–/R–: no prophylaxis/ surveillance Some centres have different strategies including longer duration of prophylaxis ≥200 days	End-organ disease: IV ganciclovir
HHV6, HHV7, HHV8	No specific antiviral preventive strategy is recommended	End-organ HHV6 disease: foscarnet

Other herpesvirus infections

HSV reinfection is one of the most common forms of viral infection after organ transplantation. The clinical manifestations of HSV infection are usually like those observed in immunocompetent patients and include oral and genital mucocutaneous vesicular rash. In highly immunocompromised patients, more extensive lesions with necrotic ulcers can be observed.

Fungal infections in lung transplantation

Invasive fungal infections are a serious complication of lung transplantation and are associated with significant morbidity and mortality. When compared to other SOT recipients, lung transplant recipients are more susceptible to fungal infections. This stems from continuous and direct contact with the environment alongside impaired clearance mechanisms caused by allograft denervation and colonization of the airways by organisms from the upper respiratory tract or from the native lung in cases of single-lung transplantation.

Aspergillus

Aspergillus infection is the most frequent fungal infection after lung transplantation; it accounts for 73% of all cases of mould infection. It generally occurs within the first year after implantation and the most common organisms are A. *fumigatus*, A. *flavus*, A. *niger*, A. *terreus*, A. *versicolor*, and others.

Aspergillus is a ubiquitous organism that is found in decaying organic matter. Exposure to airborne fungal conidia can occur during construction or renovation, gardening, composting, and farming activities. Additionally, tobacco and marijuana can be contaminated with fungi, and recreational and medical marijuana use has been associated with IA. Therefore, lung transplant recipients should be advised to avoid such environmental exposures.

The risk factors are shown in Box 32.1.

Box 32.1 Risk factors for invasive aspergillosis in lung transplant recipients

- Environmental and recreational exposure.
- Construction.
- Farming.
- Marijuana use (smoking).
- Net state of immunosuppression.
- High-dose steroids.
- Anti-lymphocytic therapy.
- Muromonab–CD3 (OKT3).
- CMV infection.
- Hypogammaglobulinaemia.

Risk factors unique to lung transplantation

- Continuous and direct contact with the environment.
- Impaired clearance mechanisms caused by allograft denervation.
- Airway colonization before transplantation.
- Airway colonization after transplantation.
- Single-lung transplantation.
- Prolonged ischaemia.
- Donor-derived infection.

Four main clinical manifestations of *Aspergillus* infection in lung transplant recipients are colonization, tracheobronchitis or bronchial anastomotic site infection, pulmonary disease, and disseminated disease. Colonization of *Aspergillus* can occur in 46% of lung transplant recipients. In most patients it occurs within 3 months and patients may be asymptomatic with diagnosis made on culture without evidence of tissue invasion. Colonization itself is not a problem; however, it may be linked to CLAD.

Management of IA requires a twofold approach: reduction of immunosuppression and selection of an appropriate antifungal agent. The choice of agent should be based on efficacy as well as toxicity with consideration of the patient's comorbid condition. Attention should be paid to special circumstances. Tracheobronchitis requires bronchoscopic debridement and inhaled antifungal therapy in addition to systemic therapy. In cases with anastomotic dehiscence, surgical intervention with stent placement may be required.

Prophylaxis

Given the risk for the development of IA following lung transplantation and the significant morbidity associated with it, many lung transplant centres implement pre-emptive or universal prophylaxis:

- Pre-emptive: targets therapy towards patients deemed to be at high risk (e.g. previous history of colonization).
- Universal: targets all transplant recipients irrespective of their risk status.

A worldwide survey reported that 58.6% of lung transplant centres use universal prophylaxis for the first 6 months. Voriconazole either alone or in combination with inhaled amphotericin is the most commonly administered agent.

Yeast

Candida species are responsible for 23% of all invasive fungal infections in lung transplant recipients. Many species can cause human disease but most infection is caused by *C. albicans*, followed by *C. glabrata*, *C. parapsilosis*, *C. tropicalis*, and *C. krusei*.

Risk factors

Risk factors include broad-spectrum antibiotics, protracted antibiotic therapy, presence of central venous lines, and renal replacement therapy.

Colonization with *Candida* is a risk factor for anastomotic infection and candidemia. Candidiasis is usually a nosocomial infection that occurs early after transplantation and the manifestations range from mucocutaneous involvement to deep organ seeding. Bronchial anastomotic involvement is the most common manifestation followed by bloodstream infection and disseminated disease. Recovery of *Candida* from a respiratory tract culture usually indicates colonization and does not require therapy. *Candida* pneumonia is rare, and its diagnosis requires demonstration of tissue invasion by histopathological examination.

Bloodstream infections are preferably treated with fluconazole or an appropriate echinocandin for at least 14 days after the first negative blood culture. Disseminated disease requires prolonged treatment until infection is cleared. *C. glabrata* demonstrates elevated minimum inhibitory concentrations to fluconazole hence high-dose fluconazole or an alternative antifungal agent should be considered. *C. krusei* is intrinsically resistant to fluconazole and should be treated with another agent. Alternative agents include echinocandin, amphotericin, and other azoles.

Despite advances in understanding of the biology and epidemiology of fungal pathogens, improvement in diagnostic modalities, and introduction of new more efficacious therapeutic agents, invasive fungal infection remains an important cause of morbidity and mortality after lung transplantation.

Bacterial infections in lung transplantation

This is the most common type of infectious complication following lung transplantation. Most episodes occur immediately with >80% occurring within the lung, mediastinum, and pleural space. Most infections are uncomplicated and respond to antibiotic therapy.

Risk factors

Preoperative factors:
- Altered anatomy.
- Aggressive immunosuppression.
- Recipients colonizing flora.

Postoperative factors:
- Decreased cough reflex.
- Decreased mucociliary clearance.
- Loss of bronchial circulation.
- Loss of lymphatic drainage.

Lung transplantation was once described as an immune state characterized by an increase in infection and an alloreactive state. The process of increasing immunosuppression to manage rejection and obliterative bronchiolitis coupled with markedly impaired lung function and mucus clearance dramatically raises the predisposition to infection in such patients.

Donor-to-host transmission is the most common source of bacterial infection post transplantation either from donor lavage or from the preservation fluid. As such, knowledge of pre-transplant airway colonization especially in the at-risk population such as CF or bronchiectasis is critical. Lung transplant recipients who are colonized with pathogens such as *Pseudomonas*, *Staphylococcus aureus*, and *Aspergillus* are at greater risk of developing post-transplantation infectious complications secondary to the presence of these organisms.

Mycobacterial infection

Mycobacterial infection after lung transplantation is uncommon. The relative risk in lung transplant recipients with tuberculous and NTM infection is greater than that in the general population. Lung transplant recipients have a higher incidence than other SOT recipients, NTM infection is rare, albeit more common than *Mycobacterium tuberculosis* infection. Lung transplant recipients are at greater risk for pulmonary infections in general because the allograft is in direct contact with the pathogen. *M. abscessus* is observed in lung transplant recipients at a higher rate than in other SOTs. It has been reported to cause skin, soft tissue, pulmonary, and disseminated disease. The most common manifestation is cutaneous lesions. Such infection has been reported throughout the post-transplant period with no increase in incidence at any specific point in that period.

Choice of antibiotic

Obtaining appropriate cultures such as blood (peripheral and line), urine, and sputum early in the infection is critical, because they are the usual sources. Early removal of central venous catheters, arterial catheters, and urinary catheters is essential. In the first month, nosocomial pathogens predominate, and empiric therapy should have broad-spectrum coverage. The emergence of multidrug-resistant pathogens has made this choice particularly challenging and susceptibility data should always guide therapeutic decisions. Some of the anti-MRSA drugs include linezolid and tigecycline. Newer agents (e.g. tedizolid, ceftobiprole, dalbavancin) have not been licensed for use in this population. The use of daptomycin is restricted to bloodstream infections as it is inactivated by pulmonary surfactant. Glycopeptide-resistant enterococci may be problematic in some regions—common infections are associated with renal tract or are central line associated. Linezolid is the drug of choice but should be used cautiously due to the risk of thrombocytopenia and peripheral neuropathy. Other significant multidrug-resistant pathogens include carbapenemase-producing Enterobacteriaceae where treatment options are very limited (e.g. IV colistin, fosfomycin, and combination treatment) based on susceptibility testing.

Burkholderia cepacia

One of the most debated areas is carriage of *B. cepacia*. The organism is associated with faster decline in patients with CF, as a result of which it is present in a disproportionately high percentage of potential transplant recipients. The strain *B. cenocepacia* is associated with extremely poor outcomes following transplantation. Many centres do not accept recipients colonized with *B. cenocepacia*, namely genomovar III.

Mycobacterium abscessus complex

M. abscessus complex is associated with rapid disease progression and multiple reports exist of postoperative recurrences with chest wall abscesses and surgical wound breakdown. Treatment needs to be well established prior to transplant and eradication can take up to 2 years. Disease that continues to progress pre transplantation should be regarded as a contraindication.

Special recipient considerations

Cystic fibrosis and bronchiectasis

Affecting approximately 1 in 3000 births in northern and western Europe, CF is a lethal disease affecting the lung via a cycle of infection and destruction of the bronchioles. As many as 98% of children show either culture or serological evidence of *Pseudomonas aeruginosa* infection by 3 years of age. Most deaths in patients with CF are from respiratory failure. In contrast, a wide range of septic lung conditions encompass bronchiectasis. The label is applied to those patients in whom dilated airways are visible on high-resolution CT scans with recurrent infections and sputum production and it is much more common in the elderly. In up to half of all patients bronchiectasis develops following a destructive infection such as pneumonia, measles, tuberculosis, or allergenic bronchopulmonary *Aspergillus*.

Both conditions can lead to inflammatory adhesions or purulent spillage at the time of transplantation. In principle, the surgical and microbiological steps taken to prevent early infection are outlined in Table 32.1 (see p. 412).

Novel emerging treatment therapies

Mycobacterium abscessus is generally considered a contraindication to lung transplantation but, in 2019, a novel case report was presented in *Nature* of a recipient aged 15 years who received a double-lung transplant colonized with *M. abscessus*. A genetically engineered bacteriophage (phage) was constructed involving a three-phage cocktail which efficiently killed the infectious *M. abscessus* strain. These transplants are high risk and mandate the use of continued IV antibiotic cocktails post transplantation but evolving gene therapy presents another string in the bow of the antimicrobial treatment arm.

Never-ending treatment: the spies

Section 7

Combined transplantation

Combined heart–lung transplantation

Introduction

Combined heart–lung transplantation (HLTx) is accepted as the only effective treatment for patients with end-stage heart and lung failure. The first HLTx was performed in 1981 in Stanford, CA, USA, on a patient with pulmonary arterial hypertension. The practice of HLTx has evolved significantly since led by improved medical therapies for end-stage cardiopulmonary failure and PH, improved outcomes following isolated heart and lung transplantation, and also driven by limited donor organ availability.

Current activity and trends over time

See Fig. 33.1.
- Global HLTx activity peaked in the year 1990 with 225 reported cases.
- Activity steadily fell to 38 in 2015, but has risen slightly since.
- HLTx only account for <1% of all cardiothoracic transplantations. The 2016 ISHLT registry reported 58 HLTx worldwide, compared with 4554 single or bilateral lung transplants and 5832 heart transplants.

Worldwide, 89 centres have reported performing HLTx since 2009:
- Of these, 56 (63%) centres average one procedure per year.
- Only five centres have performed an average of more than three per year.

Indications

In the early years, patients with end-stage lung disease with concomitant RV dysfunction tended to be considered for HLTx. However, bilateral lung transplants are now preferred in these patients since outcomes are similar or better, and right heart dysfunction commonly improves following successful lung transplantation.

Currently, the commonest indications for HLTx include:
- Congenital heart disease with Eisenmenger's syndrome—including patients with complex congenital heart disease who had previously undergone palliative surgical procedures to defer the need for transplantation.
- Idiopathic pulmonary arterial hypertension—some evidence that outcomes may be superior to bilateral lung transplantation in patients ventilated on ICU pre transplantation.
- Combined end-stage heart and lung disease—for example, due to systemic disease or pulmonary diseases with refractory RV or LV dysfunction.

HLTx used to be offered to selected patients with end-stage HF and severe secondary PH (PVR >5 Wood units or a transpulmonary gradient >15–20 mmHg) because outcomes following isolated heart transplantation were poor in these patients. However, many such patients are now offered implantable LVADs instead as a bridge to heart transplantation candidacy.

The most recent ISHLT registry report summarizes the indications for the 4054 heart–lung transplants performed worldwide (Table 33.1).

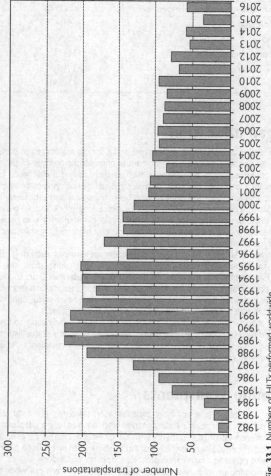

Fig. 33.1 Numbers of HLTx performed worldwide.

Table 33.1 Indications for heart–lung transplantation from 1982 to 2016

Indication	Number (%)
Congenital heart disease	1227 (37.7)
Idiopathic pulmonary arterial hypertension	962 (29.5)
Cystic fibrosis	464 (14.2)
COPD	145 (4.5)
Idiopathic pulmonary fibrosis	124 (3.8)
Alpha-1 antitrypsin deficiency	63 (1.9)
Other	272 (8.4)

Source data from ISHLT registry report.

Organ allocation

In the setting of donor organ shortages and a duty to maximize the benefits from the donated organs, it is important to consider the number of patients who could receive a transplant as well as their likely survival gains from transplantation. The combined life-years gained from carrying out one HLTx is probably less than half that of one heart transplant and a bilateral lung transplant. Therefore, whether a donor heart–lung block should be used for a single patient requiring HLTx or the organ block split for two patients, one requiring a heart transplant and the other a bilateral lung transplant, is an ethical dilemma.

In the USA, there is no allocation system for patients requiring HLTx. They must be listed separately for heart and lung transplants using the UNOS schemes. It is the heart status that usually determines organ allocation, since if donor lungs are allocated to a patient, the donor heart would only be allocated if there is no other suitable higher heart status candidate. The converse is not true if the patient is allocated the heart.

In Europe, national policies vary by country, but similarly tend to favour isolated heart or lung transplant recipients due to urgency status listing for isolated organs that is not available for potential HLTx recipients. As a result, the wait for HLTx tends to be longer.

Domino transplants

In the era before bilateral lung transplantation became fully established, some patients with normal heart function who required lung transplantation were offered HLTx (e.g. patients with CF or emphysema). In these cases, the recipient could donate their heart at the time of their HLTx to a HF patient who requires a heart transplant as a 'domino' procedure.

The domino procedure is rarely performed in the current era when such patients with normal cardiac function would more likely receive a bilateral lung transplant.

However, HLTx and domino heart donation do offer some advantages for both recipients:

- The implant time for a heart–lung block is much shorter than that of bilateral lung transplantation and, therefore, ischaemic time is significantly reduced.
- Airway complications after HLTx is infrequent compared with that following lung transplantation especially in patients with smaller stature.
- The patient scheduled to be a domino heart donor can be fully investigated beforehand and there is even the potential to consider donor–recipient HLA matching.
- The domino heart donor is essentially a living donor—the donated heart would not have been exposed to the detrimental effects of brainstem death.
- There is usually co-location of the domino heart donor and the recipient thereby minimizing donor heart ischaemic time.

Therefore, there is still a place for HLTx and domino heart donation for selected patients with lung failure and a normal heart.

Donor organ procurement

Donor assessment

Assessment of the donor is performed upon arrival at the donor hospital:
- Heart: haemodynamics, inotrope and vasopressor requirements, ECG, echocardiogram, right heart catheterization.
- Lung: arterial blood gas, bronchoscopy, CXR.

Size matching is important because oversized donor lungs can be challenging to fit inside the chest cavity of the recipient, particularly if the recipient has fibrotic lung disease. In general, it is reasonable to use a donor with a predicted total lung capacity that is within 15% of that of the recipient.

Organ procurement

There are some important differences with procurement of the heart–lung block for HLTx.
- Median sternotomy is performed, and the pericardium and pleura are opened widely including posteriorly, adjacent to the diaphragm.
- The heart is assessed visually and palpated for CAD. The lungs are palpated for nodules and atelectatic lung segments are recruited.
- The PA is separated from the ascending aorta.
- The SVC is dissected and encircled with a silk ligature cranial to the azygos vein. The azygous vein can be divided between ligatures.
- To facilitate access to the trachea at the level of the thoracic inlet, the innominate vein and artery can be divided in turn between heavy ligatures. The trachea is encircled with an umbilical tape in the space between the SVC and aortic arch.
- Following systemic heparinization, cannulas are placed in the ascending aorta and pulmonary trunk, secured with purse-string sutures, and connected to an infusion line for cardiac and lung preservation solutions respectively.
- Once all retrieval teams are ready to proceed with aortic clamping, a bolus of prostacyclin is administered into the pulmonary trunk to pre-dilate the pulmonary vascular bed.

- The SVC is ligated.
- The intrapericardial IVC is clamped and hemi-transected to vent the RA.
- The tip of the LAA is widely opened to vent the LA. The heart is allowed to beat 4–6 times until empty before the aorta is cross-clamped.
- Cardiac and lung preservation fluid infusions are commenced and the chest cavity is filled with copious cold saline for topical cooling of the thoracic organs. Since the donor heart–lung block is kept intact, lung preservation fluid is only given antegrade and not retrograde.
- Following organ preservation, the SVC and IVC are divided.
- The heart–lung block is mobilized from the posterior mediastinal attachments with sharp dissection towards the superior mediastinum, taking care not to breach the oesophageal lumen.
- Transecting the descending thoracic aorta at the level of the diaphragm and taking it with the heart–lung block helps to ensure that the dissection plane is keep well away from the posterior surface of the airways.
- Access to the posterior surface of the hilum can be improved by reflecting each lung anteriorly out of the sternotomy in turn if required.
- Superiorly, the aortic arch is mobilized by dividing the three aortic arch branches.
- At this point, the trachea is transected at the level of the thoracic inlet and the heart–lung block can be lifted out of the chest cavity.
- On the back table, a sterile endotracheal tube is reinserted into the open end of the donor trachea to inflate the lungs to a pressure of 15–20 cmH_2O to ensure that all segments are recruited.
- The trachea is then stapled 2–3 cm above the carina and the heart–lung block is packaged for transfer to the recipient centre.

Heart–lung transplant recipient procedure

Cardio-pneumonectomy

- Median sternotomy is performed; the anterior pericardium and both pleurae are opened widely.
- Throughout this procedure, great care is taken to preserve the phrenic, left recurrent laryngeal, and vagus nerves.
- Following systemic heparinization, the patient is placed onto CPB with aorto-bicaval cannulation.
- Following aortic cross-clamping, the aorta is divided above the sinotubular junction and the pulmonary trunk just proximal to its bifurcation; the SVC is transected as it enters the RA; the inferior RA is incised leaving a 2 cm cuff of atrial tissue around the IVC orifice; and the LA is divided circumferentially just anterior to the pulmonary veins and the heart is removed (Fig. 33.2).
- Lateral pericardial windows are made longitudinally on each side posterior to the phrenic nerves.

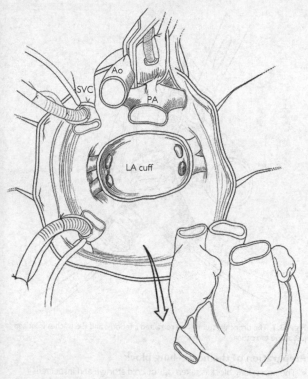

Fig. 33.2 Cardiectomy with the recipient posterior LA and PA bifurcation left behind.

- The posterior LA remnant is incised down the midline to separate the right and left pulmonary vein cuffs.
- Bilateral pneumonectomies are then performed by dissecting the lung hila and stapling the main stem bronchi.
- The vagus can be adherent to the posterior surface of each main bronchus and care should be taken to avoid their injury.
- A 1 cm patch of PA is preserved at the level of the ligamentum arteriosum to reduce risk of injuring the left recurrent laryngeal nerve.
- The two transected bronchial stumps are grasped to allow traction and dissection of the carina.
- The trachea is divided just above the take-off of the right main bronchus (Fig. 33.3).
- Meticulous haemostasis should be performed at this stage paying particular attention to the posterior mediastinum.

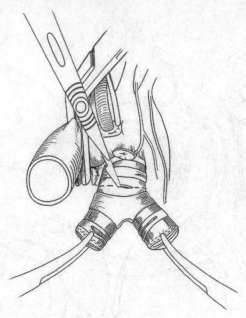

Fig. 33.3 The bronchial stumps are retracted inferiorly, and the trachea is incised just above the carina.

Preparation of the heart–lung block

- The heart–lung block is taken out of cold storage and inspected.
- Excess donor aorta and pericardium are removed.
- The paratracheal tissue should be preserved in order to maintain its blood supply.
- The donor trachea is incised one cartilaginous ring above the take-off of the right main bronchus.
- Any secretions within the airways are suctioned and a specimen sent for culture.
- The vent site on the donor LAA is now repaired.
- The donor interatrial septum is inspected through the IVC orifice and any defect repaired.

Implantation

- The heart–lung block is placed into the recipient chest cavity by passing the lungs through the laterally placed pericardial windows (Fig. 33.4).
- The tracheal anastomosis is completed with a continuous polypropylene suture; some surgeons prefer to use a continuous suture for the membranous portion only and interrupted sutures for the cartilaginous portion (Fig. 33.5).

- The peritracheal tissues are suture approximated so that the tracheal anastomosis is not in direct contact with a vascular structure and may reduce the risk of fistula formation.
- The aortic anastomosis is performed with continuous 4-0 Prolene, a de-airing cannula is secured, and the aortic cross-clamp is removed.
- A fibreoptic bronchoscopy is performed to visualize the tracheal anastomosis and for airway clearance. Ventilation of the lungs can be initiated with half tidal volume (5 mL/kg).
- The IVC and SVC anastomoses are performed while the donor heart is reperfused (Fig. 33.6).
- On completion, ventilation can be increased to full tidal volume (10 mL/kg) and the patient weaned from CPB with appropriate inotropic support and epicardial pacing as required.
- A Swan–Ganz catheter should be routinely placed for haemodynamic monitoring.

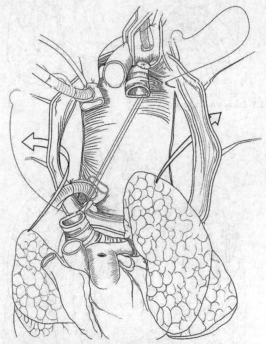

Fig. 33.4 The heart–lung block is lowered into the chest: first the left lung into the left pleural space through the incision in the pericardium behind the left phrenic nerve, then the right lung into the right pleural space through the incision in the pericardium behind the right phrenic nerve, and finally the heart into the pericardial space.

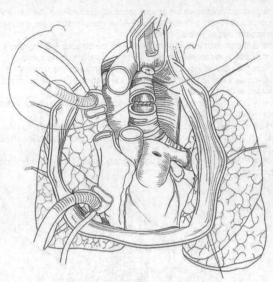

Fig. 33.5 Tracheal anastomosis.

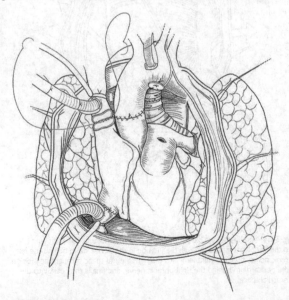

Fig. 33.6 SVC anastomosis.

Early postoperative management

Early postoperative care requires close monitoring of the haemodynamics and gas exchange. Allograft dysfunctions will manifest as they would for isolated heart or lung transplant recipients. Patients should have close monitoring of RV function with appropriate inotropic and pulmonary vasodilatory therapy. Protective ventilation should be employed to minimize the risk of barotrauma.

Early graft failure

Early graft failure resulting in death or retransplantation within the first 30 days occurs in 6.8% of HLTx. This compares unfavourable to the incidence following isolated heart or lung transplantation over the same period of 2.3%. This may be due to the combined risks of developing dysfunction of the heart or lung allografts.

Surgical complications

HLTx recipients are at risk of developing certain surgical complications less commonly encountered following isolated heart or lung transplantation:
- *Phrenic nerve dysfunction*: there is risk of injury to the phrenic nerve when opening the pericardium posteriorly and pericardial retraction while placing the lungs into the pleural cavities. Patients with phrenic nerve dysfunction require ventilation for longer periods and have prolonged ICU stays.
- *Chylothorax*: the extent of posterior mediastinal dissection to explant the diseased organs can lead to unnoticed lymphatic injury. Additionally, it is recognized that patients with congenital heart disease can have aberrant lymphatic pathways that can be injured inadvertently. This can prolong recovery and may require further surgical intervention.
- *Gastroparesis*: the vagus nerve is at risk of being injured while dissecting and performing the tracheal anastomosis. This can lead to gastroparesis which can significantly increase the risk of recurrent aspiration and is associated with the development of CLAD. It can also lead to malabsorption and malnutrition.

Immunosuppression

There is no standardized immunosuppression regimen for HLTx recipients and protocols vary between transplant centres.

Some centres advocate the use of ATG as induction therapy while other centres opt for more modern agents such as IL2RAs (e.g. basiliximab). However, the clinical benefit of induction immunosuppression remains contentious.

Maintenance immunosuppression is similar to other thoracic organ transplant recipients comprising of a combination of a CNI, a cell cycle inhibitor, and a glucocorticoid.

Allograft monitoring

Monitoring of HLTx recipients is usually lead by pulmonologists because the surveillance is primarily bronchoscopic and the majority of complications are related to the lung allografts. Regular monitoring of the patients includes:

Lung allograft:
- CXR.
- Pulmonary function testing.
- Bronchoscopy and surveillance transbronchial biopsy.

Heart allograft:
- TTE.
- Endomyocardial biopsy if evidence of dysfunction.

Acute rejection of the cardiac allograft following HLTx is uncommon with some suggesting that there may be a protective benefit of the lung allografts on the donor heart. One study focusing on endomyocardial biopsy following HLTx reported a significantly lower incidence of acute rejection compared with isolated heart transplantation. As such, most centres choose to only perform routine surveillance transbronchial biopsies unless there is specific evidence of cardiac dysfunction.

Outcomes: patient survival

ISHLT data demonstrate that operative mortality following HLTx has reduced significantly over time but remains higher than that for isolated heart or lung transplantation. Between 1982 and 1992 operative mortality was 25.4%, compared to 16.8% for 2002.

The reduction in operative mortality has been attributed to:
- Improved operative techniques.
- Improved organ preservation techniques and solutions.
- Improved patient selection.
- Greater understanding of the risk factors for adverse outcomes.
- Improvements in immunosuppressive regimens.

Median survival following HLTx has also improved over time and currently stands at 5.8 years, although this remains lower than that for isolated lung (7.1 years) and heart (10.4 years) transplantations performed over the same era. This is attributed to the fact that recipients undergoing HLTx have more complex diagnoses and have a more severe preoperative condition, the procedure being infrequently performed, and the risk of complications to both the heart and lung allografts.

However, for the recipients who survive their first year after a HLTx, median survival is significantly higher at 11.5 years for the most recent era, which is comparable to conditional survival following bilateral lung transplantation but remains shorter than that for heart transplant recipients (Fig. 33.7).

Due to the relatively small numbers performed, robust analysis is challenging, but factors that are associated with inferior survival following HLTx include:
- Recipient age ($p = 0.03$).
- Donor age ($p = 0.01$).
- More modern transplant era (hazard ratio (HR) 0.661; confidence interval (CI) 0.496–0.883; $p <0.01$).
- Donor CMV+/recipient CMV– (HR 1.438; CI 1.019–2.028; $p = 0.04$).
- Ventilator dependence preoperatively (HR 2.270; CI 1.346–3.829; $p <0.01$).

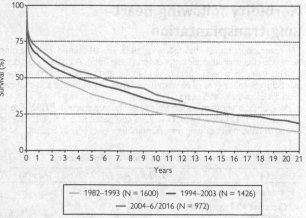

Fig. 33.7 Survival rate after HLTx.

Causes of death in heart–lung transplant recipients

The most common causes of death within the first year following HLTx include early graft failure, technical complications, and infections (Table 33.2). Beyond the first year, the commonest causes of death are infection and development of BOS.

Table 33.2 Causes of death within the first year compared to beyond the first year (ISHLT registry)

	<1 year	>1 year
BOS	14 (1.7%)	224 (21.9%)
Acute rejection	15 (1.8%)	10 (1.0%)
Malignancy	16 (1.9%)	96 (9.4%)
Infection	206 (24.8%)	246 (24.0%)
Graft failure	204 (24.5%)	157 (15.3%)
Cardiovascular	54 (6.5%)	96 (9.4%)
Technical	123 (14.8%)	13 (1.3%)
Multiple organ failure	104 (12.5%)	60 (5.9%)

Source data from ISHLT registry report.

Morbidity following heart–lung transplantation

The commonest morbidities following HLTx are associated with the long-term side effects of immunosuppression (Table 33.3). A high proportion of patients develop hypertension, dyslipidaemia, and diabetes following transplantation. Some degree of renal dysfunction is very common and observed in 45.5% of patients at 5 years.

Malignancy is another important morbidity, in particular PTLD. The incidence of PTLD following HLTx is 7.6% compared to 5.4% and 3.1% following isolated heart or lung transplantation respectively at 5 years.

Table 33.3 Cumulative post-transplant morbidity—ISHLT registry

Outcome	Within 1 year (%)	Within 5 years (%)
Severe renal dysfunction	7.1	13.7
Creatinine >2.5 mg/dL (221 µmol/L)	3.0	9.5
Chronic dialysis	3.8	3.4
Renal transplant	0.2	0.8
Diabetes	17.1	26.5
Hyperlipidaemia	28.0	70.4
CAV	2.5	6.9
BOS	7.1	31.1
Malignancy	5.7	10.5

Source data from ISHLT registry report.

Chronic allograft dysfunction

The development of chronic allograft dysfunction is a major cause of long-term morbidity and mortality following HLTx (Fig. 33.8).

Cardiac

The incidence and morbidity associated with chronic cardiac allograft dysfunction is significantly lower in HLTx recipients compared to isolated heart transplant recipients. Incidence of CAV in surviving HLTx recipients is 2.5% and 6.9% at 1 and 5 years respectively. For isolated heart transplant recipients these values are 7.7% and 30%. Following experimental investigation in animal models, this phenomenon is thought to be related to lymphoid tissue within the lung allografts localizing the recipient alloimmune response, thereby sparing the cardiac allograft from immune-mediated injury.

Lung

The incidence of CLAD/BOS is significantly higher than that of the cardiac allograft. Incidence of CLAD in surviving HLTx recipients is 7.1% and 31.1% at 1 and 5 years respectively and this is a major cause of morbidity and mortality in the heart–lung transplant population. The incidence of CLAD

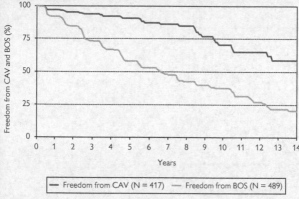

Fig. 33.8 Chronic allograft dysfunction following HLTx.

appears to be lower than that observed following isolated lung transplantation where the 1- and 5-year incidence is 9.3% and 41% respectively. It is
thought that the higher incidence of PGD in isolated lung transplant recipients may be the explanation for this observation.

Retransplantation

There have been a small number of retransplantations performed following
HLTx. However, outcomes are significantly inferior compared to first-time
HLTx recipients—with a 1-year survival of only 43% (Fig. 33.9).

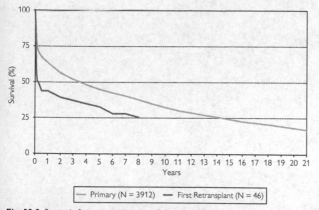

Fig. 33.9 Survival after retransplantation following HLTx.

Combined thoracoabdominal organ transplantation

Introduction

Dual thoracoabdominal organ transplantations are the most resource intensive cases in solid organ transplantation. They have unique challenges and are performed in selected patients at high-volume quaternary care centres. There are no standard indications for combined thoracoabdominal transplants, and individual centres evaluate the necessity on a case-by-case basis. The most common clinical scenarios and indications are as follows:

- *Heart–kidney*: severe HF with advanced renal disease not expected to recover following heart transplantation.
- *Lung–kidney*: lung retransplantation with concomitant nephrotoxicity from CNIs.
- *Heart–liver*: severe amyloidosis affecting both organs.
- *Lung–liver*: CF with CF-related liver disease.

At our institution, intraoperative management is performed by cardiothoracic anaesthesiologists and perfusionists who manage CPB and ECMO. In heart–kidney (HKTx) and lung–kidney transplantations (LKTx), the thoracic transplantation is finished in its entirety including chest closure, followed by a period of recovery in the ICU prior to initiating the kidney transplantation. In contrast, heart–liver and lung–liver transplantations (LLTx) are completed sequentially under the same anaesthetic.

In summary, combined thoracic/abdominal transplantations are complex endeavours. Donor and recipient selection, organ procurement, anaesthetic management, recipient surgery, and postoperative management require a multidisciplinary approach and will be discussed in detail in this chapter.

Indications and overview

Combined heart/lung–kidney transplantation

Renal failure following heart and lung transplantation is associated with an increased mortality risk, thus motivating combined HKTx or LKTx in patients with concomitant advanced renal disease.

Considerations for HKTx:

- Concomitant HF and renal insufficiency warrants consideration for HKTx when the eGFR is <60 mL/min/1.73 m^2 without necessitating dialysis dependence.
- Evidence for this approach includes a UNOS analysis demonstrating higher 5-year survival rates for HKTx recipients compared to heart transplant recipients with renal insufficiency.
- Excellent outcomes have been achieved in older patients and in sensitized patients.

Considerations for LKTx:

- The most common indication for LKTx is retransplantation for lung graft failure with concomitant CNI nephrotoxicity.

- Patient survival after LKTx at 5 years is 51.4%, similar to isolated lung transplantation, suggesting that LKTx is a feasible therapeutic option for lung transplant candidates with significant renal dysfunction.
- Combined transplantation is associated with a lower risk of rejection than single-organ transplantation.

Combined heart–liver transplantation

Less than 200 combined transplants have been performed in the USA since 1988 for the following indications:

1. Familial amyloidosis (the most common indication).
2. Familial hypercholesterolaemia.
3. Homozygous beta-thalassaemia.
4. Haemochromatosis.
5. Alcoholic cardiomyopathy.
6. Cryptogenic cirrhosis with underlying cardiomyopathy.
7. Glycogen storage disease.
8. Late-stage congenital heart disease status post previous repair.
   Considerations for heart–liver transplantation:
- Heart transplantation is performed first and the chest is left open, followed by liver transplantation and then chest closure.
- The use of MCS devices after heart transplantation can facilitate the liver implantation phase.
- Outcomes of the combined procedure are comparable to isolated heart and liver transplantations.

Combined lung–liver transplantation

Between 1990 and 2016, 131 combined LLTx were performed worldwide for the following aetiologies:

1. CF.
2. COPD.
3. Alpha-1 antitrypsin deficiency.
4. Idiopathic pulmonary fibrosis.
5. Idiopathic PA hypertension.
6. Sarcoidosis.
7. Retransplant.
   Considerations for LLTx:
- In the USA, the severity of lung disease most commonly drives organ allocation. From a liver perspective, recipient MELD scores range from 7 to 14, much lower than for patients undergoing liver transplant alone.
- The combination of high LAS and high MELD scores increases the risk of the procedure and diminishes outcomes.

Donor operation

Although the technique for organ procurement varies from centre to centre, the standard approaches to the thoracic donor operations are described in Chapter 15 (heart procurement) and Chapter 26 (lung procurement). Consideration is given to coordinate donor cross-clamp time with the recipient team to ensure optimal cold ischaemic time.

Recipient preparation and team coordination

Combined heart–kidney and lung–kidney

The logistics of combined thoracic–kidney transplantation are more flexible due to the ability of the kidney to safely tolerate prolonged cold ischaemia. In most cases, the kidney is maintained *ex situ* using hypothermic machine perfusion while the recipient is stabilized in the ICU following completion of thoracic transplantation. Typical time between the two procedures varies from 6 to 24 hours, during which time the kidney is undergoing machine perfusion. General approach:

- Thoracic transplantation completed, including chest closure.
- Recipient recovered in ICU with careful management of acid–base status, correct coagulopathy related to CPB, and stabilize thoracic graft function.
- Ideally, vasopressor support is weaned off or down to a single agent with improvement in the patient's pH and lactic acidosis, given that renal outcomes are impaired in patients who are on multiple vasopressors at the time of renal allotransplantation.
- Renal transplantation is then typically carried out in a standard retroperitoneal (heterotopic) approach although, when necessary, an intraperitoneal approach can be utilized. The renal graft is placed on the opposite side from any femoral arterial/venous catheters.

In all instances postoperative management is carried out in a multidisciplinary fashion between thoracic and abdominal transplant teams (medical and surgical). Postoperative immunosuppression is generally managed by the thoracic transplant team as recipients of thoracic organ transplants require higher levels of immunosuppression when compared to abdominal organs.

Combined heart–liver and lung–liver

This section focuses on the management and coordination of the multiorgan transplant recipient between surgical teams (thoracic and abdominal) as well as the anaesthetic team. Recipients of dual-organ transplants will typically undergo thoracic organ transplantation first, followed by abdominal organ transplantation, although a liver-first approach is more commonly being utilized for LLTx. The operative approach is typically carried out as follows:

- Once a suitable donor becomes available, procurement teams will travel to the donor hospital for evaluation and procurement of the intended organs.
- Following visualization of organs in the donor, the donor team will provide the 'go-ahead' call to the recipient team.
- The intended recipient will be anaesthetized and undergo placement of necessary intraoperative monitoring lines (arterial lines, central venous catheter, Swan–Ganz catheter, etc.) and routine TOE is performed.
- Recipient operation gets underway.
- In order to minimize cold ischaemic time, donor cross-clamp does not occur until the recipient operation is underway and progressing without complication.

- Following cross-clamp and cold preservation solution administration, the donor heart is removed first, followed by the lungs, liver, and then kidneys.
- For combined heart–liver transplantation the heart will undergo implantation first and the chest left open; the recipient will then undergo liver transplantation via a chevron incision.
- For LLTx, we favour performing a liver-first approach.

Outcomes relative to isolated transplantations

Combined thoracoabdominal organ transplantations involve significant resource utilization, and ideal allocation strategies have not been determined. In the USA, combined thoracoabdominal organ recipients receive priority over recipients on the liver-alone and kidney-alone waiting lists. The most common transplant scenario is 'thoracic-first' allocation in which the thoracic organ is allocated to a given recipient through the standard heart and lung allocation systems. By UNOS policy, the corresponding abdominal organ is then allocated to the same recipient ahead of all potential recipients on the liver alone or kidney alone waiting lists. Although there is considerable debate regarding the fairness of prioritizing dual-organ recipients in the setting of the current organ shortages, the outcomes of combined thoracoabdominal transplantations have justified the current system. The following points summarize the outcomes of combined thoracoabdominal organ transplantations in comparison to their thoracic-alone and abdominal-alone counterparts.

Heart–kidney

- Long-term outcome is comparable to heart transplantation alone with 10-year patient survival of 56.7% for heart–kidney recipients versus 53.6% for heart-alone recipients ($p = 0.13$).
- There appears to be an immunological benefit for heart–kidney recipients, with significantly reduced incidence of treatment for acute rejection in the first year (8.4% for heart–kidney recipients vs 17.4% for heart-alone recipients, $p < 0.01$).
- The 5-year kidney graft survival is comparable between heart–kidney recipients and kidney-alone recipients (72% vs 73%, $p = 0.71$).
- There does not appear to be an increased rate of futile kidney transplants in the combined heart–kidney population which lends support to the current allocation system in the USA.

Lung–kidney

- Outcomes from LKTx are the least defined.
- There appears to be a trend towards reduced patient survival compared to lung transplant alone at 1 year (71.0% vs 81.7%, $p = 0.06$); however, by 5 years patient survival was comparable (59.9% vs 51.4%, $p = 0.55$).

Heart–liver

- Long-term outcome is comparable to heart transplantation alone, with 10-year patient survival of 60.4% for combined heart–liver transplant compared to 53.6% for heart-alone (p = 0.09).
- There appears to be an immunological advantage for heart–liver recipients, with significantly decreased rates of acute rejection during the index hospitalization (3.1% vs 7.1%, p = 0.03) and during the first year post transplantation (2.1% vs 17.4%, p <0.01).
- Liver graft survival is comparable between combined heart–liver and liver transplantation alone at 1 year, 5 years, and 10 years (83.4%, 72.8%, and 71.0% vs 79.4%, 71.0%, and 65.1% for liver transplantation alone, p = 0.894).

Lung–liver

- Patient survival is comparable to lung transplantation alone and appears to be improving in the modern era.
- A UNOS analysis in the era following implementation of the LAS demonstrated a 1-year survival of 82.7% and 5-year survival of 69.0%.
- Historically, liver graft survival has been impaired in combined LLTx compared to liver transplantation alone.
- However, the favourable patient survival for LLTx in the modern era described previously indicates that this may now more closely approximate outcomes for liver transplantation alone.

Planned mechanical circulatory support for combined heart liver transplant

RV dysfunction post heart transplantation is a common problem; its likelihood is even higher following a combined heart–liver transplantation. Recently, we have performed combined heart–liver transplants with elective placement of an extracorporeal RVAD in order to protect the newly transplanted heart from high-dose inotropic support and facilitate the liver implantation (Fig. 34.1). This temporary support has maintained haemodynamic stability and prevented liver congestion from right heart dysfunction. Importantly, we use this approach in all heart–liver patients, regardless of their predisposition to RV dysfunction. The procedure is outlined as follows:

- Standard bicaval heart transplantation. Once completed, adequate de-airing is assured using TOE and the patient is separated from CPB decannulated and protamine is administrated to reverse heparinization.
- Once the patient is deemed to be stable and haemostasis is achieved, 5000 units of heparin are given IV and an extracorporeal RVAD is placed to support the circulation during the liver transplant. This enables stable haemodynamics during IVC clamping and liver reperfusion.
- A typical configuration for the RVAD is as follows:
  - RA cannula (34 Fr plastic right angle tip) is placed through purse string in the RAA.
  - Femoral venous cannula (21 Fr multiple stage) is percutaneously placed and positioned below the level of the caval anastomosis.

- These two cannulas are connected together thorough a Y connection to provide inflow to a Rotaflow centrifugal pump (MAQUET Cardiopulmonary AG, Hirrlingen, Germany) (Fig. 34.1).
- The pump outflow consists of a 19 Fr arterial cannula placed through purse-string sutures in the main PA.
- The pump speed is set to achieve about 3–4 L/min of flow. Attention must be paid to avoid volume overload of the LV.
- Midline position of the interventricular and the interatrial septa on TOE is reassuring for adequate filling of the LV.
- Inotropic support may still be required at this point for adequate function of the LV.
- Once the liver transplantation is completed, the RVAD is weaned with attention to the CVP, the cannulas are removed, and the purse strings are tied.
- An elevated CVP may warrant more prolonged RVAD support which can be achieved with just one of the venous cannulas.

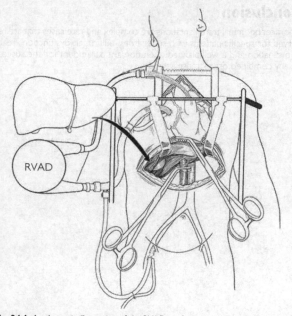

Fig. 34.1 A schematic illustration of the RVAD configuration during liver transplantation. Once the heart is transplanted and the patient is stable, the inflow to the RVAD from both the RA and the femoral vein are connected using a Y connector. The outflow Cannula to the PA is connected and the RVAD support is initiated and titrated to a speed that will support the heart, and ensure a bloodless field for the liver transplant team but will not cause overflow to the lungs and the LV. Next, the IVC is clamped below the heart and below the liver, and liver transplantation begins.

- Once the patient is stable, the chest is closed and the patient is transferred to the ICU.

Placement of an extracorporeal RVAD is safe and technically straightforward, but one should keep in mind some potential pitfalls:
- ACT should be kept around 200–250 seconds during the procedure.
- Patients may experience bleeding complications if the ACT is not kept in a tight range (we have used very low doses of heparin during RVAD support).
- The cardiac surgeon must remain involved throughout the liver transplantation to address any issues related to flow, cannulas, and haemodynamics if needed.

In our experience, elective RVAD placement in heart–liver transplantation can be performed safely and effectively. Preoperative planning involving all of the surgical and anaesthesia teams is critical to achieve a good result.

Conclusion

Thoracoabdominal transplantations are complex and rare cases that are reserved for specific patients who suffer from multiorgan dysfunction. Team coordination and a well-planned operation are paramount for the success of any combined organ transplantation.

Section 8

Anaesthetic considerations

Anaesthetic issues related to extracorporeal membrane oxygenation and ventricular assist device procedures

Extracorporeal membrane oxygenation

Indications for use: ECMO

The ELSO publishes guidelines for ECMO use (http://www.elso.org) which can include acute pulmonary and/or severe cardiac failure that may be reversible and non-responsive to current therapy. Clinical situations that may prompt the initiation of ECMO include the following:

- Severe hypoxaemic or acute respiratory failure with a PaO_2/FiO_2 ratio of <100 mmHg despite optimization of ventilation (i.e. tidal volume, PEEP, and inspiratory to expiratory (I:E) ratio).
- Hypercapnic respiratory failure with an arterial pH <7.20.
- Bridge to lung transplantation.
- Circulatory failure or refractory cardiogenic shock.
- Massive pulmonary embolism.
- Cardiac arrest.
- Inability to wean from CPB after cardiac surgery.
- Short-term bridge to cardiac or lung transplantation or placement of a VAD.

Absolute contraindication to ECMO is any pre-existing state which is incompatible with recovery (severe neurological injury, end-stage malignancy). Relative contraindications include uncontrollable bleeding and poor prognosis from the primary condition.

During ECMO, blood is drained from the native vascular system, circulated outside the body by a mechanical pump through an oxygenator and heat exchanger, and returned to the circulation. The oxygenator fully saturates haemoglobin with oxygen, while carbon dioxide is removed. Oxygenation is determined by flow rate, where elimination of carbon dioxide can be controlled by adjusting the rate of countercurrent gas flow (sweep) through the oxygenator.

There are two types of ECMO:

- *VV ECMO*: blood is extracted from the vena cava/RA and returned to the RA; provides respiratory support and requires an intact cardiovascular system to provide stable haemodynamics.
  - Venous cannulas are usually placed in one of the common femoral veins (venous drainage) and right IJ vein (arterial return). The tip of the femoral cannula should be maintained near the junction of the IVC and RA, while the tip of the IJ cannula should be maintained near the junction of the SVC and RA. Alternatively, a double-lumen cannula is available that is large enough to accommodate 4–5 L/min of blood flow. It is available in a variety of sizes, 31 Fr being the largest and most appropriate for adult males. 27 Fr being sufficient for most average sized women.
- *VA ECMO*: blood is extracted from the SVC or RA (venous drainage) and returned to the femoral arterial or aorta (arterial return), completely bypassing the heart and lungs, and thereby providing both respiratory and haemodynamic support.
  - With femoral access comes an increased risk of ischaemia of the ipsilateral lower extremity. The risks of this complication are decreased by inserting a separate arterial cannula distal to the femoral artery cannula and directing a portion of the infused blood for

perfusion of the distal extremity. In those patients transitioning from CPB, the cannulas used for bypass can be transferred from the heart/lung machine to the ECMO circuit, with blood drained from the RA and reinfused into the ascending aorta.

Once ECMO has be initiated, and blood flow and haemodynamics are stabilized, therapy is guided by blood gases and targets include:
- PaO_2 >90% for VA ECMO; >75% for VV ECMO.
- Venous oxyhaemoglobin 20–25% < arterial saturation.
- Evidence of adequate tissue perfusion (arterial blood gas, venous oxygen saturation, and blood lactate levels).

Maintenance

After haemodynamic and laboratory data demonstrate stability, blood flow rates are kept constant. Constant assessment using continuous venous oximetry via PAC or direct measures of the oxyhaemoglobin saturation of the blood in the venous limb of the ECMO circuit is performed. If venous oxyhaemoglobin saturations fall below target, increasing one or more of the following may be helpful: rate of flow, intravascular volume, or haemoglobin concentration. Some practitioners will reduce patient temperature (passive cooling) to reduce systemic oxygen uptake.

Anticoagulation

Heparin is most often used during ECMO to maintain anticoagulation and should be titrated to an ACT of 180–210 seconds. If bleeding develops, the targeted ACT is decreased. The anticoagulant effect of heparin is dependent on endogenous levels of anti-thrombin (AT3). AT3 levels should be measured if concern arises and if levels are found to be <50% of normal, then AT3 can be administered either by giving fresh frozen plasma or recombinant AT3.

Platelets

Platelet transfusions are common with ECMO use as the platelets are constantly being consumed. ECMO circuits activate platelets by constant exposure to very large surface areas of plastic. Therefore, platelet counts should be maintained at ≥50,000/mL.

Red cell transfusions

Because ECMO is providing the only source of oxygen in the setting of complete respiratory ± cardiac failure, oxygen delivery must be optimized. This is done as a balance between flow and amount of haemoglobin, which is maintained at >12 g/dL in ECMO patients.

Ventilation

Ventilation should be optimized to avoid volutrauma, barotrauma, and oxygen toxicity while preventing atelectasis. FiO_2 should be kept at <0.5 and plate pressures should be kept around 20 cmH$_2$O. Minimizing ventilator support will improve venous return and therefore cardiac output by reducing intrathoracic pressure. Tracheostomy can be performed while on ECMO with minimal risks and can improve ventilation by reducing headspace and improving patient comfort through early extubation.

Special considerations

- Blood flow should be maintained at near maximum flow rates during VV ECMO to optimize oxygen delivery. However, in VA ECMO, the flow rates should be just high enough to maintain adequate perfusion pressure and venous oxyhaemoglobin saturation, but low enough to provide sufficient preload to maintain LV output.
- Diuresis may be necessary as most patients are volume overloaded on initiation of ECMO. Ultrafiltration can be added to the ECMO circuit if patients experience renal failure.
- LV monitoring must be performed and must be continuous. LV failure may occur due to insufficient offloading of the ventricle, underlying ventricular dysfunction at baseline is now unmasked. Arterial waveform monitoring and TOE are optimal methods of ensuring continued ejection of the ventricle. If ventricular failure begins to occur, the addition of inotropic support (i.e. milrinone or dobutamine) can be started as well as mechanical support through use of IABP counterpulsation. Immediate LV decompression is essential to avoid pulmonary haemorrhage if LV ejection cannot be maintained despite IABP counter-pulsation and inotropic agents.

Weaning from ECMO

One or more trials of taking the patient off ECMO should be performed prior to discontinuing ECMO permanently:

- VV ECMO weaning trials are performed by decreasing the sweep gas through the oxygenator while maintaining blood flow at a constant. Arterial blood gases are observed for several hours during which time appropriate ventilator settings required for transition are determined.
- VA ECMO weaning trials require temporary clamping of both the drainage and infusion lines, while allowing the ECMO circuit to circulate through a bridge between the arterial and venous limbs to minimize thrombus formation within the ECMO circuit or oxygenator. Due to the heightened risk of clot formation, VA ECMO trials are shorter in duration than VV ECMO trials.

Complications of ECMO

Bleeding

- Occurs in 30–50% of patients on ECMO and can be life-threatening.
- Increased risk from continuous anticoagulation and platelet dysfunction.
- Platelet counts >50,000/microL and maintaining tight targets of ACT reduce risk of bleeding.
- Early surgical intervention if major bleeding occurs within body cavities (i.e. abdomen or pleural space).

Thromboembolism

- Systemic thromboembolism due to thrombus formation is a devastating complication that occurs in 10–20% of cases.
- VA ECMO has worse outcomes with thrombus formation than VV ECMO.
- Hypervigilance for thrombus formation within the oxygenator must be maintained and early detection can successfully prevent thromboembolism in most patients.

- Observation and inspection of all connectors and monitoring the pressure gradient across the oxygenator is critical. Any sudden change in the pressure gradient is highly suggestive that a thrombus is present.
- Large or mobile clots require immediate circuit or component exchange.
- Primed circuits should be kept at the bedside if the target ACT has been reduced due to bleeding because the risk of thrombus formation is increased.

Neurological
- Neurological injury in the ELSO registry is 10%.
- Neurological injury in cardiac failure and those in whom ECMO is administered during CPR is 50%.

Other complications
- Vessel perforation, arterial dissection, distal ischaemia may occur due to malpositioned cannula (drainage or arterial return).
- HIT can arise in patients on ECMO receiving heparin as anticoagulation.
- Pulmonary oedema and haemorrhage can occur during VA ECMO if LA pressures exceed 25 mmHg.
- Intracardiac thrombosis may form if LV ejection is not maintained during VA ECMO use.
- Cerebral or coronary hypoxia can occur from preferential perfusion of the gut and lower extremities. If unrecognized, cerebral hypoxia can result with catastrophic results.

Ventricular assist devices

Indications for use: VAD

VADs perform as an adjunct cardiac pump, taking blood returning to a failing ventricle and ejecting it downstream, either into the ascending or descending aorta in the case of a LVAD, or into the PA in the case of a RVAD. VADS can be used in the following ways:
- *Bridge to transplantation*: a VAD may be implanted in a candidate for cardiac transplantation to support a chronically failing ventricle as a stopgap until a donor organ is available.
- *Bridge to candidacy*: placed in patients who are not currently eligible for transplantation but may be able to achieve eligibility after substantial improvement in end-organ function.
- *Destination therapy*: in some patients, a long-term VAD is implanted for permanent ventricular support.
- *Bridge to recovery*: short-term use, available for rapid implantation when MCS is acutely needed for survival.

The devices used are continuous-flow pumps, which produce pulseless blood flow, that unload the failing ventricle through the action of an axial or centrifugal impeller that rotates at very high speeds. Device components include an impeller pump, and an external driveline connecting to an electrical power source. These non-pulsatile devices are placed in the thoracic cavity with blood flowing through an inflow cannula in the apex of the LV to the pump and returning it back through an outflow cannula in the ascending or descending aorta.

Pre-anaesthetic consultation

Detailed discussion with knowledgeable clinicians having training in MCS (e.g. a specialized VAD team) is extremely important. This facilitates awareness of potential patient-specific and device-specific problems and avoidance of pitfalls that may arise in the perioperative period, as well as coordination of care in the postoperative period.

Preoperative checklist-specific issues

• Understand the type of device, implantation date, pump speed, pump flow, pump power, and pulsatility index.
• Identify the location of the externalized driveline on the abdominal wall, looking for any evidence of infection.
• Is there a previous history of difficulties with the VAD function, any VAD-related complications (e.g. thromboembolism, infection, mucosal bleeding), and is the device functioning adequately for the patient's current clinical status?
• Is there any evidence of end-organ damage or impairment?
• Identify cardiovascular comorbidities (original indication for VAD implantation, current EF, presence of right HF, aortic insufficiency, arrhythmias, physical activity level):
  • Is there evidence of right HF? Right HF may be exacerbated by decreases in LV pressure and size after VAD implantation, leading to interventricular septal bowing and distortion of RV geometry and mechanics, particularly if the patient had underlying biventricular dysfunction.
• Are there any haematological abnormalities, increased risk of perioperative thrombosis or, conversely, coagulopathy? What is the risk of bleeding requiring transfusion?
• What is the anticoagulation strategy for the patient? Thromboembolism remains one of the most serious complications of VAD implantation. All types of VADs require some type of anticoagulation, which will be noted in the history, and the presence of anaemia or coagulopathy identified on preoperative laboratory tests:
  • Although the level of anticoagulation may be decreased towards the lower limit of the manufacturer's recommendation during the perioperative period, one should not completely reverse anticoagulation in VAD-supported patients for any elective surgical procedures. Exceptions include neurological procedures and some ophthalmological procedures. The anaesthesiologist, VAD management team, and surgeon should collaborate to plan a safe anticoagulation plan during the perioperative period, which may include a heparin bridge in selected patients.
• Is there a pacemaker and/or ICD? Generally, perioperative considerations regarding pacemakers and ICDs do not differ in VAD-supported patients. However, defibrillator pads must be positioned on an area of the chest that is not directly over the device or driveline. The best options are bilateral pad placement on opposite sides of the chest or anterior–posterior placement in the centre of the chest and on the back.
• Are there any pulmonary comorbidities that can be optimized (e.g. PH, pre-existing COPD, pneumonia, recent changes in oxygen requirements, or decreased activity)?

- Are there neurological comorbidities (e.g. abnormal mental status, prior cerebrovascular accident, or embolic stroke)?
- Identify any renal comorbidity (e.g. renal insufficiency, requirement for dialysis, urinary tract infection).
- Identify any hepatic comorbidity (e.g. liver insufficiency, congestive hepatopathy, coagulopathy).
- Does the patient have diabetes and difficulties with glycaemic control?
- Is the patient at risk for infectious complications (e.g. related to VAD implantation)?

Planning for postoperative care

- Planning for postoperative care should be to the most appropriate location to deliver postoperative care.
- Planning for postoperative care should begin when the case is posted.
- Postoperative care should be in an area with appropriate monitoring (telemetry) and staff specifically trained in emergency care of such patients.
- Recovery from surgery and anaesthesia in the ICU may be appropriate.

Anaesthetic technique

- Patients supported with a VAD receive general anaesthesia for most surgical interventions.
- Due to the need for anticoagulation, neuraxial anaesthetic techniques are contraindicated in most VAD patients.
- Placement of a peripheral nerve block with ultrasound guidance is relatively safe in anticoagulated patients.
- Sedation with monitored anaesthesia care is usually a good choice when feasible (e.g. endoscopy procedures).

Intraoperative management

- Intraoperative management of a patient with a VAD must include haemodynamic and VAD monitoring.
- Involvement of or consultation with a cardiac anaesthesiologist/cardiologist or surgeon with expertise in VAD management may provide additional support.
- All patients with a VAD should be transported within the hospital with the VAD under battery power, including transport to the preoperative holding area, the operating room, post-anaesthesia care unit, or ICU.
- After transport, the VAD should be promptly switched from battery power and connected to the power base unit of the device, which is connected to a wall electrical power outlet.
- Backup batteries should always be available; therefore, it is best to connect the VAD to an external power outlet to save battery power.

Intraoperative monitoring

- VAD parameters may be monitored on a console.
- Second- and third-generation non-pulsatile VADs provide continuous displays of pump speed, flow, power, and the dimensionless pulsatility index :
  - Pump speed is measured in rpm.
  - Pump flow is measured in L/min.

- Pump power is measured in watts (W).
- Pulsatility index is a dimensionless measure of the extent of LV pulsatility.

Non-invasive monitors

- Patients with non-pulsatile VADs often have no palpable pulse and minimal arterial pulse pressure; as such, automated non-invasive blood pressure monitors are only functional in approximately one-half of VAD-supported patients:
  - Hypovolaemia and/or vasodilatation further reduce pulsatility in patients with non-pulsatile devices, with consequent reduction in efficacy of non-invasive monitors.
  - Even a small pulse pressure (i.e. 10–15 mmHg) typically allows use of standard non-invasive monitoring, which may be acceptable for minor surgical procedures (e.g. colonoscopy, bronchoscopy, TOE).
- An intra-arterial catheter provides the most accurate and continuous blood pressure monitoring in VAD-supported patients:
  - Placement of an intra-arterial catheter may be difficult using palpation alone and is typically facilitated with ultrasound guidance.

Transoesophageal echocardiography

- Availability of equipment/personnel to use TOE is useful in major elective surgical procedures and serves as a partial substitute for PAC placement in selected patients.
- TOE is valuable to evaluate the following conditions, particularly in unstable patients:
  - Intravascular volume status.
  - RV function.
  - Aortic valve opening.
  - Aortic insufficiency.
  - Interventricular septal shifts.
  - Correct position of the VAD cannula.
- In the event of hypotension or cardiac arrest, TOE can be used to rapidly determine contributing factors.

Central venous or pulmonary artery catheter

- A PAC may provide information to guide intraoperative fluid management and avoid increases in PVR.
- A central venous catheter may be inserted rather than a PAC in patients without significant right heart dysfunction, with use of the CVP to monitor right heart function.
- A central venous catheter also provides large-bore access for infusion of IV fluids or blood and vasoactive infusions when these needs are anticipated.

Positioning considerations

- Surgical positioning may alter VAD function and impact haemodynamics.
- Placement of the patient in the lateral decubitus position with one-lung ventilation may result in hypoxia and/or hypercarbia increasing PVR, limiting preload to the VAD, and leading to acute RV failure.
- Reverse Trendelenburg position decreases venous return to the heart; Trendelenburg position increases venous return.

Induction/maintenance of general anaesthesia

- The decision to perform endotracheal intubation or use a supraglottic airway in a VAD-supported patient is based on the usual criteria for airway management.
- Patients supported with left-sided VADs may develop telangiectasias on mucosal surfaces, with epistaxis being a frequent complication.
- Second- and third-generation non-pulsatile VADs are relatively small in size and typically have an intrathoracic location and do not typically impair gastric emptying.
- Selection of induction drugs and dosing should take into consideration the degree of dysfunction of the unassisted ventricle.
- Maintaining adequate preload, afterload, heart rate, and rhythm are critical for haemodynamic stability.
- Reasonable targets for intraoperative MAP are within 10% of the patient's normal MAP, but no lower than 70–80 mmHg.
- A VAD will only pump what is delivered to it; maintenance of intravascular volume status is necessary to provide adequate preload for optimal VAD function:
  - Factors that decrease preload decrease pump flow and LV output and include anaesthetic agents, dehydration, haemorrhage, and lateral decubitus and reverse Trendelenburg positions.
  - If VAD flow exceeds the available LV preload, the walls of the LV near the inflow conduit can collapse and limit VAD inflow.
- VADs are 'afterload-sensitive' devices. Increases in afterload (i.e. systemic arterial hypertension) will decrease pump flow and reduce VAD output:
  - Appropriate depth of anaesthesia should be achieved prior to noxious stimuli such as laryngoscopy or skin incision, and adequate analgesia should be ensured during and after the operation has concluded.
- Arrhythmias causing clinically significant tachycardia or bradycardia interfere with optimal VAD function and can reduce pump flow. Management of arrhythmias in these patients is similar to that for patients without a VAD.
- Adequate RV function must be assured by minimizing PVR since output from the RV determines the volume ultimately ejected by a left-sided VAD. Thus, increases in PVR due to hypoxaemia, hypercarbia, pain, alpha-agonist vasopressors, hypothermia, and/or acidosis should be avoided.
- If power is normal, high flow may indicate a low SVR; thus, a vasopressor should be administered to increase vascular tone (afterload) and maintain MAP at 70–80 mmHg.
- If power is high in a hypotensive patient, the cause may be severe aortic insufficiency:
  - A sudden increase in power may indicate device thrombosis or malfunction.
  - These causes can be diagnosed with TOE examination.
- Cardiac arrest or severe hypotension (MAP ≤50 mmHg) is challenging to diagnose in a patient with a non-pulsatile VAD due to difficulty in measuring blood pressure in a patient without an arterial line.

- The first step in management is to ensure adequate airway and breathing, similar to patients without a VAD.
- In patients with a functioning non-pulsatile VAD, causes of severe hypotension include:
  - Hypovolaemia.
  - RV failure.
  - Inflow cannula obstruction.
  - Outflow cannula obstruction.
  - Tamponade.
  - Sepsis.
  - TOE can be employed to rapidly determine which of these factors is likely.

Emergence and extubation

- Extubation criteria are the same as in patients without a VAD.
- Prolonged tracheal intubation and mechanical ventilation should be avoided, if possible, to decrease the risk of respiratory infection.

Postoperative management

- Postoperative management should be conducted in a fully monitored setting. Non-invasive and invasive monitoring are continued until major bleeding, fluid shifts, and severe pain have been managed, and implanted devices have been checked.
- After transport from the operating room and upon arrival to the post-anaesthesia care unit or other monitored care setting, such as the ICU, the VAD is promptly connected to an external power outlet and the battery packs are simultaneously connected to allow recharging.
- Similar to the intraoperative period, haemodynamic stability in the postoperative period is maintained by providing adequate preload, maintaining afterload, adjusting pump speed as needed, ensuring an adequate heart rate and rhythm, and preventing any haemodynamic changes that would compromise function of the RV.
- Goals of pain management are to achieve adequate analgesia while maintaining haemodynamic stability:
  - Hypertension associated with pain should be avoided since this may increase afterload and decrease pump output.
  - Over-sedation with opioids or other sedative-analgesics must also be avoided, since this may lead to hypercarbia, hypoxia, increased PVR, and RV dysfunction.
- Reinstitution of prior pacemaker or ICD settings should be assured shortly after the patient's arrival in the post-anaesthesia care unit, ICU, or other monitored care setting:
  - Maintenance of adequate rhythm and rate is necessary for proper VAD function; patients with a pacemaker or ICD should have the device interrogated by the electrophysiology team and reprogrammed if necessary.
- Patients supported by VADs require anticoagulant and antiplatelet therapy to reduce the risk of thrombotic complications such as device thrombosis and embolic stroke. These agents are resumed when feasible (depending on the type of surgery and amount of postoperative bleeding).

Anaesthetic issues related to heart transplantation

Preoperatively

Timings

Heart transplantation is inevitably performed as an emergency procedure. One of the key aspects is timing. There is the requirement to coordinate two operations at individual sites in order to minimize the ischaemic time between cross-clamp at the donor site to reperfusion at the recipient site.

The often-complex logistics mean that timing estimates may be continually changing. It is important to allow ample time for drug and equipment preparation, patient assessment, and any procedures that are required. The timing of moving to theatre, induction of anaesthesia, and duration of surgical dissection can be critical, meaning frequent and proactive communication with all members of the multidisciplinary team is essential. Utilization of the Organ Care System (OCS) Heart (TransMedics, Andover, MA, USA) makes it possible for the beating donor heart to be preserved throughout transfer from donor to recipient, bringing increased flexibility for timings in challenging patient groups (e.g. those dependent on a LVAD).

Preoperative assessment

The preoperative status of patients undergoing heart transplantation can range from ambulatory at home on oral medications alone, to being managed as an in-patient in the ICU on MCS.

History and examination

Most of these patients will have been thoroughly investigated at the time of transplantation. However, it is important to ensure there has been no change in their health status since they were last assessed and that recent investigations are reviewed. The ECG, echocardiogram, left and right cardiac catheterization results, CXR, and pulmonary function test results should be assessed. Any concomitant organ dysfunction should be identified.

Up-to-date haematology and biochemistry results are necessary along with cross-matching of blood (4 units for transplant, 6 units if previous sternotomy or currently on mechanical support). Identification of infection or deteriorating organ function may influence patient management perioperatively or may affect their eligibility for transplantation. Assessment of the level of cardiac support the patient is currently receiving is important.

Known allergies, along with previous anaesthetic and surgical history should be reviewed. Particularly relevant is prior cardiac surgery or sternotomy, as this will influence the time required for explantation of the native heart.

Assessment of the airway and fasting status are important to ensure safe airway management intraoperatively. Clinical examination should be performed to assess volume status and explore potential difficulties with vascular access.

Medications

The use of medications for management of HF may impact management in the perioperative period. The patient may be stable on long-term HF management or may be deteriorating on escalating doses of inotropes.

Diuretic use may lead to biochemical abnormalities that may need to be corrected in the perioperative period. Any vasoactive medications should be continued until safely established on CPB and doses may need to be adjusted in order to anticipate the deleterious effects of anaesthesia and positive pressure ventilation on loading conditions and myocardial function.

ACEis, ARBS, BBs, and the angiotensin receptor–neprilysin inhibitor sacubitril/valsartan are used to control the neurohormonal changes associated with HF and prevent the remodelling that occurs. They can have pronounced effects on haemodynamics with reduced LV afterload which can improve myocardial performance. These effects can be amplified in those patients undergoing general anaesthesia, leading to severe hypotension. This may necessitate the use of vasopressors to support adequate haemodynamics intraoperatively.

The long-term use of anticoagulants in selected HF patients means that consideration needs to be given, where possible, to reversal. Ideally, patients listed for transplantation should be managed on warfarin or UFH to simplify perioperative management. Warfarin can be reversed with prothrombin complex concentrate or fresh frozen plasma along with IV vitamin K. UFH infusions may be discontinued prior to surgery or continued until CPB. Haematology involvement and advice may be required for more complex scenarios.

Preoperative implantable cardiac devices

The use of CRT devices, ICDs, and pacemakers is common in patients with advanced HF. These devices should be checked preoperatively to confirm the patient's underlying rhythm and appropriate device function. Fixed-mode pacing may be required intraoperatively to avoid interference from diathermy. ICD therapy should be disabled and transcutaneous pads applied as a replacement. Device leads will usually be cut and removed at the time of explantation and the generator box removed at the end of the procedure.

Preoperative MCS

This may include short-term MCS devices such as IABP, short-term VADs, and VA ECMO or long-term devices such as durable VADs.

In those patients with mechanical support, it is important to review device function, anticoagulation management, and complications or issues while on MCS and other organ support. They will require additional personnel and time to safely transfer to the operating room. Arterial access may be challenging (patients supported by continuous-flow devices may not have a palpable pulse) and anticoagulation will need to be reversed.

Patients on central MCS need additional planning for surgery as additional time will be required to access the chest and establish CPB. They will be at increased risk of intraoperative bleeding from adhesions and from preoperative use of anticoagulation.

Immunosuppression

Successful immunosuppression is key to long-term success of the transplant and the regimen begins in the perioperative phase. Specific regimens are largely dependent on local protocols and the potential side effect profile in each patient, but treatment may begin in the preoperative phase and be continued intraoperatively.

Surgical brief

The surgical brief should take place once the decision has been taken to proceed to surgery. It is an opportunity to introduce the perioperative care team and facilitate communication between the different specialties involved. It should include a summary of patient and donor details, proposed timings for key events, an outline of planned perioperative management including surgical approach, cardiovascular support, and immunosuppression therapy.

Intraoperatively

The time of arrival into the operating room is key. There needs to be enough time to establish vascular access, safely anaesthetize the recipient, and initiate CPB in time for the donor heart arriving in the operating room. The intraoperative time can be defined by three phases: pre CPB, CPB, and post CPB.

Pre cardiopulmonary bypass

This is the period in preparation for donor heart arrival and needs to be coordinated to ensure the recipient is established on CPB at the time the donor heart arrives. During this period, priorities are safe induction and maintenance of anaesthesia, haemodynamic stability, and end-organ perfusion and preparation for CPB.

Monitoring

Routine monitoring including continuous ECG, invasive blood pressure (non-invasive if invasive not yet established), pulse oximetry, capnography, nasopharyngeal temperature, urinary catheter, and depth of anaesthesia monitor should all be used. Additional monitoring such as CVP and PAC measurements (including PCWP and cardiac output) can be instituted as appropriate vascular devices are placed.

Induction and maintenance

No specific anaesthetic agents are mandated or preferred for induction or maintenance of anaesthesia with choice of agent dependent on experience and preference of anaesthetists involved in patient care. The goal is to achieve balanced anaesthesia without large changes in preload, afterload, contractility, rate, or rhythm. Inotropic and vasoconstrictive support is often required in the pre-CPB period. Depending on fasting status, rapid sequence induction of anaesthesia may be necessary.

In those patients established on MCS, there can be relative stability for induction of anaesthesia where the pump is performing the work of the heart. Volume replacement and vasopressor infusion may be required to maintain perfusion pressure during this time. Although there is no evidence specific to transplantation, there is no benefit to either total IV anaesthesia or volatile anaesthesia in patients undergoing cardiac surgery.

Vascular access

Vascular access can be challenging as a result of multiple previous cannulation attempts, low intravascular volume, and current implantable cardiac devices. Traditionally, the right IJ vein has been avoided in order to ensure patency of this vessel for subsequent long-term cardiac biopsies to be performed from this site. However, this is not borne out in clinical practice and any site can be used. In those with an ICD *in situ*, the left subclavian vessels may not be an option.

Given the requirement for long-term immunosuppression, a strict approach to asepsis is essential to prevent infection. Ultrasound use should be routine and a multi-lumen central venous catheter and sheath introducer, to allow insertion of a PAC, should be placed. If the PAC is used prior to heart excision, the catheter needs to be pulled back before explantation of the recipient heart and can be re-advanced later for assessment of the transplanted heart.

The decision to place vascular access before or after induction of general anaesthesia will depend on multiple factors. The perceived difficulty, patient cooperation, staff experience, cardiovascular stability, logistics, and timing will all need to be taken into account. Placing vascular access before induction of general anaesthesia may minimize the time from induction and intubation to initiation of CPB and may assist in delivery of vasopressor and inotropic support during induction. Significant delays to induction of anaesthesia should be avoided and alternative strategies such as surgical cutdown for vascular access should be discussed if difficulties are encountered.

Immunosuppression

High doses of corticosteroids may be administered at induction of anaesthesia and/or prior to reperfusion of the donor heart based on institutional protocol.

Microbiology

Antimicrobials are essential and should be guided by local protocols and patient microbiological history. Prophylactic antibiotics should be administered prior to commencing surgery and re-administered during the case as required.

Surgical pause

This should take place prior to surgical incision and ensure that the donor heart has been retrieved at the donor site and that it is appropriate for the transplant operation to proceed. Any additional concerns of the implanting team should be identified and addressed.

Repeat sternotomy

In those patients who are having a repeat surgery or who are on MCS, planning needs to take place as accessing the chest and establishing the patient on CPB will be more challenging. Prolonged time to access the chest should be accounted for, cross-matched blood should be available, and external defibrillation pads should be placed. It is not uncommon for CPB to be established through femoral venous, and femoral or axillary arterial cannulation.

Blood and coagulation

Cross-matched blood should be available for commencement of surgery. Antifibrinolytics such as tranexamic acid or epsilon-aminocaproic acid are used to minimize perioperative bleeding. When ready for CPB, heparin is administered and ACT is monitored. Further dosing is targeted to ACT during bypass.

HIT is a major challenge for cardiac transplantation and, where appropriate, transplantation may need to be delayed until >3 months since previous heparin exposure. In cases where this is not possible, alternative agents such as the direct thrombin inhibitor bivalirudin can be used and exposure to heparin in the perioperative period avoided. Other options for patients with current or remote HIT and positive HIT antibodies for whom surgery cannot be postponed include (1) preoperative plasmapheresis and intraoperative administration of heparin, (2) preoperative administration of IVIG and intraoperative anticoagulation using heparin, and (3) co-administration of epoprostenol intraoperatively with heparin.

Cardiopulmonary bypass

This period involves recipient heart explantation and donor heart implantation. Priorities are to ensure immunosuppression is administered according to the agreed perioperative plan, coagulation monitoring is continued, and that preparations are made for coming off CPB.

Haemodynamic priorities include identifying and managing low SVR and preparing for the post-CPB period. Vasoplegia is common following cardiac transplantation, may manifest during CPB through low MAP with poor end-organ perfusion, and requires the administration of vasopressors.

It is common practice to continue low tidal volume ventilation with or without inhaled NO during the CPB period in a bid to minimize bypass-induced lung ischaemia and mitigate the elevation in RV afterload following transplantation.

Post cardiopulmonary bypass

This period includes weaning from CPB and establishing the new heart in the recipient circulation. This involves continually assessing heart function, and instituting and adjusting vasopressor and inotropic support as appropriate.

Weaning from CPB

Reperfusion time is required prior to weaning from CPB. The longer the ischaemic period, the longer this reperfusion should be. Low-dose infusions of inotrope and vasoconstrictor can be commenced at this time and titrated according to cardiovascular response. Temporary epicardial atrial and ventricular pacing wires are placed and a heart rate of 90–110 bpm targeted.

A PAC can be floated with transient reduction in flows to monitor pulmonary pressures and cardiac output during separation from CPB.

Weaning should not commence until this reperfusion period is complete, the patient is normothermic, there is no acidaemia, blood glucose is under control (<10 mmol/L), haemoglobin concentration >7.5 g/dL, and potassium normalized.

The weaning process should be gradual and performed under continuous assessment of haemodynamic parameters, TOE, and visual inspection. This information should be integrated to assess overall graft function and cardiovascular status. The well-functioning heart should be able to support the circulation with a MAP >60 mmHg, a CVP <16 cmH$_2$O, and a cardiac index >2.2 L/min/m^2 with low or moderate doses of vasopressors and inotropes. If initial evaluation reveals inadequate graft function, the graft should be further rested on CPB and changes made to cardiovascular management.

TOE

Intraoperative TOE is an invaluable diagnostic and monitoring tool in patients undergoing heart transplantation. TOE is employed for (1) intraoperative monitoring in the pre-transplantation period, (2) evaluation of cardiac allograft function and surgical anastomoses in the immediate post-transplantation period, and (3) diagnosis and management of haemodynamic abnormalities.

In the pre-CPB phase, the future anastomotic sites, ascending aorta, PA, and caval veins should be evaluated for the presence of atherosclerosis or thrombus, respectively. Also, the presence of thrombus at sites of low blood flow and stasis should be evaluated, as clot can be dislodged during surgical manipulation.

Following CPB, a comprehensive evaluation of the newly transplanted heart should be performed, including LV and RV function, as well as complete evaluation of valve function by two-dimensional and colour flow Doppler imaging. In addition, the anastomotic sites of the ascending aorta, main PA, IVC, and SVC should show no discrete areas of narrowing by two-dimensional and have laminar flow by colour flow Doppler. Moreover, throughout the post-CPB and in the immediate postoperative period, TOE is paramount in haemodynamic management, aiding in the decision to escalate haemodynamic support or to further deploy MCS.

Ongoing cardiovascular management

The main cardiovascular issues following heart transplantation are related to PGD, often predominantly RV dysfunction, and vasoplegia. These features rarely exist in isolation and the failing graft following transplantation can result from varying degrees of each. Monitoring of clinical and echocardiographic parameters will allow diagnosis and targeted treatment.

Primary graft dysfunction

PGD is likely responsible for the majority of early transplant deaths. It is characterized by the transplanted heart being unable to support recipient circulation due to predominantly LV or RV dysfunction or a combination of both. Risk factors which include donor, recipient, and surgical factors should be identified by the perioperative team to facilitate early diagnosis and intervention. Management comprises a spectrum of cardiovascular support ranging from low- to high-dose inotropes and the use of MCS. Devices including IABP, VA ECMO, or short-term VAD (LVAD, RVAD, or BiVAD) should be considered early in the context of persistent graft dysfunction despite high-dose inotropic support. PGD is covered in more detail in Chapter 17.

RV dysfunction

RV dysfunction is common following heart transplantation and is a cause of major morbidity and mortality. It results from a combination of factors; the recipient often has a degree of PH resulting from end-stage HF. In addition, the donor heart has undergone a series of insults from donor brain death, cardioplegia, ischaemic-reperfusion injury, and CPB. In the early post-transplant setting it may be classified as PGD or secondary graft dysfunction where there is a discernible cause (e.g. PH).

The diagnosis is challenging and a combination of clinical and echocardiographic parameters, along with clinical judgement is used. The RV may appear dilated or poorly functioning on visual inspection. Invasive monitoring may demonstrate an elevated CVP, an elevated CVP:PA wedge pressure ratio, and a low cardiac index. Echocardiography findings may include increased RV volume and reduced RV contractility by reduced longitudinal contractility (tricuspid annular plane systolic excursion) or reduced fractional area change with or without a reduced LV end-diastolic volume.

Ventricular interdependence means that any approach to management of RV failure needs to target both ventricles. Goals include optimizing RV preload, minimizing RV afterload, optimizing inotropic support, and maintaining systemic blood pressure. A faster heart rate (90–110 bpm) may help prevent RV distension. Sinus rhythm or AV sequential pacing maintains AV synchrony and consistent RV filling.

Although the RV is usually preload tolerant, in the dilated and failing RV, fluid administration can have deleterious effects causing a deterioration in global cardiac function by ventricular interdependence. In a response to a small fluid challenge, if there are increased filling pressures along with a minimal or even negative response to cardiac output, volume overload of the RV should be considered. Volume reduction can be targeted by diuretic bolus and/or infusion and management should focus on the other factors that can impact RV performance.

Minimizing RV afterload comes from the use of selective pulmonary vasodilators (such as inhaled NO, often started pre-emptively as described previously) and avoidance of factors that increase RV afterload such as hypoxia, acidaemia, hypercarbia, and high airway pressures.

The ideal inotropic agent would improve RV contractility, reduce RV afterload, and have minimal effects on the systemic vasculature. This can improve the coupling of the RV to the pulmonary circulation without lowering systemic blood pressure, which is essential to maintain RV perfusion. Similarly, any vasopressors used should increase systemic pressure while having minimal effect on the pulmonary vasculature. Combinations of inotropes and vasopressors are often used with all of these factors in mind.

IABP should be considered particularly in the context of LV systolic dysfunction with the goal of reducing PCWP, RV afterload, and improving coronary perfusion. If these measures are insufficient to support the newly transplanted graft, short-term RVAD (RV support only) or VA ECMO (biventricular support) should be considered early.

Vasoplegia

Vasoplegia in this setting lacks a universal diagnosis but is clinically evident when a patient has low systemic blood pressure, low SVR, and normal cardiac output. It is often refractory to high doses of vasopressors.

It is associated with postoperative morbidity and mortality with risk factors including the pre-transplant use of mechanical circulatory and prolonged CPB times. Vasoplegia can be managed with vasopressors such as vasopressin and/or norepinephrine (noradrenaline) along with methylene blue in resistant cases. Agents such as inodilators and anaesthetic agents need to be titrated as clinically indicated.

Bleeding/coagulation

Bleeding can be problematic following cardiac transplantation and can be as a result of prolonged CPB times, hypothermia, haemodilution, preoperative antiplatelet/anticoagulant use, and inflammatory activation. Bleeding risk is increased in those who have been on preoperative mechanical support. Requirement for blood products can be determined by laboratory tests including full blood count, laboratory coagulation screen, and point-of-care testing such as TEG.

Once cardiovascular parameters are stable and bleeding is controlled, the chest is closed and the patient is transferred back to the ICU.

Postoperatively

Once the patient is stable, they should be transferred to the ICU for ongoing management. Depending on the support instituted in the operating room, this may require additional personnel to ensure it occurs safely. All cardiovascular monitoring should be continued during this period. In selected patients, the TOE probe may be left *in situ* for continued monitoring, but should be removed as soon as cardiovascular stability is confirmed and the risk of tamponade has reduced.

It is important that a detailed structured handover is given to the ICU team who will continue ongoing care. Anaesthetic, surgical, and perfusion representatives should be present. Checklists ensure that salient points are covered including postoperative immunosuppression.

The early problems in the ICU will largely be similar to those in the post-CPB period. Cardiovascular issues remain such as PGD, RV failure, and vasoplegia. Haemodynamic instability should prompt careful clinical assessment and institution of support as appropriate. Patients are at ongoing risk of bleeding and any clinical deterioration may require prompt echocardiography to identify potential cardiac tamponade. In addition, recipients are at risk of hypothermia, acute kidney injury, and acid–base disturbance, all of which should be actively corrected.

In those patients on minimal cardiovascular and respiratory support who are warm, not bleeding, and neurologically appropriate, tracheal extubation should be considered as soon as possible.

Anaesthetic issues related to lung transplantation

Introduction

Preoperative evaluation for lung transplantation should include a comprehensive review of medical and surgical history, medications, and available testing. While testing is often comprehensive and available at the time of listing, optimization remains challenging in the setting of end-stage cardiopulmonary disease given the narrow time frame of the 'transplant window'.

Review of history

Indications for lung transplantation are organized by four primary diagnoses of end-stage pulmonary disease, including (1) *obstructive lung disease*, (2) *restrictive lung disease*, (3) *CF* or *immunodeficiency disorders*, and (4) *pulmonary vascular disease*. Comorbid conditions that exist by indication may influence anaesthetic choice and surgical planning (Table 37.1).

Both medical and surgical complexity continue to expand through increased acceptance of donation after circulatory death and high risk donors, wider adoption of bridging with mechanical cardiopulmonary support. Although the LAS reflects urgency of transplantation, there has not yet been a surgical scoring system for this population that predicts outcomes, particularly that includes functional status and frailty. These are associated with worsened outcomes in lung transplantation, but are difficult to routinely quantify and optimize prior to transplantation.

Table 37.1 Common indications for lung transplantation with associated comorbidities

Indication for transplantation	Common clinical presentation
CF	Younger age, suppurative secretions, empyema, antibiotic-resistant infections, pleural adhesions, indwelling ports
	Malnutrition, malabsorption, and vitamin K deficiency; pancreatic insufficiency
	Diabetes, hepatic dysfunction, bowel dysfunction (obstruction)
Fibrotic disease	Older age, small chest cavity, concomitant cardiovascular disease (CAD, pulmonary vascular disease, carotid disease)
	Steroid dependency, chronic immunosuppression, association with systemic immune disease (Sjögren's syndrome, rheumatoid arthritis), inflammatory myositis, hepatic dysfunction
Obstructive disease	Older age, concomitant cardiovascular disease (CAD, pulmonary vascular disease, carotid disease), steroid dependency, bullous disease
Pulmonary vascular disease	Vascularized adhesions, RV dysfunction, venous congestion of the liver and kidneys
	Impingement of the recurrent laryngeal nerve by enlarged PAs
	Clotting or bleeding disorders, indwelling ports or lines for ongoing pulmonary vasodilators

Review of medications

Preoperative medications such as bronchodilators, antibiotics, pulmonary vasodilators, and immunosuppressants should be continued until transplantation. Inhaled or IV pulmonary vasodilators should be replaced by IV or inhaled therapies, or discontinued after initiation of VA ECMO or CPB.

Anxiety, depression, and pre-existing pain conditions are predictive of poor pain outcomes following lung transplantation, and should be optimized preoperatively if possible. Medications with respiratory depressant or sedative effects should be minimized.

Some lung transplant patients require systemic anticoagulation until transplantation for thromboprophylaxis of atrial fibrillation or thromboembolic conditions, which may require reversal once in the operating room. UFH and low-molecular-weight heparin, warfarin, and more recently direct-acting oral anticoagulants have been described in the perioperative period for lung transplantation. Timing and dosing of reversal agents should be considered in the context of MCS.

Steroid-dependent and immunosuppressed patients are at increased risk for steroid-dependent diabetes. This warrants evaluation of glycaemic control (HbA1c), as well as reviewing markers of any comorbid known endocrine disorders.

Fasting status and previous anaesthetic records should be reviewed. The consent process includes risks of the anaesthetic, death, intraoperative recall, invasive line and TOE placement, and review of the pain management plan and postoperative recovery. Use of anxiolytics and narcotics such as benzodiazepines or opiates in the preoperative area is not recommended unless absolutely necessary.

Physical examination

Physical examination should focus on the airway, heart, lungs, neurological system and spine, and extremities for evidence of cardiopulmonary failure, and evaluating ease of intravascular access.

Laboratory testing and Imaging

Pulmonary function tests, blood gases, and V/Q scans help predict ability to tolerate one-lung ventilation and inform the sequence of recipient native pneumonectomy. If the non-operative lung has little perfusion, or the room air PaO_2 is <45 mmHg, intraoperative mechanical circulatory support, or MCS, may be necessary.

Cardiac testing assists in identifying candidacy, urgency of transplantation, and planning intraoperative pulmonary support (e.g. VV ECMO), or cardiopulmonary MCS. ECG, resting TTE, and right heart catheterization; CI; CVP; and pulmonary pressures are key diagnostic modalities to identify patients at risk for intraoperative haemodynamic instability. Older patients may have CAD established by left heart catheterization. Cardiac MRI is helpful to identify irrecoverable cardiac scarring and to quantify RV function for patients with long-standing congenital heart disease or PH.

Oesophageal imaging and function tests may demonstrate evidence of stricture, dysfunction, or aspiration. If aspiration is present, a rapid sequence intubation must be considered. If oesophageal stricture is found, the risk of placing a TOE probe should be weighed carefully. The presence of oesophageal dysfunction may alter the route of enteral feeding, nutrition, and recovery.

Certain disease states raise suspicion for liver or renal dysfunction (e.g. CF) or RV dysfunction (e.g. idiopathic pulmonary fibrosis, Table 37.1). Complete blood counts, chemistry panels, liver and renal function tests, as well as coagulation studies should be reviewed. Preoperatively, avoidance of transfusion is desirable to mitigate risks of alloimmunization. However, blood products are commonly needed for lung transplantation, and blood type, screen, and cross-match should be performed in advance.

Intraoperative medication management

The anaesthesia team will often administer induction immunosuppression. Awareness of drug mechanism, dosing, metabolism, and drug compatibility is necessary. Expensive monoclonal antibody therapies should be dosed after assurance that MCS and/or plasmapheresis are not needed, so the drug reaches therapeutic blood concentrations.

Gram-positive coverage with both a cephalosporin and vancomycin in the setting of immunosuppression is warranted. For recipients with significant, long-standing resistant microbial burden, a specialized antibiotic regimen will be designed. Dosing and re-dosing of both immunosuppression and antibiotics should be adjusted accordingly if MCS is utilized.

Surgical strategies and anaesthetic considerations

Anaesthesia for particular surgical strategies: MCS

Cardiopulmonary MCS may be present preoperatively, or planned for patients with (1) severe PH or anticipated RV failure as a result of PA clamping and recipient native pneumonectomy; (2) concomitant cardiac procedures (e.g. intracardiac shunts, coronary bypass or valve repair); (3) complex airway resulting in inability to safely and adequately achieve lung isolation; (4) small donor lung size relative to the recipient, to avoid full cardiac output through a small vascular bed; and (5) fragile LA tissue in the recipient or inadequate donor LA cuff that prohibits clamping of the atria and completion of the pulmonary venous anastomoses. Recently, some centers have demonstrated a perioperative outcome benefit with an elective VA strategy for intraoperative support.

Intraoperative teams must communicate prior to induction to confirm the surgical plan. This includes review of the surgical approach, single or bilateral procedure, positioning, cannulation sites and type of MCS. VV ECMO, VA ECMO, or CPB may be cannulated centrally or peripherally. If the patient is on preoperative VV ECMO, it may be continued into the postoperative phase. Patients requiring peripheral VA ECMO should have a right upper extremity arterial line to monitor oxygenation to the head and upper body to monitor for potential Harlequen (North-South) syndrome, where deoxygenated, inadequately mixed blood is pumped from the left ventricle to the upper body. Urgent MCS may be needed due to unanticipated haemorrhage, RV failure, or poor function of the newly implanted allograft.

The surgical team and perfusionist should be present in the room on induction of anaesthesia, especially for high-risk patients such as those with severe pulmonary hypertension. The need for MCS is possible at any stage, and teams, equipment (appropriately sized cannulas, circuits, and pumps), and systemic heparin doses should be prepared.

Anaesthetic planning

Intraoperative monitoring

Standard monitoring includes a five-lead ECG, blood pressure, central and peripheral temperature, end-tidal carbon dioxide monitoring, pulse oximetry, and urine output. Pulse oximeters placed on the extremities will often lose signal during the procedure due to positioning, vasoconstriction, or poor distal perfusion related to surgical manipulation or loss of pulsatile flow. Fluid warmers and warming devices should be utilized, as it is difficult to maintain body temperature with a large amount of exposed body surface and extracorporeal MCS.

Invasive haemodynamic monitoring is necessary for lung transplantation. Cannula position for MCS may influence the site of arterial line placement. Radial arterial lines may become dampened during the case and a femoral arterial line may be needed. Monitoring CVP, pulmonary pressures, cardiac output, and mixed venous oxygenation is extremely useful in guiding volume resuscitation and haemodynamic management. The choice of central line site may be influenced by VV ECMO choice of cannulation site.

Equipment

Single- and double-lumen tubes of various sizes should be available for lung isolation. A single-lumen tube may be placed for pre-transplant bronchoscopy for management of secretions, and may remain in place if the procedure will be performed completely on VA ECMO or CPB. Fibreoptic bronchoscopy confirms lung isolation and allows for bronchopulmonary toilet. During bronchial anastomosis, the anaesthesia team should avoid inserting suction catheters or bronchoscopes in the operative lung, while the surgical team carefully avoids balloon puncture of the bronchial cuff during dissection and native lung pneumonectomy. Insertion of airway exchange catheters for exchange of double- to single-lumen tubes at the completion of the procedure should be carefully performed in light of the fresh bronchial anastomoses.

Intraoperative management

Anaesthesia induction and maintenance

Induction is a key time of potential haemodynamic instability, particularly in the setting of PH or underlying RV dysfunction, and MCS should be immediately available. Although prophylactic IABP placement has been described, there is little evidence to support its use in this setting. Usually, ECMO or CPB are prepared. A rapid sequence intubation with use of rapid-acting neuromuscular blockers may be chosen if the patient is not appropriately NPO prior to induction. Induction agents should include those that avoid myocardial depression and reduction of SVR. Drugs or manoeuvres that increase pulmonary vascular tone (i.e. PVR) should also be avoided, as this may precipitate right heart decompensation in patients with borderline RV function. Importantly, surgical stimulation, poor pain control, or shivering may all precipitate increases in PVR that may be poorly tolerated in a patient with severe PH or borderline RV function. MCS circuits can absorb significant amounts of medication used for pain control and sedation (e.g. lipophilic or highly protein-bound drugs), due to an increased volume of distribution and decreased drug clearance. Similarly, absorption binding of fentanyl to pulmonary endothelium results in significant reductions in plasma concentrations following initial native pneumonectomy and may require redosing.

Inotropic and vasopressor support should be available for support of the RV in the setting of PA clamping. Inhaled pulmonary vasodilators (e.g. inhaled NO and prostaglandins) are thought to reduce mean pulmonary pressures, improve V/Q matching and thereby the PaO_2/FiO_2 ratio, and RV function in lung transplant patients. Randomized controlled studies have failed to show benefit for inhaled NO for prevention of ischaemia-reperfusion injury or demonstrate any clear perioperative or long-term benefits. A recent randomized controlled trial recently demonstrated non-inferiority when comparing iNO to inhaled epoprostenol in the lung transplant population.

Positioning

For a SOLT, a posterior thoracotomy incision is typically performed, and the patient will be positioned laterally with the operative side up. For a midline sternotomy approach, the patient is typically supine with arms tucked. In the bilateral thoracotomy or thoracosternotomy ('clamshell') approach, the patient will be positioned supine with arms tucked, or arms lifted anteriorly, flexed slightly at the level of the elbow, and abducted carefully, with the forearms resting on cushioned support. Avoidance of direct nerve compression or over-abduction is critical to avoid peripheral nerve injury. Careful padding of the axillary and ulnar nerves is recommended.

Ventilation strategies

Supporting oxygenation, ventilation, and avoiding acidosis during one-lung ventilation is a challenge in patients with end-stage disease. In patients with suppurative disease, it is helpful to achieve early lung isolation and avoid cross-contamination from the chronically infected native lung into the surgical field, chest cavity, and newly transplanted lungs.

Positive pressure ventilation, high inspiratory pressures, or high PEEP exacerbates haemodynamic instability by intrathoracic venous compression. Patients with increased lung compliance and expiratory obstruction are at risk for dynamic lung hyperinflation, or 'breath stacking', and permissive hypercapnia may be necessary. Recipient pneumonectomy typically begins with to the lung with less perfusion to minimize hypoxaemia due to shunting in the deflated lung. If hypoxaemia due to shunting occurs, this improves dramatically with PA clamping and recipient pneumonectomy. Avoidance of drugs that interfere with hypoxic pulmonary vasoconstriction is important during this stage. Protective strategies should always be employed for any native lung not being explanted, and the newly transplanted lungs. This includes a low FiO_2 <40%, driving pressures not to exceed 15 cmH_2O, 5–10 cmH_2O PEEP with low tidal volumes. Most centres use 6 cc/kg of predicted body weight as a starting strategy to reduce barotrauma. There is significant institutional variability on how these goals are achieved, with little information about the donor lungs being provided to the care team in order to tailor the ventilation strategy. After a SOLT, significant differences in compliance between the native and transplanted lungs may exist, which rarely may require differential ventilation.

Haemodynamic instability is encountered with intravascular volume loss, surgical manipulation of the heart, PA clamping and unclamping, as well as reperfusion of the pulmonary allograft (Table 37.2). Communication between teams during these steps is critical.

Fluid management

The newly transplanted lung is susceptible to developing pulmonary oedema due to disrupted lymphatic drainage, which can lead to increased extravascular lung water. Additional injury is incurred due to ischaemia-reperfusion, endothelial disruption, and subsequent primary graft dysfunction, which makes fluid management particularly challenging.

Table 37.2 Anticipating anaesthetic interventions by surgical step

Surgical step	Anaesthetic steps
Exposure and dissection	Evaluate oxygenation, ventilation, and haemodynamic performance on one-lung ventilation
	Bleeding during dissection may require early resuscitation and inotrope/pressor support
PA clamp	Assess RV function frequently via TOE, CI, mixed venous saturation
	If RV failure ensues, consider MCS
Recipient pneumonectomy	When organ arrives in room, second check for organ compatability is performed
	Heparin is administered to achieve and maintain a suitable ACT for planned level of MCS
Implantation of donor lung: bronchial anastomosis	Avoid airway suctioning. Surgical team prompts the anaesthesia team to test for bronchial leak/integrity via slow manual inflation with room air.
Implantation of donor lung: PA anastomosis	Maintain anticoagulation goals, prepare for reperfusion
Implantation of donor lung: LA anastomosis	Potential for volume loss. Volume, inotropic, and pressor support may be required
	Steroids and mannitol are given just after posterior anastomosis complete
De-airing of the graft	Partial release of PA clamp and full removal of LA clamp prior to finishing anterior LA anastomosis
	Assess for air on TOE
	Aortic venting with needle if left sided air observed
	Notify any available team members of reperfusion (next step)
Reperfusion	Gradual release of PA clamp by surgical team
	Potential for haemodynamic instability, volume loss. May require inotropic or pressor support
	Teams coordinate manual ventilation post reperfusion with low FiO_2, and initiate mechanical ventilation with inhaled pulmonary vasodilators, and lung protective settings

Lung transplant patients are volume resuscitated with balanced crystalloids or colloid if they do not require transfusion. In an off pump population, each litre of intraoperative fluid increases grade 3 PGD by 13% after adjusting for patient weight. With each litre of colloid administered, a decreased PaO_2/FiO_2 ratio at 12 hours and delay in extubation was observed. An elevated CVP has been associated with delayed extubation due to early graft dysfunction, with the proposed mechanism being increased hydrostatic pressure through the pulmonary vasculature, leading to increased alveolar fluid.

On the other hand, avoidance of volume resuscitation in lieu of high-dose vasopressors or inotropes to support the haemodynamics risks ensuing end-organ malperfusion and injury. Lung transplant patients carry a significant risk of acute kidney injury, amplified by perioperative immuno-suppressants, antibiotics, diuretics, and high-dose vasoactive drug use. We recommend a goal-directed approach to volume replacement using invasive monitoring, for example, cardiac output, mixed venous, invasive pressures, and TOE to guide volume resuscitation to optimize perfusion, oxygen delivery, and lactate clearance.

Bleeding and transfusion

Transfusion is commonly required during lung transplantation, particularly after the blood loss associated with graft de-airing and reperfusion. Bleeding risks include a bilateral procedure, previous thoracic surgery, known pleural adhesions, and CPB. Literature describing transfusion-related outcomes in lung transplantation is derived from small, retrospective, observational trials from single centres, and confounded by risk factors for bleeding and the use of MCS. A few studies suggest a transfusion-related immunomodulatory effect in lung transplantation, but more recent studies indicate that peri-operative transfusion is associated with worsened PGD, CLAD, and overall graft and patient survival in lung transplantation.

Transfusion has been implicated in allograft rejection and poor outcomes. Some centers ensure all lung transplant patients receive EBV and CMV negative products, particularly when the recipient and the donor are also EBV and CMV negative, although this is challenging if massive transfusion is needed or blood shortages are encountered. Leucoreduction of products for SOT is widely accepted. However, if patients have had a prior bone marrow transplant, or are receiving rATG, irradiated products are required. High-volume red blood cell transfusion is associated with morbidity and mortality in lung transplantation, while platelet transfusion has been implicated in the development of post-lung transplant anti-HLA antibodies, with worsened graft and patient survival. *Preoperative* transfusion is linked to the development of new HLA antibodies, challenges in organ matching, and worsened lung transplantation outcomes, it remains unclear how or if *intraoperative* allogeneic red blood cell or platelet transfusion affects HLA alloimmunization and allograft function.

Antifibrinolytics have been described for lung transplantation. Aprotinin reduces bleeding and transfusion requirements, but is associated with acute kidney injury and death in cardiac surgical patients and no longer available in the US. Tranexamic acid and aminocaproic acid reduce bleeding and transfusion requirements in cardiac and non-cardiac surgery, but these have not been well studied in lung transplantation.

Prothrombin complex concentrates allow for rapid replacement of clotting factors without transfusion of fresh frozen plasma, albeit with the problems of limited availability, significant cost, and associated risk of thromboembolism. In non-surgical populations, the risk of thromboembolism associated with prothrombin complex concentrate administration for warfarin reversal is similar to those receiving fresh frozen plasma, approximating 7%. Off-label use of prothrombin complex concentrates as well as activated factor VII has been described for postoperative haemorrhage in lung transplantation. Extreme caution should be taken in administering these medications in the setting of MCS, as catastrophic thromboembolism may occur.

Transoesophageal echocardiography

TOE allows for evaluation of intracardiac shunting, monitoring of LV and RV function, and preload optimization, and procedural guidance for cannulae placement. During the dynamic phases of lung transplantation, guide thorough deairing during reperfusion, and evaluation of both PA and pulmonary vein anastomoses post lung transplantation. Despite the utility of real-time evaluation, there remains no consensus about routine use of TOE during lung transplantation, which carries a class 2b indication according to the American College of Cardiology/American Heart Association/American Society of Echocardiography guidelines. Fig. 37.1a shows a normal pulmonary vein tracing with pulsed wave Doppler, with peak systolic pulmonary vein velocities well below 100 cm/s, while Fig. 37.1b shows an isolated elevated peak systolic pulmonary vein velocity exceeding 100 cm/s suggestive of pulmonary vein stenosis or kinking. Fig. 37.2 shows RV dilation, hypertrophy, and dysfunction during lung transplantation in a mid-oesophageal four-chamber view (Fig. 37.2a) and transgastric short-axis view (Fig. 37.2b), with a 'D-shaped' LV indicating both volume and pressure overload.

Acute pain management

Good perioperative pain management provides physiological benefits and improved graft function, extubation times, patient satisfaction, and reduced ICU length of stay during hospitalization. The evidence in lung transplantation is limited to small, single-centre studies that highlight both individual and institutional practice variability.

Thoracic epidural catheters are identified as a gold standard for pain control. Timing of catheter placement, choice of local anaesthetic solution, and adjunct use makes comparing outcomes difficult. An ideal strategy employs catheter placement prior to weaning the ventilator, and such that it covers both the incision and chest tubes. In the setting of systemic anticoagulation or coagulopathy, epidural catheter placement or removal should be avoided to avoid the risk of epidural haematoma. Regional catheters, e.g. paravertebral, thoracic fascial plane blocks, and catheters and local wound infiltration with and without intermittent bolus techniques have been described as effective alternatives. Adjuncts such as acetaminophen, gabapentin, lidocaine, ketamine and dexmedetomidine may be employed as non-narcotic adjuncts, while non-steroidal anti-inflammatory drugs are typically avoided due to renal toxicity issues. It remains unclear how or if these strategies translate into improved long-term pain outcomes.

(a)

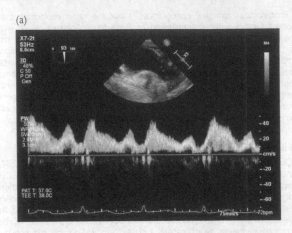

(b)

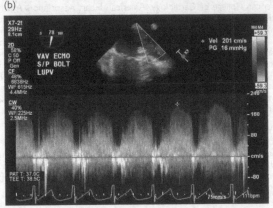

Fig. 37.1 (a) Pulsed wave Doppler of the left superior pulmonary vein in the mid-oesophageal, two-chamber view. Systolic dominance of a normal pulmonary vein tracing, with velocities <100 cm/s and without turbulence is noted (colour flow Doppler not shown). (b) Abnormal continuous-wave Doppler of the left superior pulmonary vein in the mid-oesophageal, two-chamber view. Here velocities throughout systole and diastole exceed 200 cm/s, and pulsed wave Doppler is not possible because the velocities are too high. See plate section.

Chronic pain management

Chronic pain after lung transplantation is estimated at approximately 10–49%. Post-thoracotomy pain syndrome and post-sternotomy pain are well-described, significant problems in the general thoracic and cardiac surgical population with 25–80% attributed to extensive nerve damage. Risk

(a)

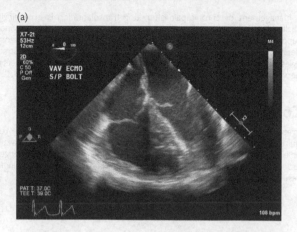

(b)

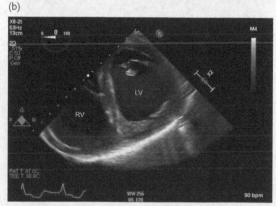

Fig. 37.2 (a) TOE demonstrating RV dilation and dysfunction in the mid-oesophageal, four-chamber view. This patient required VAV ECMO for support during lung transplantation. (b) TOE demonstrating RV dilation, hypertrophy, and dysfunction in the transgastric, short-axis view of the RV. This patient has the classically described 'D-shaped left ventricle' suggestive of both pressure and volume overload, and required VAV ECMO for support during lung transplantation. See plate section.

factors in thoracic surgery include youth, female sex, and the presence of preoperative pain. In patients undergoing clamshell incisions, the incidence is not described. In lung transplant patients undergoing various surgical approaches, about half of survey respondents describe their pain as significantly compromising their quality of life. The source of pain is multifactorial and related to pre-existing pain conditions, CNIs, and pain at incision and thoracostomy tube sites.

Management of chronic pain after lung transplantation is exceedingly challenging due to potential drug interactions, interference with immuno-suppression regimens, and the potentially catastrophic risk of respiratory depression associated with opioids. Multimodal pain management strategies, cognitive behavioural therapy, non-narcotic adjuncts, and therapeutic nerve blocks or ablations should be considered whenever possible.

Conclusion

Preparing a comprehensive anaesthetic plan for lung transplantation requires an in-depth evaluation of pre-existing conditions, medications, available testing, and understanding of the surgical plan. Anaesthetic challenges include intraoperative management of anaesthesia haemodynamics, volume resuscitation, bleeding, and pain.

Index

For the benefit of digital users, indexed terms that span two pages (e.g., 52–53) may, on occasion,
appear on only one of those pages.
Tables, figures, and boxes are indicated by t, f, and b following the page number